FACTS ABOUT NURSING 80-81

PREPARED BY AMERICAN NURSES' ASSOCIATION

PUBLISHED BY AMERICAN JOURNAL OF NURSING COMPANY

TABLE OF CONTENTS

List of Charts

Chart

PREFACE

The first edition of *Facts About Nursing* was published by the American Nurses' Association in 1935. The volumes published since that time, including this 1980-81 edition give current statistics from reliable sources on nurses—their distribution, education, and related information. These continuous records reflect the growth and changes in nursing in response to the health needs of all people. They also contain information that can be used by health planners and researchers to improve health care delivery.

Because of ANA's commitment to provide additional data as it becomes relevant to nursing, two new sections are included in this volume for the first time: minority nurses and nurses in expanded roles. Both sections are part of ANA's resolve to provide statistics on contemporary nursing.

This publication was prepared in the Statistics Unit of the Research and Policy Analysis Department of the American Nurses' Association. The editor of this edition of *Facts About Nursing* was Aleda V. Roth. Carol Johnson, Research Associate, compiled and directed the preparation of tabular material and the final production of this volume, with the assistance of Barbara Lane, Statistical Assistant. We also acknowledge the numerous contributions made by other ANA staff.

We are grateful to the many individuals and agencies who have contributed material for this edition, including: National League for Nursing; National Student Nurses' Association; Department of Health and Human Services, formerly Department of Health, Education, and Welfare; Department of Labor; other federal agencies; state boards of nursing; state nurses' associations; American Hospital Association; The American Red Cross; International Council of Nurses; Health Insurance Institute; National Education Association; National Federation of Licensed Practical Nurses; American Medical Association; and American Osteopathic Hospital Association. Their continued cooperation makes this statistical summary possible.

Pauline F. Brimmer, Ph.D., R.N.
Director
Research and Policy Analysis Department
American Nurses' Association

Chapter I, Section A
NURSE RESOURCES

Government agencies, health care organizations, and educational institutions have relied heavily on comprehensive health manpower information. Indeed, the availability of complete and accurate data is a requisite for effective health planning and evaluation. Since registered nurses constitute the largest group of health care professionals, timely data on their numbers, distribution, and characteristics are essential for monitering trends in the health care delivery system.

The role of the nurse within the changing health care system is becoming increasingly complex. For this reason, health planning agencies, professional associations, and federal, state, and local governments have all been involved in determining and obtaining information on nursing resources. The primary source for information on the registered nurse population has been the American Nurses' Association. Since 1949, ANA has conducted periodic censuses of registered nurses. The latest study, the 1977-78 inventory of registered nurses, was partially supported by the National Center for Health Statistics (NCHS) of the U.S. Department of Health and Human Services. The NCHS contract helped defray much of the cost of data processing and tabulation of more than 1.5 million records.

The inventory provides an enumeration of all registered nurses licensed and living or working in the United States. It provides broad scale statistics on the characteristics of the nurse supply, including demographic data and other information related to employment and educational preparation. Since the relative proportions of such a large group of persons change slowly, especially from one year to the next, and because of the substantial expense associated with such a massive survey endeavor, annual inventories are not deemed necessary. Furthermore, the periodicity of the study is limited to a 3-year cycle at the minimum because the inventory data is collected through the state licensing systems. Individual state licensing periods are not uniform and cover about a 3-year time span overall. The primary strength of the inventory is that it is the sole source of complete registered nurse enumeration on the national, state, and local level. A sizeable number of nurses hold multiple licenses. In the inventory, licenses of nurses throughout the country are unduplicated. Since some nurses are located in states where they may not hold a license but do hold an active license to practice in another state, the inventory counts the nurse in the state of employment if employed in nursing, and, if not so employed, in the state of residence. Hence, the inventory reflects the actual numbers of nurses and each state's complement. Data for the latest inventory were collected over the period 1976 to 1979.

The 1977 national sample survey conducted by the American Nurses' Association under contract with the Division of Nursing of the Public Health Service was developed as a mechanism to complement the inventory by providing annual estimates of the nurse population as well as more specialized information on nurses than that available from the inventory. The target population for the study consisted of all registered nurses possessing an active license to practice nursing in one of the 50 states and the District of Columbia between October 1976 and May 1977. Actual survey results reflect the cohort of this group surveyed and licensed in September 1977. Samples were drawn from the individual state boards of nursing registration files, and duplicate records were purged so that each nurse was assigned a unique probability of selection. The advantage of the sample survey approach is that it is an appropriate mechanism for obtaining detailed estimates on mobility of nurses, annual estimates of change in activity rates, and more in-depth information collected uniformly than that available through the inventories. The major limitation of the sample survey is that survey results are estimates of the population parameters, and hence, are subject to sampling errors. The effective response rate to the sample survey was 82.2 percent. Disparities between the findings of the sample survey and the inventory can be attributed to intrinsic methodologic differences, differential response rates, and reference dates.

In addition to the periodic studies of nurses, annual estimates of the nurse population have been made. For 1976 and previous years, the estimates were obtained from the Interagency Conference on Nursing Statistics, a group of statisticians representing the American Nurses' Association, the National League for Nursing, the Division of Nursing, and other agencies. In subsequent years, the annual estimates were prepared by the Division of Health Professions Analysis of the Public Health Service. The 1980 preliminary estimate of the total registered nurse supply was 1,119,100, which can be translated into 945,700 full-time equivalents (full-time equivalents are computed by adding one-half of nurses employed part-time to all nurses employed full-time). Increases in the nurse supply have more than kept pace with concomitant population growth. There were 506 nurses per 100,000 population, or 427 full-time equivalent nurses per 100,000 population, in 1980. Contrasted to the corresponding statistics in 1976, these ratios reflected 12.7 percent and 11.2 percent gains, respectively.

The 1977-78 inventory of registered nurses indicated there were 1,375,208 registered nurses holding an active license to practice nursing. Of that number, 958,308 nurses, or 69.7 percent, reported employment in nursing; 323,483 nurses, or 23.5 percent, were not employed in nursing; and 93,417, or 6.8 percent, failed to report employment status. Adjustments for nonresponse were made to the questions on employment status and county of employment, and the corresponding totals are presented in the table showing the ratios of nurses to population by state and region. All other tables incorporate the unadjusted counts.

Using the adjusted data, it was estimated there were 1,028,003 nurses, or 74.8 percent of the registered nurse population, employed in nursing in 1977. This figure represented a 29.3 percent increase in the number of employed nurses since the 1972 inventory. Of the state and regional tabulations adjusted for nonresponse to employment status and county of employment, the District of Columbia showed the highest nurse-population ratio (885 nurses per 100,000 residents), followed by New Hampshire (782 nurses per 100,000 population). The lowest ratio (268 per 100,000 population) was observed in Arkansas, which traditionally had reported the lowest ratios. In general, the New England states had the most favorable ratios, and the South Central regions maintained the lowest nurse-population ratios. In terms of the total number of active nurses in each state, New York ranked first, with an estimated 101,443 nurses, and California was second, with 89,692 active nurses.

The preponderance of active nurses worked in institutional settings, predominantly hospitals. Almost two-thirds (65.0 percent) of all employed nurses were employed in hospitals. The second largest area was the nursing home sector, where 7.6 percent were working. With respect to the noninstitutional settings, 6.2 percent of the employed nurses were employed in physician's and dentist's offices; 5.5 percent were in general community health; 3.5 percent were school nurses; 3.4 percent were in schools of nursing; 2.8 percent were in private duty nursing; and 2.2 percent were in occupational health. Less than one percent (3,672 nurses) reported they were self-employed (other than private duty). About 2.2 percent reported some other field of employment, and 1.3 percent failed to report their employment setting.

The nursing home and community health fields recorded the largest growth in the number of active nurses since 1972, 34.6 percent and 35.2 percent, respectively. On the other hand, private duty nursing continued to decline as a career choice for nurses, down 32 percent since 1972.

When queried regarding the primary clinical practice area, more nurses marked medical-surgical nursing (39.2 percent) than any other area. There has been an upward trend in the proportion selecting medical-surgical nursing since 1966, when 33.7 percent reported this area. General nursing practice was the area cited by the next largest group, 14.8 percent, followed by geriatric nursing practice (8.0 percent).

There was a direct correspondence between age of the nurse and employment in nursing, reflecting a typical pattern observed in previous studies of nurses. Those in the youngest age groups showed higher activity rates, with a slight decline notable during the childbearing ages of 25-39 years, a slight resurgence in employment from 40-54 years, and a general decline thereafter. The 1977 data, in contrast to that of 1972, suggested that younger nurses were staying employed longer and older nurses were dropping out of nursing at a much higher rate.

Nurses are predominantly women. Only 27,301 of the nation's nurses in 1977 were men. While the number of men in nursing has increased by 86.7 percent since 1972, their relative proportion in the population showed only slight gains. In 1972, men comprised 1.3 percent of the nurse population, and in 1977, 2.0 percent.

A review of the data by marital status showed 65.5 percent overall were married. Activity rates varied by marital status. Of those employed in nursing, married nurses had a greater proclivity toward part-time work. About 57.7 percent of the full-time and 83.6 percent of the part-time complement were married. Of those not employed in nursing, 79.2 percent were married.

Trends in the highest educational preparation of the nurses are important statistics to monitor, since demands for improvement in the health care delivery system as well as certain positions often require additional educational preparation beyond the initial nursing preparation. According to the 1977-78 inventory, 59.8 percent of the registered nurse population hold a nursing diploma as their highest credential; 12.2 percent, an associate degree; 18.1 percent, a baccalaureate; and 4.0 percent, a master's degree or doctorate. In contrast, the 1972 ANA inventory reported 71.1 percent holding a diploma; 4.3 percent, an associate degree; 14.0 percent, a baccalaureate; and 3.0 percent, a master's degree or doctorate as their highest educational preparation.

The 1977 national sample survey estimated there were 1,401,633 nurses licensed in September 1977, of whom 978,234 nurses, or almost 70 percent, were employed in nursing. An estimated 423,400 nurses were not employed in the nursing field. Of the total nurse population, 3.0 were not employed in nursing but were seeking employment in the field. About 27.2 percent of the total number were neither active in nursing nor seeking a nursing position. About 56,870 nurses, or 4.1 percent of the nurse population, were in non-nursing positions. Slightly more than one-third of that group were engaged in health-related employment.

Of the 323,980 inactive nurses out of the labor force at the time of the study, the majority tended to be over 50 years of age. Those in the younger age brackets were more likely to have children present in the home than not. About 90.7 percent of those inactive nurses less than 40 years of age reported having children at home, and 82.8 percent of the group in the 40-49 year age bracket indicated the presence of children in the household.

Selected data from the 1977 national sample survey recorded detailed information with respect to the highest educational preparation of employed nurses. The survey data revealed nurses in certain leadership positions were most likely to hold less than a baccalaureate as their highest educational credential, as were those holding positions primarily involving direct patient care activities.

Nurses who spent at least some portion of their time in direct patient care were queried regarding specific activities carried out during the course of their job. Several tasks were performed more often by nurses with baccalaureates than those with lesser education. These activities included obtaining health histories, performing some portion of physical examinations, selecting a plan of treatment as a result of interpreting laboratory test results, developing therapeutic plans, instructing patients in management of a defined illness, instructing and counseling patients and families in health promotion and maintenance, implementing therapy, and having primary responsibility for follow-through on patient care. Furthermore, significantly more nurses with master's and doctoral degrees than nurses without graduate education reported performing each of the tasks associated with the development of health care plans (selection of treatment plans, development and modification of medications, development of therapeutic plans, instruction and counseling of patients and families in health promotion and maintenance, and primary responsibility for follow-through on patient care) on a routine or often basis. On the other hand, two activities performed more often by registered nurses with associate degrees and diplomas in contrast with those with higher degrees were assisting the physician during physical examinations and administering medications.

The Bureau of Labor Statistics calculates annual estimates of unemployment rates for registered nurses. The 1979 rate was 1.8 percent, which was invariant from the previous year.The average annual unemployment rate for nurses is substantially lower than for females generally, and more closely approximates the rate of pharmacists and other health professionals than it does the rates of those in other selected health occupations.

The National League for Nursing annually surveys newly licensed nurses 6 months after licensure. The 1978 study included new licensees from each state and the District of Columbia, excluding Iowa and Oklahoma. Nationally, 95.1 percent of the newly licensed nurses were employed in nursing, 0.7 percent were employed in another field, 1.9 percent were not employed but were seeking a nursing position, and 2.3 percent were entirely out of the labor force. The proportion of nurses actively seeking a nursing job ranged from none in Alaska to 4.0 percent in New York.

Data from the 1977 national sample survey of registered nurses was the first to provide estimates of the number and distribution of nurses whose basic nursing education was received in a foreign country and who were licensed in the United States. Out of the total registered nurse population in 1977, an estimated 3.7 percent, or 52,436 nurses, were foreign nurse graduates. Almost four-fifths (77.9 percent) of the foreign nurse graduates were employed in nursing. There were marked regional differences in the geographic distribution of foreign nurse graduates. The largest proportions, 28.1 percent and 26.5 percent, respectively, were located in the Middle Atlantic and Pacific regions.

Data from the U.S. Department of Justice, Immigration and Naturalization Service on professional and student nurses admitted as immigrants are included in this section. From 1976 to 1978 the number of professional nurses and health trainees immigrating to the United States has declined by more than 40 percent. In 1976 there were 6,444 professional nurses and health trainees from foreign countries entering the United States; by 1978, the comparable count was 3,817 nurses and health trainees. A decline in the relative proportions of professional nurses from Asia was observed. In 1976 almost 70 percent of the total number came from Asia, with those from the Philippines, India, and Korea accounting for the majority of this group. In 1977 and 1978 about 56.0 percent and 57.0 percent of the nurses, respectively, were from Asia. There was a substantial drop in the number of nurses from India and Korea in the past 2 years.

Table I-A-1. Estimated Number of Registered Nurses in Relation to Population, 1971-1980

Year	Resident population (in thousands)	Number of nurses in practice		Nurses per 100,000 population	FTE per 100,000 population
		Total nurses	Full-time equivalent		
1980[1]	221,227	1,119,100	945,700	506	427
1979[1]	219,213	1,074,500	907,500	490	414
1978[1]	217,391	1,028,400	868,300	473	399
1977[1]	215,585	981,500	828,300	455	384
1976	214,047	961,000	821,650	449	384
1975	212,318	906,000	774,500	427	365
1974	210,674	857,000	732,500	407	348
1973	209,118	815,000	696,500	390	333
1972	207,364	780,000	664,000	376	320
1971	205,056	750,000	642,000	366	313

[1]Preliminary estimates.

SOURCES: U.S. Department of Health and Human Services, Public Health Service, Health Resources Administration, Bureau of Health Professions, Division of Health Professions Analysis. Unpublished data, 1980. Interagency Conference on Nursing Statistics, 1976 and previous years.

Table I-A-2. Estimated Number of Employed Registered Nurses by Highest Educational Preparation, 1971-1980

Year	Total	Highest educational preparation							
		Diploma		Associate degree		Baccalaureate		Master's and above	
		Number	Percent	Number	Percent	Number	Percent	Number	Percent
1980[1]	1,119,100	833,800	74.5	(2)	(2)	232,100	20.7	53,200	4.8
1979[1]	1,074,500	810,800	75.5	(2)	(2)	214,600	20.0	49,100	4.6
1978[1]	1,028,400	785,700	76.4	(2)	(2)	197,500	19.2	45,200	4.4
1977[1]	981,500	760,600	77.5	(2)	(2)	178,900	18.2	42,000	4.3
1976	961,000	765,000	79.6	(2)	(2)	163,000	17.0	33,000	3.4
1975	906,000	731,500	80.7	(2)	(2)	144,000	15.9	30,500	3.4
1974	857,000	647,000	75.5	51,600	6.0	130,400	15.2	28,000	3.3
1973	815,000	627,500	77.0	43,200	5.3	118,200	14.5	26,100	3.2
1972	780,000	613,400	78.6	35,200	4.5	107,200	13.7	24,200	3.1
1971	750,000	603,100	80.4	27,800	3.7	96,600	12.9	22,500	3.0

[1]Preliminary estimates.
[2]Nurses with associate degrees as highest educational preparation are included with diploma.

SOURCES: U.S. Department of Health and Human Services, Public Health Service, Health Resources Administration, Bureau of Health Professions, Division of Health Professions Analysis. Unpublished data, 1980. U.S. Department of Health, Education, and Welfare, Public Health Service, Health Resources Administration, Bureau of Health Manpower, Division of Nursing, *First Report to the Congress, February 1, 1977*, p. 18; Interagency Conference on Nursing Statistics, 1976, and previous years.

Table I-A-3. Adjusted Totals for Employed Registered Nurses and Ratio per 100,000 Population, by State and Region, 1977-78

State and region	Employed nurses[1] (adjusted figure)	Nurse-population ratio[2]	State and region	Employed nurses[1] (adjusted figure)	Nurse-population ratio[2]
United States, total .	1,028,003	- 472			
New England.....	88,427	718	East North Central .	199,077	484
Connecticut	20,789	662	Illinois..........	58,043	515
Maine..........	6,263	574	Indiana	22,909	429
Massachusetts ...	45,165	776	Michigan.........	41,533	454
New Hampshire .	6,628	782	Ohio	52,969	494
Rhode Island	6,188	661	Wisconsin........	23,623	505
Vermont	3,394	698			
			West North Central .	91,293	536
Middle Atlantic...	209,337	561	Iowa	15,499	530
New Jersey	35,284	480	Kansas	11,848	506
New York.......	101,443	561	Minnesota	26,159	652
Pennsylvania	72,610	611	Missouri	21,542	449
			Nebraska	8,874	562
South Atlantic....	151,682	438	North Dakota	3,775	577
Delaware	3,553	602	South Dakota.....	3,596	512
Dist. of Columbia	6,136	885			
Florida	41,120	475	Mountain.........	50,111	492
Georgia.........	18,153	361	Arizona..........	13,795	590
Maryland	19,672	471	Colorado.........	15,492	583
North Carolina...	23,897	429	Idaho............	3,516	404
South Carolina...	10,087	348	Montana.........	3,957	510
Virginia.........	21,648	420	Nevada..........	2,709	422
West Virginia....	7,416	398	New Mexico	4,468	368
			Utah	4,350	340
East South Central	43,793	315	Wyoming	1,824	440
Alabama........	10,828	291			
Kentucky	11,677	333	Pacific...........	128,461	436
Mississippi......	6,512	273	Alaska...........	1,776	422
Tennessee.......	14,776	344	California........	89,692	407
			Hawaii	3,979	440
West South Central	65,822	302	Oregon	12,793	532
Arkansas	5,776	267	Washington	20,221	547
Louisiana	11,459	291			
Oklahoma.......	8,845	312			
Texas	39,742	309			

[1] Adjusted for nonresponse to questions on employment status and county of employment.
[2] Ratios based on 1977 population, Market Statistics.

SOURCE: American Nurses' Association, Research and Policy Analysis Department, Statistics Unit, 1977-78 inventory of registered nurses. Pre-publication data. 1980.

CHART 1. RATIO OF EMPLOYED NURSES TO POPULATION,¹ 1977-78

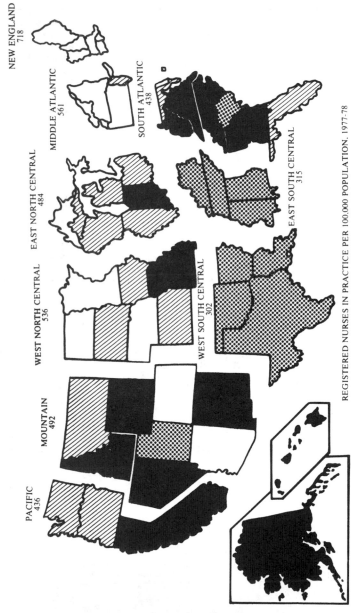

NEW ENGLAND
718

MIDDLE ATLANTIC
561

SOUTH ATLANTIC
438

EAST NORTH CENTRAL
484

EAST SOUTH CENTRAL
315

WEST NORTH CENTRAL
536

WEST SOUTH CENTRAL
302

MOUNTAIN
492

PACIFIC
436

REGISTERED NURSES IN PRACTICE PER 100,000 POPULATION, 1977-78

885-561 (15 STATES)   449-361 (13 STATES)
547-454 (13 STATES)   348-268 (10 STATES)

¹Excludes armed forces overseas.

SOURCE: American Nurses' Association. Research and Policy Analysis Department Statistics Unit. 1977-78 inventory of registered nurses. Prepublication data. 1980.

Table I-A-4. Number and Percent[1] of Registered Nurses, Employed or Resident in each State, by Employment Status, 1977-78

State	Total number	Employed in nursing		Not employed in nursing		Employment status not reported	
		Number	Percent	Number	Percent	Number	Percent
Total	1,375,208	958,308	69.7	323,483	23.5	93,417	6.8
Alabama	13,372	10,599	79.3	2,500	18.7	273	2.0
Alaska	2,474	1,670	67.5	658	26.6	146	5.9
Arizona	19,139	12,825	67.0	4,978	26.0	1,336	7.0
Arkansas	8,253	5,714	69.2	1,928	23.4	611	7.4
California	125,308	80,372	64.1	32,078	25.6	12,858	10.3
Colorado	20,801	15,138	72.8	5,200	25.0	463	2.2
Connecticut	27,851	16,712	60.0	5,253	18.9	5,886	21.1
Delaware	4,993	3,454	69.2	1,408	28.2	131	2.6
District of Columbia	6,613	5,625	85.1	434	6.6	554	8.4
Florida	55,368	37,517	67.8	12,398	22.4	5,453	9.8
Georgia	23,628	16,674	70.6	5,157	21.8	1,797	7.6
Hawaii	5,174	3,190	61.7	958	18.5	1,026	19.8
Idaho	4,962	3,463	69.8	1,432	28.9	67	1.4
Illinois	74,262	49,626	66.8	14,422	19.4	10,214	13.8
Indiana	28,069	20,891	74.4	4,682	16.7	2,496	8.9
Iowa	20,171	15,083	74.8	4,402	21.8	686	3.4
Kansas	16,143	10,721	66.4	3,878	24.0	1,544	9.6
Kentucky	15,583	11,020	70.7	3,682	23.6	881	5.7
Louisiana	14,298	11,234	78.6	2,782	19.5	282	2.0
Maine	8,966	5,922	66.0	2,565	28.6	479	5.3
Maryland	28,117	18,246	64.9	7,727	27.5	2,144	7.6
Massachusetts	61,664	42,463	68.9	15,411	25.0	3,790	6.1
Michigan	56,888	40,035	70.4	15,025	26.4	1,828	3.2
Minnesota	31,299	22,087	70.6	4,670	14.9	4,542	14.5
Mississippi	8,243	6,474	78.5	1,701	20.6	68	0.8
Missouri	26,662	19,844	74.4	4,179	15.7	2,639	9.9
Montana	5,326	3,869	72.6	1,336	25.1	121	2.3
Nebraska	12,002	8,601	71.7	3,068	25.6	333	2.8
Nevada	3,586	2,615	72.9	851	23.7	120	3.3
New Hampshire	9,457	6,445	68.2	2,727	28.8	285	3.0
New Jersey	49,969	31,418	62.9	13,533	27.1	5,018	10.0
New Mexico	6,281	4,321	68.8	1,668	26.6	292	4.6
New York	132,209	98,667	74.6	29,940	22.6	3,602	2.7
North Carolina	30,125	23,718	78.7	5,949	19.7	458	1.5
North Dakota	4,735	3,670	77.5	935	19.7	130	2.7
Ohio	69,620	51,127	73.4	16,104	23.1	2,389	3.4
Oklahoma	11,949	8,107	67.8	2,587	21.7	1,255	10.5
Oregon	15,199	12,538	82.5	2,359	15.5	302	2.0
Pennsylvania	107,153	65,781	61.4	33,198	31.0	8,174	7.6
Rhode Island	7,991	5,986	74.9	1,729	21.6	276	3.5
South Carolina	12,982	9,967	76.8	2,832	21.8	183	1.4
South Dakota	4,617	3,504	75.9	995	21.6	118	2.6
Tennessee	18,569	13,989	75.3	3,483	18.8	1,097	5.9
Texas	54,549	38,902	71.3	14,471	26.5	1,176	2.2
Utah	6,164	4,276	69.4	1,793	29.1	95	1.5
Vermont	4,750	3,287	69.2	1,299	27.3	164	3.5
Virginia	30,204	21,239	70.3	8,307	27.5	658	2.2
Washington	29,165	17,097	58.6	7,453	25.6	4,615	15.8
West Virginia	9,440	7,364	78.0	2,009	21.3	67	0.7
Wisconsin	28,359	23,461	82.7	4,692	16.5	206	0.7
Wyoming	2,506	1,760	70.2	657	26.2	89	3.6

[1]Percentages may not add to 100.0 due to rounding.

SOURCE: American Nurses' Association, Research and Policy Analysis Department, Statistics Unit, 1977-78 inventory of registered nurses. Pre-publication data, 1980.

Table I-A-5. Number and Percent[1] of Registered Nurses, Employed in Nursing, by Field of Employment and Type of Position, 1977-78

Type of position	Total		Hospital		Nursing home		School of nursing		Private duty		Community health	
	Number	Percent	Number	Percent	Number	Percent	Number	Percent	Number	Percent	Number	Percent
Total	958,308	100.0	622,804	100.0	72,692	100.0	32,199	100.0	26,410	100.0	52,864	100.0
Administrator/assistant	34,881	3.6	14,796	2.4	8,052	11.1	2,755	8.6	...	...	3,998	7.6
Consultant	7,609	0.8	1,236	0.2	1,273	1.8	125	0.4	...	...	1,778	3.4
Supervisor/assistant	91,862	9.6	56,734	9.1	17,456	24.0	289	0.9	...	...	7,470	14.1
Instructor	42,775	4.5	10,266	1.6	1,612	2.2	26,272	81.6	...	...	878	1.7
Head nurse/assistant	133,426	13.9	96,019	15.4	17,273	23.8	179	0.6	...	...	3,389	6.4
General duty/staff	543,782	56.7	408,443	65.6	24,233	33.3	807	2.5	...	...	27,964	52.9
Nurse practitioner	13,625	1.4	4,378	0.7	194	0.3	180	0.6	...	...	2,582	4.9
Clinical nursing specialist	5,472	0.6	3,276	0.5	44	0.1	437	1.4	...	...	728	1.4
Other specified type	68,311	7.1	21,817	3.5	1,400	1.9	734	2.3	26,410	100.0	2,966	5.6
Not reported	16,565	1.7	5,839	0.9	1,155	1.6	421	1.3	...		1,111	2.1

Type of position	School nurse		Occupational health nurse		Office nurse (physician's or dentist's)		Self-employed		Other specified field		Field of employment not reported	
	Number	Percent	Number	Percent	Number	Percent	Number	Percent	Number	Percent	Number	Percent
Total	33,530	100.0	20,736	100.0	59,553	100.0	3,672	100.0	21,112	100.0	12,736	100.0
Administrator/assistant	1,099	3.3	756	3.6	1,213	2.0	247	6.7	1,608	7.6	357	2.8
Consultant	807	2.4	298	1.4	191	0.3	363	9.9	1,345	6.4	193	1.5
Supervisor/assistant	1,816	5.4	2,375	11.5	2,839	4.8	93	2.5	2,101	10.0	689	5.4
Instructor	...	...	324	1.6	232	0.4	533	14.5	2,264	10.7	394	3.1
Head nurse/assistant	2,507	7.5	3,865	18.6	7,653	12.9	61	1.7	1,777	8.4	703	5.5
General duty/staff	23,840	71.1	11,594	55.9	38,764	65.1	521	14.2	4,948	23.4	2,668	20.9
Nurse practitioner	915	2.7	404	1.9	3,384	5.7	253	6.9	1,103	5.2	232	1.8
Clinical nursing specialist	157	0.5	35	0.2	212	0.4	182	5.0	299	1.4	102	0.8
Other specified type	2,389	7.1	1,085	5.2	5,065	8.5	1,109	30.2	4,713	22.3	623	4.9
Not reported	...		...		...		310	8.4	954	4.5	6,775	53.2

[1]Percentages may not add to 100.0 due to rounding.

SOURCE: American Nurses' Association, Research and Policy Analysis Department, Statistics Unit, 1977-78 inventory of registered nurses. Pre-publication data, 1980.

Table I-A-6. Number and Percent¹ of Registered Nurses, Employed in Nursing, by Field of Employment and Area of Clinical Practice, 1977-78

Area of clinical practice	Total		Hospital		Nursing home		School of nursing		Private duty		Community health	
	Number	Percent	Number	Percent	Number	Percent	Number	Percent	Number	Percent	Number	Percent
Total	958,308	100.0	622,804	100.0	72,692	100.0	32,199	100.0	26,410	100.0	52,864	100.0
Community health	61,059	6.4	4,581	0.7	373	0.5	1,952	6.1	423	1.6	31,656	59.9
General practice	142,205	14.8	78,976	12.7	3,733	5.1	3,100	9.6	9,973	37.8	3,586	6.8
Geriatric	76,606	8.0	9,147	1.5	58,578	80.6	634	2.0	2,716	10.3	2,345	4.4
Obstetric/gynecologic	76,057	7.9	59,519	9.6	303	0.4	3,487	10.8	364	1.4	2,127	4.0
Medical/surgical	375,361	39.2	332,077	53.3	1,455	2.0	13,397	41.6	7,195	27.2	1,563	3.0
Pediatric/maternal-child health	59,928	6.3	41,559	6.7	434	0.6	2,983	9.3	337	1.3	2,348	4.4
Psychiatric/mental health	51,564	5.4	35,823	5.8	1,747	2.4	3,280	10.2	345	1.3	5,456	10.3
Other clinical areas	47,078	4.9	27,847	4.5	627	0.9	1,892	5.9	614	2.3	1,460	2.8
Not reported	68,450	7.1	33,275	5.3	5,442	7.5	1,474	4.6	4,443	16.8	2,323	4.4

Area of clinical practice	School nurse		Occupational health nurse		Office nurse (physician's or dentist's)		Self-employed		Other specified field		Field of employment not reported	
	Number	Percent	Number	Percent	Number	Percent	Number	Percent	Number	Percent	Number	Percent
Total	33,530	100.0	20,736	100.0	59,553	100.0	3,672	100.0	21,112	100.0	12,736	100.0
Community health	15,425	46.0	2,806	13.5	843	1.4	232	6.3	1,585	7.5	1,183	9.3
General practice	5,050	15.1	11,110	53.6	21,504	36.1	638	17.4	3,242	15.4	1,293	10.2
Geriatric	153	0.5	152	0.7	423	0.7	312	8.5	1,444	6.8	702	5.5
Obstetric/gynecologic	401	1.2	122	0.6	7,349	12.3	672	18.3	1,229	5.8	484	3.8
Medical/surgical	919	2.7	1,053	5.1	12,610	21.2	474	12.9	2,745	13.0	1,873	14.7
Pediatric/maternal-child health	4,539	13.5	102	0.5	6,004	10.1	105	2.9	1,103	5.2	414	3.3
Psychiatric/mental health	517	1.5	279	1.3	484	0.8	395	10.8	2,357	11.2	881	6.9
Other clinical areas	2,338	7.0	1,907	9.2	4,211	7.1	480	13.1	5,165	24.5	537	4.2
Not reported	4,188	12.5	3,205	15.5	6,125	10.3	364	9.9	2,242	10.6	5,369	42.2

¹Percentages may not add to 100.0 due to rounding.

SOURCE: American Nurses' Association, Research and Policy Analysis Department, Statistics Unit, 1977-78 inventory of registered nurses. Pre-publication data, 1980.

Table I-A-7. Number of Registered Nurses, by Age Group, Sex, and Employment Status, 1977-78

Sex and employment status	Total number	Age group										
		Under 25 years	25-29	30-34	35-39	40-44	45-49	50-54	55-59	60-64	65 years and over	Age not reported
Total	*1,375,208*	*100,359*	*212,009*	*193,269*	*162,355*	*142,206*	*124,767*	*125,920*	*95,353*	*64,871*	*70,698*	*83,401*
Employed in nursing	958,308	92,791	177,311	141,977	115,850	104,606	92,654	90,144	63,902	36,362	20,365	22,346
Not employed in nursing	323,483	5,517	29,178	46,012	41,952	33,502	28,568	32,032	28,231	25,635	44,768	8,088
Employment status not reported	93,417	2,051	5,520	5,280	4,553	4,098	3,545	3,744	3,220	2,874	5,565	52,967
Female	*1,273,034*	*95,450*	*197,453*	*181,092*	*153,879*	*135,370*	*118,995*	*120,652*	*91,605*	*62,260*	*67,823*	*48,455*
Employed in nursing	907,928	88,516	165,928	133,135	110,182	100,088	88,806	86,785	61,717	35,088	19,621	18,062
Not employed in nursing .	314,277	5,276	28,025	44,685	40,872	32,615	27,862	31,364	27,639	24,998	43,630	7,311
Employment status not reported	50,829	1,658	3,500	3,272	2,825	2,667	2,327	2,503	2,249	2,174	4,572	23,082
Male	*27,301*	*1,826*	*6,727*	*6,031*	*3,462*	*2,345*	*1,934*	*1,380*	*1,084*	*761*	*654*	*1,097*
Employed in nursing	22,855	1,667	6,059	5,357	3,028	1,995	1,637	1,149	798	461	223	481
Not employed in nursing ..	3,300	113	511	524	352	301	259	204	252	273	402	109
Employment status not reported	1,146	46	157	150	82	49	38	27	34	27	29	507
Sex not reported	*74,873*	*3,083*	*7,829*	*6,146*	*5,014*	*4,491*	*3,838*	*3,888*	*2,664*	*1,850*	*2,221*	*33,849*
Employed in nursing	27,525	2,608	5,324	3,485	2,640	2,523	2,211	2,210	1,387	813	521	3,803
Not employed in nursing ...	5,906	128	642	803	728	586	447	464	340	364	736	668
Employment status not reported	41,442	347	1,863	1,858	1,646	1,382	1,180	1,214	937	673	964	29,378

SOURCE: American Nurses' Association, Research and Policy Analysis Department, Statistics Unit, 1977-78 inventory of registered nurses. Pre-publication data, 1980.

Table I-A-8. Percent[1] of Registered Nurses, by Age Group, Sex, and Employment Status, 1977-78

Sex and employment status	Total number	Age group										
		Under 25 years	25-29	30-34	35-39	40-44	45-49	50-54	55-59	60-64	65 years and over	Age not reported
Total	100.0	100.0	100.0	100.0	100.0	100.0	100.0	100.0	100.0	100.0	100.0	100.0
Employed in nursing	69.7	92.5	83.6	73.5	71.4	73.6	74.3	71.6	67.0	56.1	28.8	26.8
Not employed in nursing	23.5	5.5	13.8	23.8	25.8	23.6	22.9	25.4	29.6	39.5	63.3	9.7
Employment status not reported	6.8	2.0	2.6	2.7	2.8	2.9	2.8	3.0	3.4	4.4	7.9	63.5
Female	92.6	95.1	93.1	93.7	94.8	95.2	95.4	95.8	96.1	96.0	95.9	58.1
Employed in nursing	71.3	88.2	78.3	68.9	67.9	70.4	71.2	68.9	64.7	54.1	27.8	21.7
Not employed in nursing	24.7	5.3	13.2	23.1	25.2	22.9	22.3	24.9	29.0	38.5	61.7	8.8
Employment status not reported	4.0	1.7	1.7	1.7	1.7	1.9	1.9	2.0	2.4	3.4	6.5	27.7
Male	2.0	1.8	3.2	3.1	2.1	1.6	1.6	1.1	1.1	1.2	0.9	1.3
Employed in nursing	1.7	1.7	2.9	2.8	1.9	1.4	1.3	0.9	0.8	0.7	0.3	0.6
Not employed in nursing	0.2	0.1	0.2	0.3	0.2	0.2	0.2	0.2	0.3	0.4	0.6	0.1
Employment status not reported	0.1	(²)	0.1	(²)	(²)	(²)	0.2	(²)	(²)	(²)	(²)	0.6
Sex not reported	5.4	3.1	3.7	3.2	3.1	3.2	3.1	3.1	2.8	2.9	3.1	40.6
Employed in nursing	2.0	2.6	2.5	1.8	1.6	1.8	1.8	1.8	1.5	1.3	0.7	4.6
Not employed in nursing	0.4	0.1	0.3	0.4	0.4	0.4	0.4	0.4	0.4	0.6	1.0	0.8
Employment status not reported	3.0	0.3	0.9	0.9	1.0	1.0	0.9	1.0	1.0	1.0	1.4	35.2

[1]Percentages may not add to 100.0 due to rounding.
[2]Less than 0.1 percent.

SOURCE: American Nurses' Association, Research and Policy Analysis Department, Statistics Unit, 1977-78 inventory of registered nurses. Pre-publication data, 1980.

Table I-A-9. Number and Percent¹ of Registered Nurses, Employed in Nursing, by Highest Educational Preparation and Field of Employment, 1977-78

Field of employment	Total nurses		Highest educational preparation													
			Less than baccalaureate		Baccalaureate in nursing		Baccalaureate in other field		Master's in nursing		Master's in other field		Doctorate		Not reported	
	Number	Per cent	Number	Per cent	Number	Per cent	Number	Per cent	Number	Per cent	Number	Per cent	Number	Per cent	Number	Per cent
Total	958,308	100.0	722,861	75.4	158,086	16.5	31,262	3.3	26,608	2.8	13,162	1.4	1,846	0.2	4,483	0.5
Hospital	622,804	100.0	485,855	78.0	102,823	16.5	18,079	2.9	9,291	1.5	4,099	0.7	276	(2)	2,381	0.4
Nursing home	72,692	100.0	63,328	87.1	6,188	8.5	1,853	2.5	533	0.7	423	0.6	37	0.1	330	0.5
School of nursing	32,199	100.0	4,849	15.1	9,526	29.6	2,116	6.6	10,679	33.2	3,766	11.7	1,197	3.7	66	0.2
Private duty	26,410	100.0	22,842	86.5	2,087	7.9	748	2.8	227	0.9	200	0.8	25	0.1	281	1.1
Community health	52,864	100.0	30,872	58.4	15,553	29.4	2,097	4.0	2,606	4.9	1,488	2.8	64	0.1	184	0.3
School nurse	33,530	100.0	19,122	57.0	8,358	24.9	3,290	9.8	800	2.4	1,770	5.3	33	0.1	157	0.5
Occupational health nurse	20,736	100.0	18,400	88.7	1,455	7.0	573	2.8	81	0.4	118	0.6	6	(2)	103	0.5
Office nurse	59,553	100.0	52,203	87.7	5,631	9.5	944	1.6	272	0.5	148	0.2	9	(2)	346	0.6
Self-employed	3,672	100.0	2,321	63.2	630	17.2	171	4.7	354	9.6	141	3.8	33	0.9	22	0.6
Other specified field	21,112	100.0	13,829	65.5	3,916	18.5	980	4.6	1,391	6.6	770	3.6	133	0.6	93	0.4
Not reported	12,736	100.0	9,240	72.6	1,919	15.1	411	3.2	374	2.9	239	1.9	33	0.3	520	4.1

¹Percentages may not add to 100.0 due to rounding.

²Less than 0.1 percent.

SOURCE: American Nurses' Association, Research and Policy Analysis Department, Statistics Unit, 1977-78 inventory of registered nurses. Pre-publication data, 1980.

Table I-A-10. Number and Percent¹ of Registered Nurses by Employment Status, Marital Status and Sex, 1977-78

Marital status and sex	Total		Employed in nursing										Not employed in nursing		Employment status not reported	
			Total		Full-time		Part-time (regular)		Part-time (irregular)		Full or part-time not reported					
	Number	Percent	Number	Percent	Number	Percent	Number	Percent	Number	Percent	Number	Percent	Number	Percent	Number	Percent
All nurses	1,375,208	100.0	958,308	100.0	667,709	100.0	186,751	100.0	99,764	100.0	4,084	100.0	323,483	100.0	93,417	100.0
Never married	192,704	14.0	167,656	17.5	153,487	23.0	7,823	4.2	5,843	5.9	503	12.3	21,591	6.7	3,457	3.7
Married	901,206	65.5	627,568	65.5	385,143	57.7	159,570	85.4	80,067	80.3	2,788	68.3	256,133	79.2	17,505	18.7
Widowed	60,327	4.4	36,700	3.8	26,768	4.0	4,557	2.4	5,120	5.1	255	6.2	21,460	6.6	2,167	2.3
Divorced/separated	104,457	7.6	88,306	9.2	77,026	11.5	6,635	3.6	4,342	4.4	303	7.4	13,783	4.3	2,368	2.5
Marital status not reported	116,514	8.5	38,078	4.0	25,285	3.8	8,166	4.4	4,392	4.4	235	5.8	10,516	3.3	67,920	72.7
Female	1,273,034	100.0	907,928	100.0	629,801	100.0	178,646	100.0	95,616	100.0	3,865	100.0	314,277	100.0	50,829	100.0
Never married	186,607	14.7	162,302	17.9	148,662	23.6	7,531	4.2	5,629	5.9	480	12.4	20,980	6.7	3,325	6.5
Married	880,742	69.2	610,668	67.3	370,139	58.8	158,506	88.7	79,320	83.0	2,703	69.9	253,121	80.5	16,953	33.4
Widowed	59,587	4.7	36,247	4.0	26,433	4.2	4,507	2.5	5,055	5.3	252	6.5	21,223	6.8	2,117	4.2
Divorced/separated	101,923	8.0	86,178	9.5	75,106	11.9	6,528	3.7	4,250	4.4	294	7.6	13,469	4.3	2,276	4.5
Marital status not reported	44,175	3.5	12,533	1.4	9,461	1.5	1,574	0.9	1,362	1.4	136	3.5	5,484	1.7	26,158	51.5
Male	27,301	100.0	22,855	100.0	20,743	100.0	1,187	100.0	842	100.0	83	100.0	3,300	100.0	1,146	100.0
Never married	5,739	21.0	5,092	22.3	4,615	22.2	268	22.6	196	23.3	13	15.7	536	16.2	111	9.7
Married	17,982	65.9	15,270	66.8	13,887	66.9	794	66.9	530	62.9	59	71.1	2,318	70.2	394	34.4
Widowed	322	1.2	217	0.9	178	0.9	22	1.9	17	2.0	...	...	91	2.8	14	1.2
Divorced/separated	2,040	7.5	1,724	7.5	1,562	7.5	85	7.2	70	8.3	7	8.4	254	7.7	62	5.4
Marital status not reported	1,218	4.5	552	2.4	501	2.4	18	1.5	29	3.4	4	4.8	101	3.1	565	49.3
Sex not reported	74,873	100.0	27,525	100.0	17,165	100.0	6,918	100.0	3,306	100.0	136	100.0	5,906	100.0	41,442	100.0
Never married	358	0.5	262	1.0	210	1.2	24	0.3	18	0.5	10	7.4	75	1.3	21	0.1
Married	2,482	3.3	1,630	5.9	1,117	6.5	270	3.9	217	6.6	26	19.1	694	11.8	158	0.4
Widowed	418	0.6	236	0.9	157	0.9	28	0.4	48	1.5	3	2.2	146	2.5	158	0.4
Divorced/separated	494	0.7	404	1.5	358	2.1	22	0.3	22	0.7	2	1.5	60	1.0	30	0.1
Marital status not reported	71,121	95.0	24,993	90.8	15,323	89.3	6,574	95.0	3,001	90.8	95	69.9	4,931	83.5	41,197	99.4

¹Percentages may not add to 100.0 due to rounding.

SOURCE: American Nurses' Association, Research and Policy Analysis Department, Statistics Unit, 1977-78 inventory of registered nurses. Pre-publication data, 1980.

Table I-A-11. Number and Percent¹ of Male Registered Nurses, Employed in Nursing, by Field of Employment and Type of Position, 1977-78

Type of position	Total		Hospital		Nursing home		School of nursing		Private duty		Community health	
	Number	Percent	Number	Percent	Number	Percent	Number	Percent	Number	Percent	Number	Percent
Total	22,855	100.0	18,594	100.0	851	100.0	473	100.0	338	100.0	688	100.0
Administrator/assistant	1,374	6.0	818	4.4	218	25.6	68	14.4	...	...	92	13.4
Consultant	180	0.8	53	0.3	6	0.7	1	0.2	...	...	47	6.8
Supervisor/assistant ...	2,543	11.1	1,994	10.7	223	26.2	5	1.1	...	...	108	15.7
Instructor	735	3.2	293	1.6	23	2.7	347	73.4	...	...	13	1.9
Head nurse/assistant ..	2,969	13.0	2,568	13.8	145	17.0	3	0.6	...	...	70	10.2
General duty/staff	10,148	44.4	9,106	49.0	209	24.6	12	2.5	...	...	244	35.5
Nurse practitioner	541	2.4	336	1.8	8	0.9	4	0.8	...	...	47	6.8
Clinical nursing specialist	167	0.7	107	0.6	3	0.4	13	2.7	...	...	11	1.6
Other specified type ...	3,819	16.7	3,131	16.8	8	0.9	14	3.0	338	100.0	43	6.3
Not reported	379	1.7	188	1.0	8	0.9	6	1.3	...		13	1.9

Type of position	School nurse		Occupational health nurse		Office nurse (physician's or dentist's)		Self-employed		Other specified field		Field of employment not reported	
	Number	Percent	Number	Percent	Number	Percent	Number	Percent	Number	Percent	Number	Percent
Total	146	100.0	427	100.0	285	100.0	173	100.0	618	100.0	262	100.0
Administrator/assistant	15	10.3	41	9.6	10	3.5	16	9.2	80	12.9	16	6.1
Consultant	2	1.4	11	2.6	4	1.4	13	7.5	39	6.3	4	1.5
Supervisor/assistant ...	14	9.6	74	17.3	27	9.5	4	2.3	76	12.3	18	6.9
Instructor	...	...	3	0.7	3	1.1	4	2.3	42	6.8	7	2.7
Head nurse/assistant ..	12	8.2	64	15.0	32	11.2	4	2.3	60	9.7	11	4.2
General duty/staff	84	57.5	204	47.8	123	43.2	17	9.8	109	17.6	40	15.3
Nurse practitioner	7	4.8	11	2.6	50	17.5	22	12.7	46	7.4	10	3.8
Clinical nursing specialist	1	0.7	1	0.2	5	1.8	9	5.2	14	2.3	3	1.1
Other specified type ...	11	7.5	18	4.2	31	10.9	77	44.5	133	21.5	15	5.7
Not reported	...		...		...		7	4.0	19	3.1	138	52.7

¹Percentages may not add to 100.0 due to rounding.

Statistics Unit, 1977-78 inventory of registered nurses. Pre-publication data 1980.

Table I-A-12. Number and Percent[1] of Registered Nurses, Not Employed in Nursing, by Marital Status and Age Group, 1977-78

Age group	Total		Marital status									
			Never married		Married		Widowed		Divorced/separated		Not reported	
	Number	Percent	Number	Percent	Number	Percent	Number	Percent	Number	Percent	Number	Percent
Total	323,483	100.0	21,591	100.0	256,133	100.0	21,460	100.0	13,783	100.0	10,516	100.0
Under 25 years	5,517	1.7	1,500	6.9	3,686	1.4	11	0.1	91	0.7	229	2.2
25-29	29,178	9.0	2,587	12.0	24,921	9.7	83	0.4	724	5.3	863	8.2
30-34	46,012	14.2	1,540	7.1	41,928	16.4	193	0.9	1,224	8.9	1,127	10.7
35-39	41,952	13.0	1,051	4.9	38,249	14.9	297	1.4	1,358	9.9	997	9.5
40-44	33,502	10.4	882	4.1	30,061	11.7	433	2.0	1,262	9.2	864	8.2
45-49	28,568	8.8	1,050	4.9	24,929	9.7	664	3.1	1,176	8.5	749	7.1
50-54	32,032	9.9	1,453	6.7	27,183	10.6	1,227	5.7	1,418	10.3	751	7.1
55-59	28,231	8.7	1,706	7.9	22,700	8.9	1,904	8.9	1,271	9.2	650	6.2
60-64	25,635	7.9	2,320	10.7	17,637	6.9	3,476	16.2	1,509	10.9	693	6.6
65 years and over ...	44,768	13.8	6,966	32.3	20,081	7.8	12,462	58.1	3,401	24.7	1,858	17.7
Not reported	8,088	2.5	536	2.5	4,758	1.9	710	3.3	349	2.5	1,735	16.5

[1]Percentages may not add to 100.0 due to rounding.

SOURCE: American Nurses' Association, Research and Policy Analysis Department, Statistics Unit, 1977-78 inventory of registered nurses. Pre-publication data, 1980.

**Table I-A-13. Estimated Number and Percent of Registered Nurses[1]
Not Employed in Nursing, by Selected Characteristics, September 1977**

Characteristics	Number	Percent
	N=423,400	
Actively seeking nursing employment	*42,028*	*9.9*
Employed in non-nursing field	*56,870*	*13.4*
Not employed and not seeking employment	*323,980*	*76.5*
Less than 40 years of age	*111,995*	*26.5*
With children under 6 years of age	42,432	10.0
With children 6-17 years	59,176	14.0
No children	10,000	2.4
Not reported	387	0.1
40-49 years	*53,663*	*12.7*
With children	44,454	10.5
No children	9,016	2.1
Not reported	193	(2)
50 years and over	*155,104*	*36.6*
50-59 years	57,854	13.7
60 years and over	97,250	23.0
Age not reported	*3,218*	*0.8*
Not employed-seeking not reported	*522*	*0.1*

[1]Includes only registered nurses actively licensed and living in the United States in September 1977.
[2]Less than 0.1 percent.

SOURCE: Roth, Aleda V., et al. *1977 National Sample Survey of Registered Nurses: A Report on the Nurse Population and Factors Affecting Their Supply*, final report on Contract No. (HRA 231-76-0085) between the American Nurses' Association and the Division of Nursing, U.S. Department of Health and Human Services, NTIS Publication No. HRP-0900603, 1979. Unpublished data.

Table I-A-14. Estimated Percent of Registered Nurses[1] Employed in Selected "Leadership" Positions in Nursing Service Settings, by Highest Nursing-Related Educational Preparation, September 1977

"Leadership" positions	Highest nursing-related educational preparation				
	Diploma	Associate degree	Baccalaureate	Master's	Doctorate
Hospital director or assistant director of nursing services	53.1	8.8	20.8	16.0	1.3
Public health administrator or supervisor	47.6	9.4	33.3	8.6	1.1
Nursing home administrator or director of nursing services	78.2	7.4	9.1	5.3	...
In-service education director or instructor..	41.8	8.6	35.8	13.9	...
Hospital supervisor or assistant	69.3	11.1	17.0	2.6	...
Nursing home supervisor or assistant	76.2	8.8	13.7	1.4	...
Hospital head nurse or assistant	66.2	15.5	17.4	0.9	...

[1]Includes only registered nurses actively licensed and working in the United States in September 1977.

SOURCE: Roth, Aleda V., et al. *1977 National Sample Survey of Registered Nurses: A Report on the Nurse Population and Factors Affecting Their Supply*, final report on Contract No. (HRA 231-76-0085) between the American Nurses' Association and the Division of Nursing, U.S. Department of Health and Human Services, NTIS Publication No. HRP-0900603, 1979. Unpublished data.

Table I-A-15. Estimated Percent of Registered Nurses[1] Employed in Selected "Direct Patient Care" Positions, by Highest Nursing-Related Educational Preparation, September 1977

	Highest nursing-related educational preparation[2]			
"Direct patient care" positions	*Diploma*	*Associate degree*	*Baccalaureate*	*Master's*
Clinical nursing specialist	39.7	13.8	17.4	29.1
Nurse clinician	61.5	8.6	18.9	11.0
Nurse practitioner/midwife	47.5	4.1	29.2	19.1
Public health nurse	53.3	8.1	36.2	2.4
Staff nurse in public health agency	67.0	8.8	22.6	1.5
School nurse	52.7	4.7	36.5	6.1
Occupational health staff nurse	85.8	3.1	10.6	...
Hospital general duty/staff nurse	65.4	17.1	16.8	0.7
Nursing home general duty/staff nurse	81.4	7.3	10.1	0.8
Physician's office staff nurse ...	80.7	11.0	7.0	0.4

[1]Includes only registered nurses actively licensed and working in the United States in September 1977.

[2]No registered nurses in "direct patient care" positions with doctoral degrees.

SOURCE: Roth, Aleda V., et al. *1977 National Sample Survey of Registered Nurses: A Report on the Nurse Population and Factors Affecting Their Supply*, final report on Contract No. (HRA 231-76-0085) between the American Nurses' Association and the Division of Nursing, U.S. Department of Health and Human Services, NTIS Publication No. HRP-0900603, 1979. Unpublished data.

Table I-A-16. Estimated Percent of Registered Nurses[1] Spending Some Time in Direct Patient Care Who Performed Activities Routinely or Often by Highest Nursing-Related Educational Preparation and Activity in Primary Nursing Job, September 1977

Activity	Total	Highest nursing-related educational preparation		
		Less than baccalaureate	Baccalaureate	Master's degree and above
	(n =[2] 10,110) (N =[3] 857,765)	(n = 8,048) (N = 685,658)	(n = 1,822) (N = 151,032)	(n = 221) (N = 19,170)
Assessment				
Obtain health histories	56.7	55.4	61.9	61.7
Perform complete physical examinations	11.6	11.4	12.1	16.0
Perform some portion of physical examination	30.2	29.2	34.8	31.8
Assist during patient examinations	59.5	62.5	50.1	26.7
Devising a plan of health care				
Select plans of treatment	17.2	16.3	19.7	30.0
Develop and modify medication	27.7	27.2	29.0	36.5
Develop therapeutic plans	41.3	38.9	50.1	61.9
Implementing/evaluating a plan of health care				
Perform medical management	34.6	34.0	37.2	37.4
Instruct patients in management of defined illness	63.6	62.4	69.0	64.0
Instruct patients in health maintenance	60.1	57.7	69.4	76.8
Implement therapy	52.2	50.4	60.1	57.2
Administer medication	79.0	81.0	74.9	42.0
Sustain and support persons during diagnosis or therapy	64.4	64.1	67.0	57.0
Have primary responsibility for follow-through on patient care	41.6	40.5	45.4	52.9
Have primary responsibility for normal mothers	5.5	5.7	4.4	7.3

[1]Includes only registered nurses actively licensed and working in the United States in September 1977.

[2]Includes 19 registered nurses who did not report highest nursing-related educational preparation.

[3]Includes 1,904 (weighted) registered nurses who did not report highest nursing-related educational preparation.

NOTE: "N" corresponds to the weighted population estimate derived from the sample and "n" refers to the actual number of surveys upon which the estimate was based.

SOURCE: Roth, Aleda V., et al. *1977 National Sample Survey of Registered Nurses: A Report on the Nurse Population and Factors Affecting Their Supply*, final report on Contract No. (HRA 231-76-0085) between the American Nurses' Association and the Division of Nursing, U.S. Department of Health and Human Services, NTIS Publication No. HRP-0900603, 1979.

**Table I-A-17. Unemployment Rates for Registered Nurses and Others,
1970-1979**

Year	Annual averages				
	Registered nurses[1]	*Licensed practical nurses*[1]	*Total 16 years and over*	*Female 16 years and over*	*Female 25-54 years*
1979	1.8	4.2	5.8	6.8	5.2
1978	1.8	3.4	6.0	7.2	5.4
1977	2.6	3.9	7.0	8.2	6.4
1976	2.6	5.2	7.7	8.6	6.8
1975	2.3	4.8	8.5	9.3	7.5
1974	1.9	3.8	5.6	6.7	4.9
1973	1.9	3.1	4.9	6.0	4.4
1972	2.0	3.6	5.6	6.6	4.9
1971	2.0	3.0	5.9	6.9	5.3
1970	1.9	2.6	4.9	5.9	4.5

[1]In 90 cases out of 100, on the average, the standard error falls within the following ranges: RN, ±.44; LPN, ±1.00.

SOURCE: U.S. Department of Labor, Bureau of Labor Statistics, *Employment and Earnings*, and unpublished data, 1980.

Table I-A-18. Average Annual Unemployment Rates for Civilian Workers and Selected Health Occupations, 1971-1979

Occupations	1979	1978	1977	1976	1975	1974	1973	1972	1971
All civilian workers	5.8	6.0	7.0	7.7	8.5	5.6	4.9	5.6	5.9
Health occupations									
Physicians (M.D. and D.O.)	0.5	0.3	0.5	0.4	0.5	0.5	0.3	0.1	0.4
Dentists	0.1	0.5	0.8	0.6	. . .	0.3	0.2	. . .	0.5
Pharmacists	1.7	1.3	2.2	1.6	1.9	1.1	0.4	0.8	1.1
Registered nurses	1.8	1.8	2.6	2.6	2.3	1.9	1.9	2.0	2.0
Licensed practical nurses	4.2	3.4	3.9	5.2	4.8	3.8	3.1	3.6	3.0
Nurses' aides, orderlies, attendants . . .	7.7	8.3	8.5	9.3	8.7	6.2	6.4	5.7	6.1
Therapists	2.6	4.3	3.4	3.3	3.5	3.2	1.2	1.6	5.0
Clinical laboratory technologists, technicians	3.6	4.3	2.5	3.1	4.5	3.8	2.3	2.3	4.1
Health aides, except nursing	4.4	4.2	4.9	5.5	6.5	4.5	2.9	5.5	5.2
Dental assistants	6.3	5.6	8.7	8.3	7.0	6.3	5.2	3.9	5.0

SOURCE: U.S. Department of Labor, Bureau of Labor Statistics, *Employment and Earnings*, and unpublished data, 1980.

Table I-A-19. Employment of Newly Licensed Registered Nurses, Six Months After Licensure, by State of Residence, 1978

			Employment status		
				Not employed in nursing		
State	Total number	Employed in nursing	Employed in other field	Looking for work	Not looking for work
		Percent	Percent	Percent	Percent
Total	53,143	95.1	0.7	1.9	2.3
Alabama	908	96.0	0.6	2.1	1.3
Alaska	48	97.9	...	...	2.1
Arizona	533	93.4	0.9	2.1	3.6
Arkansas	411	95.4	0.5	1.7	2.4
California	3,950	94.5	0.7	2.2	2.5
Colorado	581	94.5	1.0	1.9	2.6
Connecticut	819	94.3	0.6	2.9	2.2
Delaware	182	94.0	...	3.3	2.7
District of Columbia	130	96.9	1.5	0.8	0.8
Florida	1,888	94.6	0.7	2.2	2.5
Georgia	1,089	96.1	1.2	1.2	1.6
Hawaii	141	87.2	2.8	3.5	6.4
Idaho	182	96.2	0.5	1.1	2.2
Illinois	2,689	96.7	0.4	1.3	1.6
Indiana	1,349	96.4	0.4	1.3	1.9
Iowa[1]	...	...	...	...	...
Kansas	683	96.5	0.7	0.3	2.5
Kentucky	928	95.3	1.0	1.6	2.2
Louisiana	813	94.8	0.9	2.2	2.1
Maine	299	96.3	1.3	0.7	1.7
Maryland	1,221	95.9	0.3	1.5	2.3
Massachusetts	1,974	95.9	0.9	1.6	1.6
Michigan	2,300	95.7	0.5	1.8	2.0
Minnesota	1,332	96.5	0.9	1.0	1.7
Mississippi	414	94.4	0.5	1.0	4.1
Missouri	1,406	96.7	0.4	1.1	1.8
Montana	210	95.2	1.0	1.4	2.4
Nebraska	470	94.9	0.2	1.1	3.8
Nevada	107	93.5	1.9	1.9	2.8
New Hampshire	271	96.7	1.1	1.5	0.7
New Jersey	2,047	94.7	0.5	2.3	2.5
New Mexico	262	94.7	0.4	3.4	1.5
New York	5,294	91.2	1.4	4.0	3.5
North Carolina	1,211	95.0	0.7	1.8	2.4
North Dakota	257	95.7	0.8	2.7	0.8
Ohio	2,981	96.7	0.4	1.5	1.4
Oklahoma[1]	...	...	...	...	...
Oregon	709	96.2	0.3	1.6	2.0
Pennsylvania	3,439	96.9	0.4	1.2	1.6
Rhode Island	239	96.7	0.8	1.3	1.3
South Carolina	585	94.9	1.0	1.7	2.4
South Dakota	231	96.5	1.7	0.4	1.3
Tennessee	993	95.7	0.4	1.2	2.7
Texas	2,983	95.0	0.5	1.6	2.8
Utah	341	94.1	0.6	0.9	4.4
Vermont	111	91.0	...	3.6	5.4
Virginia	1,291	94.9	1.1	1.9	2.1
Washington	1,007	91.8	1.6	3.3	3.4
West Virginia	429	93.0	0.5	1.9	4.7
Wisconsin	1,355	98.0	0.2	0.7	1.1
Wyoming	50	86.0	2.0	2.0	10.0

[1]Did not participate in survey.

SOURCE: National League for Nursing, *Employment, Mobility, and Personal Characteristics of Nurses Newly Licensed in 1978*, State Summaries, Volume 1, Publication No. 19-2050 (DS 8001), 1980.

Table I-A-20. Estimated Number and Percent of Registered Nurses[1] Who Received Their Basic Nursing Educational Preparation in a Foreign Country by Employment Status and Region,[2] September 1977

			Employment status			
			Employed in nursing		Not employed in nursing	
Region	Total					
	N	Percent	N	Percent	N	Percent
Total	52,436	100.0	40,851	77.9	11,585	22.1
Pacific	13,884	100.0	11,157	80.4	2,727	19.6
Mountain	1,719	100.0	1,208	70.3	511	29.7
West North Central	1,133	100.0	562	49.6	571	50.4
East North Central	8,897	100.0	6,816	76.6	2,081	23.4
West South Central	3,757	100.0	3,299	87.8	458	12.2
East South Central	267	100.0	267	100.0	...	...
South Atlantic	6,089	100.0	4,330	71.1	1,760	28.9
Middle Atlantic	14,739	100.0	11,724	79.5	3,016	20.5
New England	1,951	100.0	1,489	76.3	462	23.7

[1] Includes only registered nurses actively licensed in September 1977 who worked in the United States if employed in nursing, or lived in the United States if not employed in nursing.

[2] Region of employment if employed in nursing or region of residence if not employed in nursing. States included in each region are: *New England*—Connecticut, Maine, Massachusetts, New Hampshire, Rhode Island, Vermont; *Middle Atlantic*—New Jersey, New York, Pennsylvania; *South Atlantic*—Delaware, District of Columbia, Florida, Georgia, Maryland, North Carolina, South Carolina, Virginia, West Virginia; *East South Central*—Alabama, Kentucky, Mississippi, Tennessee; *West South Central*—Arkansas, Louisiana, Oklahoma, Texas; *East North Central*—Illinois, Indiana, Michigan, Ohio, Wisconsin; *West North Central*—Iowa, Kansas, Minnesota, Missouri, Nebraska, North Dakota, South Dakota; *Mountain*—Arizona, Colorado, Idaho, Montana, Nevada, New Mexico, Utah, Wyoming; *Pacific*—Alaska, California, Hawaii, Oregon, Washington.

NOTE: "N" corresponds to the weighted population estimate derived from the sample. Because of rounding, sums of estimated numbers (N) and estimated percents may not add to totals.

SOURCE: Roth, Aleda V., et al. *1977 National Sample Survey of Registered Nurses: A Report on the Nurse Population and Factors Affecting Their Supply*, final report on Contract No. (HRA 231-76-0085) between the American Nurses' Association and the Division of Nursing, U.S. Department of Health and Human Services, NTIS Publication No. HRP-0900603, 1979.

Table I-A-21. Estimated Number and Percent of Registered Nurses[1] Who Received Their Basic Nursing Educational Preparation in a Foreign Country (September 1977) and Foreign Stock[2] in the United States Population (April 1970), by Region[3]

Region	Estimated foreign stock in United States population		Estimated registered nurses				Ratio of foreign nurse graduates per 1,000 RNs
			Foreign nurse graduates		Total U.S. RN population		
	N	Percent	N	Percent	N	Percent	
Total	33,500,000	100.0	52,436	100.0	1,401,633	100.0	37.4
Pacific	6,200,000	18.5	13,884	26.5	202,767	14.5	68.5
Mountain	1,100,000	3.3	1,719	3.3	64,751	4.6	26.5
West North Central	1,940,000	5.8	1,133	2.2	115,035	8.2	9.8
East North Central	6,270,000	18.7	8,897	17.0	253,132	18.1	35.1
West South Central	1,470,000	4.4	3,757	7.2	88,280	6.3	42.6
East South Central	230,000	0.7	267	0.5	56,093	4.0	4.8
South Atlantic	2,410,000	7.2	6,089	11.6	193,556	13.8	31.5
Middle Atlantic	10,210,000	30.6	14,739	28.1	308,375	22.0	47.8
New England	3,620,000	10.8	1,951	3.7	119,643	8.5	16.3

[1]Includes only registered nurses actively licensed in September 1977 who worked in the United States if employed in nursing, or lived in the United States if not employed in nursing.

[2]U.S. Department of Commerce, Bureau of the Census, *County and City Data Book 1977*, p. 16. Includes the foreign-born population and the native population of foreign or mixed parentage.

[3]For the registered nurses, region indicates region of employment if employed in nursing, or region of residence if not employed in nursing. For the United States population, region is region of residence. For states included in each region, see Table I-A-20.

NOTE: "N" corresponds to the weighted population estimate derived from the sample. Because of rounding, sums of estimated numbers (N) and estimated percents may not add to totals.

SOURCE: Roth, Aleda V., et al. *1977 National Sample Survey of Registered Nurses: A Report on the Nurse Population and Factors Affecting Their Supply*, final report on Contract No. (HRA 231-76-0085) between the American Nurses' Association and the Division of Nursing, U.S. Department of Health and Human Services, NTIS Publication No. HRP-0900603, 1979.

Table I-A-22. Registered Nurses and Health Trainees Admitted as Immigrants, by Country or Region of Last Permanent Residence, Fiscal Year 1978

Country or region of last permanent residence	Number admitted	Registered nurses	Health trainees[1]	Country or region of last permanent residence	Number admitted	Registered nurses	Health trainees[1]
All countries	3,817	3,779	38	Africa (continued)			
				Cape Verde Islands	1	1	...
Europe	652	646	6	Egypt	5	5	...
Albania	1	1	...	Ethiopia	4	4	...
Austria	5	5	...	Ghana	9	9	...
Belgium	2	2	...	Kenya	3	3	...
Bulgaria	1	1	...	Lesotho	1	1	...
Czechoslovakia	3	3	...	Liberia	2	2	...
Denmark	6	6	...	Libya	5	5	...
Finland	3	3	...	Mauritius	2	2	...
France	10	9	1	Nigeria	10	9	1
Germany	145	145	...	Sierra Leone	2	1	1
Greece	3	3	...	South Africa, Rep. of	8	8	...
Hungary	5	5	...	Southern Rhodesia	1	1	...
Ireland	12	12	...	Sudan	1	1	...
Italy	11	11	...	Zambia	5	5	...
Malta	1	1	...				
Netherlands	10	9	1	Oceania	37	36	1
Norway	7	6	1	Australia	17	17	...
Poland	31	31	...	Fiji	4	4	...
Portugal	12	12	...	New Zealand	14	14	...
Romania	6	6	...	Papua New Guinea	1	1	...
Spain	12	12	...	Western Samoa	1	...	1
Sweden	6	5	1				
Switzerland	13	13	...	North America	792	781	11
U.S.S.R.	26	26	...	Canada	403	399	4
United Kingdom	314	312	2	Mexico	45	42	3
Yugoslavia	7	7	...	West Indies	290	287	3
				Anguilla	1	1	...
Asia	2,169	2,153	16	Antigua	2	2	...
Afghanistan	1	1	...	Bahamas	5	5	...
Bahrain	1	1	...	Barbados	23	23	...
Bangladesh	1	1	...	Bermuda	1	1	...
Burma	7	7	...	British Virgin Is.	2	2	...
Cambodia	2	2	...	Cuba	29	29	...
China	111	111	...	Dominica	7	5	2
Mainland	9	9	...	Dominican Republic ...	33	33	...
Taiwan	102	102	...	Grenada	10	10	...
Hong Kong	46	46	...	Haiti	13	13	...
India	80	79	1	Jamaica	125	124	1
Indonesia	1	1	...	Martinique	1	1	...
Iran	18	18	...	St. Christopher	9	9	...
Israel	19	19	...	Nevis	1	1	...
Japan	10	10	...	St. Christopher	8	8	...
Jordan	11	11	...	St. Vincent	7	7	...
Jordan	10	10	...	Trinidad & Tobago	22	22	...
Palestine	1	1	...	Central America	54	53	1
Korea	319	319	...	Belize	10	10	...
Kuwait	11	11	...	Costa Rica	4	4	...
Laos	6	5	1	El Salvador	7	6	1
Lebanon	16	16	...	Guatemala	4	4	...
Macao	1	1	...	Honduras	8	8	...
Malaysia	6	6	...	Nicaragua	6	6	...
Nepal	1	1	...	Panama	15	15	...
Pakistan	7	7	...				
Philippines	1,375	1,372	3	South America	107	105	2
Saudi Arabia	10	10	...	Argentina	11	11	...
Singapore	1	1	...	Bolivia	5	5	...
Sri Lanka	1	1	...	Brazil	2	2	...
Syria	1	1	...	Chile	7	7	...
Thailand	33	33	...	Colombia	18	18	...
United Arab Emirates ...	1	1	...	Ecuador	4	4	...
Vietnam	71	60	11	Guyana	37	36	1
Yemen (Aden)	1	1	...	Paraguay	1	1	...
				Peru	15	14	1
Africa	60	58	2	Uruguay	3	3	...
Cameroon	1	1	...	Venezuela	4	4	...

[1]Includes student nurses.

SOURCE: U.S. Department of Justice, Immigration and Naturalization Service, 1980. Unpublished data.

Chapter I, Section B
MINORITY NURSES

Interest in the numbers, distribution, and characteristics of minorities in nursing has increased significantly. Such data is required for effective affirmative action in nursing services and education as well as for evaluation of programs geared toward recruitment and retention of minorities in the nursing profession. The 1977 national sample survey conducted by the American Nurses' Association under contract with the Division of Nursing, U.S. Department of Health and Human Services, provided detailed data on the racial/ethnic composition of the registered nurse population. The reader is referred to the source publication for discussion of the study methods and associated sampling errors. It was estimated that 6.2 percent, or 87,386 nurses, had minority racial/ethnic backgrounds. In contrast, 1976 data from the U.S. Department of Commerce, Bureau of the Census, showed 13.2 percent of the total U.S. resident population of 214,669,000 persons were racial/ethnic minorities.

Further delineation of the 1977 national sample survey revealed 2.5 percent of the total registered nurse population reported being black; 1.4 percent, Hispanic; 0.2 percent, American Indian; and 2.1 percent, Asian. About 3.0 percent of the minority nurses were male and 97.0 percent female. The median age of minority nurses was 37.3 years.

With respect to employment status, minority nurses exhibited higher employment patterns than their non-minority counterparts. The nurse labor force consists of those actively engaged in nursing as well as those not employed but seeking a nursing position. Overall, 83.2 percent of the minority nurses were employed in nursing and 86.0 percent were in the nurse labor force. On the other hand, non-minority nurses reported 68.8 percent working in the field of nursing and 71.9 percent in the nurse labor force. Although nurses tend generally to have much higher labor force participation rates than other comparably educated women, the disparity between participation rates of minorities and non-minorities is consistent with data reported by the Bureau of Labor Statistics for women in general. In 1975, the labor force participation rate for women with one or more years of college was 67 percent for minorities versus 57 percent for the corresponding non-minority population.

The majority of the minority nurses (60.9 percent) received their basic nursing education in diploma programs; 19.8 percent, from associate degree programs; and 18.8 percent, from baccalaureate programs; however, a higher percentage of non-minority nurses earned a diploma as their initial nursing credential than minority nurses. About 75.9 percent of the non-minority nurses held a diploma, 10.7 percent an associate degree and 13.4 percent a baccalaureate. Differences were noted in initial nursing education programs between black and Asian nurses. About 30 percent of the black nurses initially had graduated from associate degree programs, and only 12.2 percent received their basic nursing education in baccalaureate program. In contrast, 9.9 percent of the Asian nurses were initially prepared in associate degree programs and 29.9 percent received their preparation in a baccalaureate program.

Similar differences were apparent in the highest educational preparation of minority registered nurses. About 72 percent of the minority nurses had as their highest nursing-related educational preparation an associate degree or diploma; 23 percent had a baccalaureate; and 5 percent, a master's or doctorate. Among the non-minority nurses the corresponding percentages were 79 percent, 17 percent, and 4 percent, respectively.

Examination of the data by geographic region showed half of the nurses with minority backgrounds were located in the Pacific states (24.8 percent) and Middle Atlantic states (24.6 percent). The East North Central and South Atlantic states accounted for 14.5 percent and 13.9 percent, respectively, the next largest numbers of minority nurses.

Table I-B-1. Estimated Number of Racial/Ethnic Minorities in U.S. Population (1976) and in the Registered Nurse Population (1977)[1] by Sex

	Black and other races[2]				
		Registered nurses			
		Total		Employed in nursing	
Sex	U.S. resident population	(n)	N	(n)	N
Total	28,442,000	882	87,386	738	72,688
Female	14,871,000	862	84,771	721	70,661
Male	13,571,000	20	2,615	17	2,027

[1] Includes only registered nurses actively licensed in September 1977 who worked in the United States if employed in nursing, or lived in the United States if not employed in nursing.

[2] The term "Black and other races" describes persons of all races other than white.

NOTE: "N" corresponds to the weighted population estimate derived from the sample and "n" refers to the actual number of surveys upon which the estimate was based.

SOURCES: U.S. Department of Health, Education, and Welfare, Public Health Service, Health Resources Administration, *Minorities and Women in the Health Fields: Applicants, Students, and Workers*, DHEW Publication No. (HRA) 79-33, October 1978. Roth, Aleda V., et al. *1977 National Sample Survey of Registered Nurses: A Report on the Nurse Population and Factors Affecting Their Supply*, final report on Contract No. (HRA 231-76-0085) between the American Nurses' Association and the Division of Nursing, U.S. Department of Health and Human Services, NTIS Publication No. HRP-0900603, 1979.

Table I-B-2. Estimated Number and Percent of Registered Nurses[1] With Minority Racial/Ethnic Background by Employment Status, September 1977

| | | | | Employment status | | | | | |
| | Total | | | Employed in nursing | | | Not employed in nursing | | |
Racial/ethnic background	(n)	N	Per-cent	(n)	N	Per-cent	(n)	N	Per-cent
Total	882	87,386	100.0	738	72,688	83.2	144	14,699	16.8
Black	329	35,476	100.0	282	30,170	85.0	47	5,307	15.0
Hispanic ...	208	19,652	100.0	171	16,340	83.1	37	3,312	16.9
American Indian ...	43	3,296	100.0	31	2,094	63.5	12	1,201	36.4
Asian	302	28,962	100.0	254	24,084	83.2	48	4,879	16.8

[1] Includes only registered nurses actively licensed in September 1977 who worked in the United States if employed in nursing, or lived in the United States if not employed in nursing.

NOTE: "N" corresponds to the weighted population estimate derived from the sample and "n" refers to the actual number of surveys upon which the estimate was based. Because of rounding, sums of estimated numbers (N) and estimated percents may not add to totals.

SOURCE: Roth, Aleda V., et al. *1977 National Sample Survey of Registered Nurses: A Report on the Nurse Population and Factors Affecting Their Supply*, final report on Contract No. (HRA 231-76-0085) between the American Nurses' Association and the Division of Nursing, U.S. Department of Health and Human Services, NTIS Publication No. HRP-0900603, 1979.

CHART 2. ESTIMATED PERCENT OF REGISTERED NURSES[1]
WITH MINORITY RACIAL/ETHNIC BACKGROUND, 1977

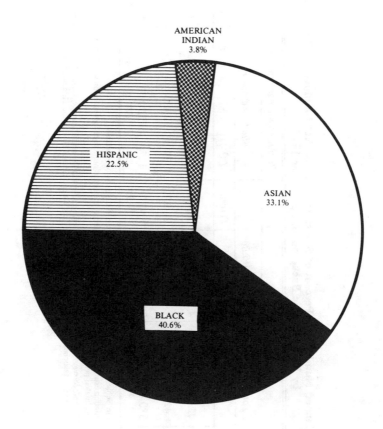

AMERICAN
INDIAN
3.8%

HISPANIC
22.5%

ASIAN
33.1%

BLACK
40.6%

[1]Includes only registered nurses actively licensed in September 1977 who worked in the United States if employed in nursing, or lived in the United States if not employed in nursing and who reported racial/ethnic background.

SOURCE: Roth, Aleda, V., et al. *1977 National Sample Survey of Registered Nurses: A Report on the Nurse Population and Factors Affecting Their Supply*, final report on Contract No. (HRA 231-76-0085) between the American Nurses' Association and the Division of Nursing, U.S. Department of Health and Human Services, NTIS Publication No. HRP-0900603, 1979.

Table I-B-3. Estimated Number and Percent of Registered Nurses[1] Not Employed in Nursing, by Racial/Ethnic Background, September 1977

| Employment status | Total | | | Racial/ethnic background | | | | | | | | |
| | | | | White | | | Black and other | | | Not reported | | |
	(n)	N	Percent	(n)	N	Percent	(n)	N	Percent	(n)	N	Percent
Total, not employed in nursing	4,533	423,400	100.0	4,327	403,203	100.0	144	14,697	100.0	62	5,499	100.0
Seeking position in nursing	470	42,028	9.9	438	39,170	9.7	27	2,493	17.0	5	365	6.6
Not seeking position in nursing	4,057	380,875	90.0	3,883	363,536	90.2	117	12,204	83.0	57	5,134	93.4
Not reported	6	497	0.1	6	497	0.1	...	...	...	...	...	...

[1]Includes only registered nurses actively licensed in September 1977 who lived in the United States if not employed in nursing.

NOTE: "N" corresponds to the weighted population estimate derived from the sample and "'n'" refers to the actual number of surveys upon which the estimate was based. Because of rounding, sums of estimated numbers (N) and estimated percents may not add to totals.

SOURCE: Roth, Aleda V., et al. *1977 National Sample Survey of Registered Nurses: A Report on the Nurse Population and Factors Affecting Their Supply*, final report on Contract No. (HRA 231-76-0085) between the American Nurses' Association and the Division of Nursing, U.S. Department of Health and Human Services, NTIS Publication No. HRP-0900603, 1979.

Table I-B-4. Estimated Number[1] and Median Age of Minority Registered Nurses[2] by Employment Status and Marital Status, September 1977

Marital status	Total			Employment status					
				Employed in nursing			Not employed in nursing		
	(n)	N	Median age	(n)	N	Median age	(n)	N	Median age
Total, minority nurses	882	87,386	37.3	738	72,688	36.5	144	14,699	45.0
Never married	162	17,847	30.1	152	16,705	29.6	10	1,142	(3)
Married	588	57,994	38.0	486	47,570	37.5	102	10,424	42.2
Widowed	37	2,642	53.9	19	875	(3)	18	1,767	(3)
Divorced/separated	94	8,669	41.4	80	7,304	40.3	14	1,365	(3)
Not reported	1	233		1	233		...	...	...

[1]Includes nurses who did not report age.

[2]Includes only registered nurses actively licensed in September 1977 who worked in the United States if employed in nursing, or lived in the United States if not employed in nursing.

[3]Insufficient number of cases to compute median.

NOTE: "N" corresponds to the weighted population estimate derived from the sample and "n" refers to the actual number of surveys upon which the estimate was based. Because of rounding, sums of estimated numbers (N) may not add to totals.

SOURCE: Roth, Aleda V., et al. *1977 National Sample Survey of Registered Nurses: A Report on the Nurse Population and Factors Affecting Their Supply*, final report on Contract No. (HRA 231-76-0085) between the American Nurses' Association and the Division of Nursing, U.S. Department of Health and Human Services, NTIS Publication No. HRP-0900603, 1979.

Table I-B-5. Estimated Number and Percent of Minority Registered Nurses[1] by Racial/Ethnic Background and Basic Nursing Educational Preparation, September 1977

Basic nursing educational preparation	Total minorities			Racial/ethnic background								
				Black			Asian			Other		
	(n)	N	Percent	(n)	N	Percent	(n)	N	Percent	(n)	N	Percent
Total	882	87,386	100.0	329	35,476	40.6	302	28,962	33.1	251	22,948	26.3
Diploma	555	53,232	100.0	186	20,402	38.3	182	17,186	32.3	187	15,644	29.4
Associate degree ...	160	17,323	100.0	90	10,669	61.6	33	2,856	16.5	37	3,798	21.9
Baccalaureate and above ...	163	16,469	100.0	51	4,311	26.2	85	8,652	52.5	27	3,506	21.3
Not reported	4	363	100.0	2	94	25.9	2	269	74.1	...	...	...

[1]Includes only registered nurses actively licensed in September 1977 who worked in the United States if employed in nursing, or lived in the United States if not employed in nursing and who reported racial/ethnic background.

NOTE: "N" corresponds to the weighted population estimate derived from the sample and "n" refers to the actual number of surveys upon which the estimate was based. Because of rounding, sums of estimated numbers (N) and estimated percents may not add to totals.

SOURCE: Roth, Aleda V., et al. *1977 National Sample Survey of Registered Nurses: A Report on the Nurse Population and Factors Affecting Their Supply*, final report on Contract No. (HRA 231-76-0085) between the American Nurses' Association and the Division of Nursing, U.S. Department of Health and Human Services, NTIS Publication No. HRP-0900603, 1979.

Table I-B-6. Estimated Number and Percent of Minority Registered Nurses[1] by Highest Nursing-Related Educational Preparation, Basic Nursing Educational Preparation, and Racial/Ethnic Background, September 1977

Basic nursing educational preparation and racial/ethnic background	Total			Highest nursing-related educational preparation														
				Diploma			Associate degree			Baccalaureate			Master's degree and above			Not reported		
	(n)	N	Per-cent	(n)	N	Per-cent	(n)	N	Per-cent	(n)	N	Per-cent	(n)	N	Per-cent	(n)	N	Per-cent
Total	882	87,386	100.0	481	46,173	100.0	152	16,144	100.0	203	20,314	100.0	42	4,393	100.0	4	363	100.0
Black	329	35,476	40.6	148	16,679	36.1	82	9,650	59.8	76	6,803	33.5	21	2,250	51.2	2	94	25.9
Asian	302	28,962	33.1	156	14,636	31.7	35	2,866	17.8	94	9,736	47.9	15	1,456	33.1	2	269	74.1
Other	251	22,948	26.3	177	14,858	32.2	35	3,628	22.5	33	3,775	18.6	6	687	15.6	...	...	...
Diploma	555	53,232	60.9	481	46,173	100.0	6	644	4.0	46	4,215	20.7	22	2,198	50.0	...	...	...
Black	186	20,402	23.3	148	16,679	36.1	3	403	2.5	22	1,995	9.8	13	1,324	30.1	...	...	...
Asian	182	17,186	19.7	156	14,636	31.7	3	241	1.5	17	1,700	8.4	6	608	13.8	...	...	...
Other	187	15,644	17.9	177	14,858	32.2	...	...	...	7	520	2.6	3	266	6.1	...	...	...
Associate degree	160	17,323	19.8	...	...	...	146	15,500	96.0	9	1,110	5.5	5	714	16.3	...	...	...
Black	90	10,669	12.2	...	...	...	79	9,247	57.3	7	837	4.1	4	586	13.3	...	...	...
Asian	33	2,856	3.3	...	...	...	32	2,625	16.3	1	231	1.1	...	...	...	...	...	...
Other	37	3,798	4.3	...	...	...	35	3,628	22.5	1	42	0.2	1	128	2.9	...	...	...
Baccalaureate and above	163	16,469	18.8	...	...	...	...	...	...	148	14,990	73.8	15	1,480	33.7	...	...	...
Black	51	4,311	4.9	...	...	...	...	...	...	47	3,971	19.5	4	340	7.7	...	...	...
Asian	85	8,652	9.9	...	...	...	...	...	...	76	7,805	38.4	9	847	19.3	...	...	...
Other	27	3,506	4.0	...	...	...	...	...	...	25	3,214	15.8	2	293	6.7	...	...	...
Not reported	4	363	0.4	...	...	...	...	...	...	...	...	...	...	...	...	4	363	100.0
Black	2	94	0.1	...	...	...	...	...	...	...	...	...	...	...	...	2	94	25.9
Asian	2	269	0.3	...	...	...	...	...	...	...	...	...	...	...	...	2	269	74.1
Other	...	...	...	...	...	...	...	...	...	...	...	...	...	...	...	...	...	...

[1] Includes only registered nurses actively licensed in September 1977 who worked in the United States if employed in nursing, or lived in the United States if not employed in nursing and reported racial/ethnic background.

NOTE: "N" corresponds to the weighted population estimate derived from the sample and "n" refers to the actual number of surveys upon which the estimate was based. Because of rounding, sums of estimated numbers (N) and estimated percents may not add to totals.

SOURCE: Roth, Aleda V., et al. 1977 National Sample Survey of Registered Nurses: A Report on the Nurse Population and Factors Affecting Their Supply, final report on Contract No. (HRA 231-76-0085) between the American Nurses' Association and the Division of Nursing. U.S. Department of Health and Human Services, NTIS Publication No. HRP-0900603, 1979.

CHART 3. ESTIMATED PERCENT OF REGISTERED NURSES[1] BY HIGHEST NURSING-RELATED EDUCATIONAL PREPARATION AND RACIAL/ETHNIC BACKGROUND, SEPTEMBER 1977

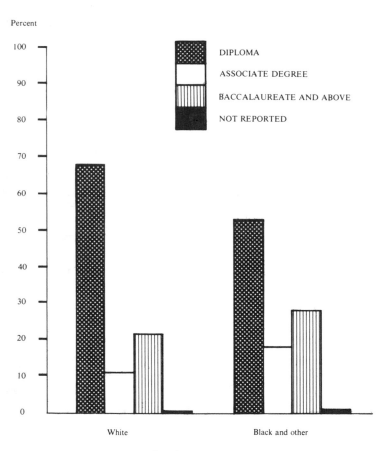

Percent

DIPLOMA

ASSOCIATE DEGREE

BACCALAUREATE AND ABOVE

NOT REPORTED

White   Black and other

Racial/ethnic background

[1]Includes only registered nurses actively licensed in September 1977 who worked in the United States if employed in nursing, or lived in the United States if not employed in nursing.

SOURCE: Roth, Aleda V., et al. *1977 National Sample Survey of Registered Nurses: A Report on the Nurse Population and Factors Affecting Their Supply*, final report on Contract No. (HRA 231-76-0085) between the American Nurses' Association and the Division of Nursing, U.S. Department of Health and Human Services, NTIS Publication No. HRP-0900603, 1979.

Chapter 1, Section C
NURSES IN EXPANDED ROLES

Since the mid-1960s there has been a growing trend in the utilization of nurses in expanded roles of health care, particularly that of the nurse practitioner. Present emphasis on preventive health sciences and the focus on primary health care needs of the population signal a continuing need for such nurses. Data on their educational preparation, their employment, and the impact of the health care delivered by nurses in expanded roles is essential for future planning of educational and service programs.

The 1977 national sample survey conducted by the American Nurses' Association under contract with the Division of Nursing collected data on the estimated total U.S. registered nurse population. According to the ANA study, there were an estimated 9,634 nurses holding titles of nurse practitioner or nurse-midwife (576 were nurse-midwives in 1977). An estimated 8,065 held a position title of clinical nursing specialist, and 13,046 were nurse anesthetists.

Five activities included in the 1977 national sample survey related to primary expanded role tasks. Nurses were asked to indicate how often they performed these tasks. The activities were performing complete physical examinations, selecting a plan of treatment as a result of interpreting laboratory test results, developing and modifying medication requirements, performing medical management for selected health conditions, and having primary responsibility for follow-through on patient care. More than two-thirds of the nurses with position titles of nurse practitioner/nurse-midwife reported performing these activities on a routine basis or frequently.

A longitudinal study of nurse practitioners was initiated in 1973 by the State University of New York at Buffalo under contract with the Division of Nursing, U.S. Department of Health, Education, and Welfare (renamed U.S. Department of Health and Human Services in 1980). This study, describing the circumstances of nurse practitioners' education and employment, was divided into three phases. The purpose of the study was essentially to identify nurse practitioner programs and to follow selected cohorts of nurse practitioner students one year after graduation. In Phase I, 133 programs meeting predetermined criteria for offering education of nurses in expanded roles were identified. All students in expanded role programs in 1973 who would graduate between May 1974 and June 1975 and who responded to the initial question-naire constituted the cohort of nurse practitioners to be followed in Phase II of the study. The Phase I response rates were 99 percent for certificate programs and 98 percent for master's programs. For the questionnaire sent to 1,297 students querying about their background, experience, income, previous func-tions in the nursing role, and other measures of role satisfaction and expec-tations, the response rates were 85 percent for those in certificate programs and 84 percent for those in master's programs.

Phase II consisted of two surveys: a one-year after graduation follow-up of the 1,099 nurse practitioners identified in the Phase I cohort and a survey of employers of these nurse practitioners. The employers were contacted a minimum of 6 months following the expected completion of the nurse practitioner program. The Phase II response rates were 68.5 percent for the student cohort and 82.8 percent for the employers.

Phase III entailed the updating of programs initiated between January 1, 1974, and December 31, 1976, resulting in the identification of 110 new nurse practitioner programs and 88 old programs still active. Current program information was sought from each of the 198 programs identified. The overall response rates from the program survey were 94.4 percent for the certificate programs and 82.4 percent for the master's programs.

Only students enrolled in the new nurse practitioner programs responding to the program questionnaire were eligible to receive the Phase III student survey. Out of this group, those expected to graduate between March 1977 and July 1978 were mailed the student survey. About 89 percent responded to the Phase III student mailings. The study design called for follow-up mailings to students at least 6 months after graduation. In Phase III, those students who actually graduated between March and September 1977 constituted the cohort of nurse practitioners who received a follow-up survey. The response rate for this group was 64 percent. Employers of those nurses who were determined to be engaged in primary care in nurse practitioner positions were surveyed 6 months following the nurses' graduations. About 78.5 percent of the employers responded.

There were differences in the geographic distribution of nurse practitioner programs, the largest number (61) being located in the Southern states in 1977. Each region of the country exhibited growth from 1973 to 1977 in the number of nurse practitioner programs; however, the relative proportions of programs remained fairly stable. Only the Midwestern states declined five percentage points, from about 20 percent to 15 percent.

The preponderance (90 percent) of nurse practitioner graduates surveyed were employed in nursing. There were disparities in employment patterns according to demographic characteristics between Phase II and Phase III cohorts. The Phase II group appeared to have lower proportions of nurse practitioners employed in the under-35-year-age-at-graduation category and among the married nurses. In Phase III more white nurses were employed than black nurses. The observed differences in employment status between the two cohorts were generally not great, however, and may partially be due to varying magnitudes of response rates in each of the studies.

In terms of their professional backgrounds, most nurse practitioner graduates had more than 5 years experience in professional nursing; the majority had previous work experience in hospitals. About half had a baccalaureate or master's as their highest nursing education prior to their nurse practitioner training. Of the nurse practitioner graduates who were not employed, the largest proportions in both Phase II and Phase III cohorts indicated they were not seeking employment.

Graduates who were providing primary care were asked to indicate the one setting in which they spent the majority of their time as a nurse practitioner. About two-thirds reported they were practicing in ambulatory clinical practice areas. About one-third of the Phase II and one-fifth of the Phase III respondents were in practice settings located in the inner city area.

Phase II graduates reported the percentage of time they spent in nurse practitioner functions by major employment setting. The proportion of time in the nurse practitioner role varied by settings, as expected. About two-thirds of those in ambulatory practice and three-fifths of those in hospital practice spent 100 percent of their time as nurse practitioners.

A demographic study of nurse anesthetists was conducted jointly by the American Society of Anesthesiologists and the American Association of Nurse Anesthetists. There were 12,162 active nurse anesthetists in the United States in 1972. The Manpower Analysis Branch of the Bureau of Health Manpower developed two models for estimating the 1980 supply of and need for nurse anesthetists. The Manpower Analysis Branch estimated that in 1980 the number of nurse anesthetists would be between 15,835 and 16,080, while the corresponding 1980 requirements were estimated to range from 22,267 to 25,530 nurse anesthetists.

The American College of Nurse-Midwives presented data on the 623 nurse-midwives in clinical practice in the United States in late 1976. The majority (85 percent) of clinical nurse-midwives held one position, and 15 percent held two concurrent positions. On the average, nurse-midwives spent almost three-quarters of their time in direct patient care and clinical instruction associated with patient care. About 45.6 percent worked in hospital settings. The second and third most common employers of clinical nurse-midwives were public health agencies and physicians in private practice, accounting for 13.8 percent and 12.9, respectively. About 84 percent of the clinical nurse-midwives reported the management of normal deliveries as a routine function. These 521 nurses delivered a total of 33,613 babies during the 12 months prior to completion of the survey.

**Table I-C-1. Estimated Number and Percent of Registered Nurses[1]
Employed in Nursing, by Selected Types of Positions,
September 1977**

Type of position	(n)	N	Percent
Total	401	30,745	100.0
Nurse practitioner/midwife	131	9,634	31.3
Clinical nursing specialist	94	8,065	26.2
Nurse anesthetist	176	13,046	42.4

[1]Includes only registered nurses actively licensed and working in the United States in September 1977.

NOTE: "N" corresponds to the weighted population estimate derived from the sample and "n" refers to the actual number of surveys upon which the estimate was based.

SOURCE: Roth, Aleda V., et al. *1977 National Sample Survey of Registered Nurses: A Report on the Nurse Population and Factors Affecting Their Supply,* final report on Contract No. (HRA 231-76-0085) between the American Nurses' Association and the Division of Nursing, U.S. Department of Health and Human Services, NTIS Publication No. HRP-0900603, 1979.

Table I-C-2. Estimated Percent of Registered Nurses[1] Spending Some Time in Direct Patient Care Who Performed Activities Routinely or Often by Position/Title and Activity in Primary Nursing Job, September 1977

Activity	*Type of position/title*		
	Nurse practitioner/ midwife	*Clinical nursing specialist*[2]	*Nurse anesthetist*[3]
	(n=131) (N=9,634)	(n=90) (N=7,803)	(n=170) (N=12,552)
Assessment			
Obtain health histories	87.3	69.2	72.0
Perform complete physical examinations ...	72.8	18.0	19.5
Perform some portion of physical examinations	71.8	31.9	28.8
Assist during patient examinations	31.6	46.6	7.3
Devising a plan of health care			
Select plans of treatment	66.4	23.2	47.3
Develop and modify medication	71.0	38.0	51.8
Develop therapeutic plans	80.1	58.7	29.3
Implementing/evaluating a plan of health care			
Perform medical management	70.7	46.0	37.5
Instruct patients in management of defined illness	77.8	79.2	12.0
Instruct patients in health maintenance	88.2	68.1	13.4
Implement therapy	82.6	69.5	38.0
Administer medication	47.1	65.1	85.8
Sustain and support persons during diagnosis or therapy	56.0	81.8	43.1
Have primary responsibility for follow-through on patient care	75.1	56.2	21.6
Have primary responsibility for normal mothers	14.8	4.4	13.4

[1] Includes only registered nurses actively licensed and working in the United States in September 1977.

[2] Excludes (n=4) nurses or an estimated N=262 nurses who did not respond to the question.

[3] Excludes (n=6) nurses or an estimated N=494 nurses who did not respond to the question.

NOTE: "N" corresponds to the weighted population estimate derived from the sample and "n" refers to the actual number of surveys upon which the estimate is based.

SOURCE: Roth, Aleda V., et al. *1977 National Sample Survey of Registered Nurses: A Report on the Nurse Population and Factors Affecting Their Supply*, final report on Contract No. (HRA 231-76-0085) between the American Nurses' Association and the Division of Nursing, U.S. Department of Health and Human Services, NTIS Publication No. HRP-0900603, 1979.

Table I-C-3. Selected Demographic Characteristics of Nurse Practitioner Graduate Respondents and Nonrespondents, Phase II and Phase III

Demographic characteristics	Phase II[1] Total Number	Percent	Respondents Number	Percent	Nonrespondents Number	Percent	Phase III Total Number	Percent	Respondents Number	Percent	Nonrespondents Number	Percent
Sex	1,099	100.0	753	100.0	346	100.0	655	100.0	420	100.0	235	100.0
Male	22	2.0	14	1.9	8	2.3	20	3.1	13	3.1	7	3.0
Female	1,077	98.0	739	98.1	338	97.7	635	96.9	407	96.9	228	97.0
Racial/ethnic background[2]	1,090	100.0	748	100.0	342	100.0	651	100.0	418	100.0	233	100.0
White	981	90.0	690	92.2	291	85.1	589	90.5	383	91.6	206	88.5
Black	74	6.8	38	5.1	36	10.5	39	6.0	22	5.3	17	7.3
Asian	19	1.7	14	1.9	5	1.5	7	1.1	2	0.5	5	2.1
American Indian	3	0.3	2	0.3	1	0.3	2	0.3	2	0.5	...	...
Hispanic	13	1.2	4	0.5	9	2.6	14	2.1	9	2.1	5	2.1
Marital status[2]	1,083	100.0	743	100.0	340	100.0	646	100.0	412	100.0	234	100.0
Unmarried	485	44.8	335	45.1	150	44.1	275	42.6	160	38.8	115	49.1
Married	598	55.2	408	54.9	190	55.9	371	57.4	252	61.2	119	50.9
Age[2]	990	100.0	683	100.0	307	100.0	648	100.0	416	100.0	232	100.0
Less than 25 years	33	3.3	21	3.1	12	3.9	32	4.9	19	4.6	13	5.6
25-34	528	53.3	363	53.1	165	53.7	331	51.1	204	49.0	127	54.8
35-44	259	26.2	181	26.5	78	25.4	186	28.7	120	28.9	66	28.4
45-54	139	14.1	94	13.8	45	14.7	87	13.4	65	15.6	22	9.5
55 or more	31	3.1	24	3.5	7	2.3	12	1.9	8	1.9	4	1.7
Region[3] of program	1,099	100.0	753	100.0	346	100.0	655	100.0	420	100.0	235	100.0
Northeast	316	28.8	205	27.2	111	32.1	211	32.2	127	30.2	84	35.7
South	306	27.8	208	27.6	98	28.3	219	33.5	144	34.3	75	31.9
Midwest	203	18.5	139	18.5	64	18.5	65	9.9	47	11.2	18	7.7
West	274	24.9	201	26.7	73	21.1	160	24.4	102	24.3	58	24.7

[1] Demographic data was obtained during Phase I of project.

[2] Includes only those graduates who responded to item.

[3] States included in each region are: *Northeast*—Connecticut, Delaware, District of Columbia, Maine, Massachusetts, New Hampshire, New Jersey, New York, Pennsylvania, Rhode Island, and Vermont; *South*—Alabama, Arkansas, Florida, Georgia, Kentucky, Louisiana, Maryland, Mississippi, North Carolina, Oklahoma, South Carolina, Tennessee, Texas, Virginia, and West Virginia; *Midwest*—Illinois, Indiana, Iowa, Kansas, Michigan, Minnesota, Missouri, Nebraska, North Dakota, Ohio, South Dakota, and Wisconsin; *West*—Alaska, Arizona, California, Colorado, Hawaii, Idaho, Montana, Nevada, New Mexico, Oregon, Washington, and Wyoming.

SOURCE: U.S. Department of Health, Education, and Welfare, Public Health Service, Health Resources Administration, Division of Nursing, *Longitudinal Study of Nurse Practitioners, Phase II*, DHEW Publication No. 78-92, September, 1978, p. 32, and *Longitudinal Study of Nurse Practitioners, Phase III*, DHEW Publication No. HRA 80-2, May, 1980, p. 41.

Table I-C-4. Selected Professional Characteristics of Nurse Practitioner Graduate Respondents and Nonrespondents, Phase II and Phase III

Professional characteristics	Phase II[1]						Phase III					
	Total		Respondents		Nonrespondents		Total		Respondents		Nonrespondents	
	Number	Percent	Number	Percent	Number	Percent	Number	Percent	Number	Percent	Number	Percent
Years in professional nursing[2]	1,090	100.0	745	100.0	354	100.0	652	100.0	418	100.0	234	100.0
Less than one	27	2.5	17	2.3	10	2.9	9	1.4	5	1.2	4	1.7
1-5	391	35.9	272	36.5	119	34.5	247	37.9	147	35.2	100	42.8
6-10	300	27.5	199	26.7	101	29.3	190	29.1	127	30.4	63	26.9
11-15	166	15.2	119	16.0	47	13.6	89	13.6	55	13.1	34	14.5
16-20	114	10.5	72	9.7	42	12.2	67	10.3	46	11.0	21	9.0
21 or more	92	8.4	66	8.8	26	7.5	50	7.7	38	9.1	12	5.1
Prior nursing preparation[2]	1,098	100.0	753	100.0	345	100.0	655	100.0	420	100.0	235	100.0
Diploma	381	34.7	252	33.5	129	37.4	227	34.7	153	36.4	74	31.5
Associate degree	72	6.5	41	5.4	31	9.0	84	12.8	49	11.7	35	14.9
Baccalaureate	585	53.3	409	54.3	176	51.0	309	47.2	200	47.6	109	46.4
Master's	60	5.5	51	6.8	9	2.6	35	5.3	18	4.3	17	7.2
Degree in field other than nursing[2]	1,098	100.0	753	100.0	345	100.0	655	100.0	420	100.0	235	100.0
None	998	90.9	677	89.9	321	93.1	581	88.7	363	86.4	218	92.8
Associate degree	9	0.8	9	1.2	...	...	13	2.0	10	2.4	3	1.3
Baccalaureate	58	5.3	42	5.6	16	4.6	37	5.6	29	6.9	8	3.4
Master's	29	2.6	22	2.9	7	2.0	23	3.5	17	4.1	6	2.5
Doctorate	1	0.1	1	0.1	...	...	1	0.2	1	0.2	...	...
Other[3]	3	0.3	2	0.3	1	0.3	...	...	...	...	...	...

Employment status²	*1,023*	*100.0*	*753*	*100.0*	*270*	*100.0*	*(5)*	*(5)*	*(5)*	*(5)*	*(5)*	*(5)*
Employed as nurse practitioner⁴ ...	770	75.3	532	70.3	238	88.1	(5)	(5)	(5)	(5)	(5)	(5)
Employed, not as nurse practitioner ...	143	14.0	122	16.1	21	7.8	(5)	(5)	(5)	(5)	(5)	(5)
Not employed ...	77	7.5	70	9.2	7	2.6	(5)	(5)	(5)	(5)	(5)	(5)
Not graduated ...	31	3.0	27	3.6	4	1.5	(5)	(5)	(5)	(5)	(5)	(5)
Deceased	2	0.2	2	0.8	...	...	(5)	(5)	(5)	(5)	(5)	(5)
Number of years in job just prior to entering nurse practitioner program²	*1,049*	*100.0*	*720*	*100.0*	*329*	*100.0*	*639*	*100.0*	*411*	*100.0*	*228*	*100.0*
Less than 2 ...	286	27.2	203	28.2	83	25.2	171	26.8	110	26.8	61	26.8
2	284	27.1	194	27.0	90	27.4	176	27.6	115	28.0	61	26.8
3-5	234	22.3	162	22.5	72	21.9	165	25.8	101	24.6	64	28.0
6-10	154	14.7	103	14.3	51	15.5	87	13.6	59	14.3	28	12.3
11-15	66	6.3	39	5.4	27	8.2	27	4.2	16	3.9	11	4.8
16 or more ...	25	2.4	19	2.6	6	1.8	13	2.0	10	2.4	3	1.3

¹With the exception of employment status, professional data was obtained during Phase I of project.
²Includes only those graduates who responded to item.
³Includes preparation not leading to a degree.
⁴Includes respondents functioning wholly or in part as nurse practitioners.
⁵Information not available.

SOURCE: U.S. Department of Health, Education, and Welfare, Public Health Service, Health Resources Administration, Division of Nursing, *Longitudinal Study of Nurse Practitioners, Phase II*, DHEW Publication No. 78-92, September, 1978, p. 33, and *Longitudinal Study of Nurse Practitioners, Phase III*, DHEW Publication No. HRA 80-2, May, 1980, p. 42.

**Table I-C-5. Selected Demographic Characteristics of Nurse
Practitioner Graduates, by Employment Status, Phase II**

Demographic characteristics	Total		Employment status			
			Employed		Not employed	
	Number	Percent	Number	Percent	Number	Percent
Sex[1]	724	100.0	654	100.0	70	100.0
Male	14	1.9	13	2.0	1	1.4
Female	710	98.1	641	98.0	69	98.6
Racial/ethnic background[1]	721	100.0	651	100.0	70	100.0
White	665	92.2	599	92.0	66	94.3
Black	37	5.1	34	5.2	3	4.3
Other[2]	19	2.6	18	2.8	1	1.4
Marital status[1] ...	716	100.0	646	100.0	70	100.0
Unmarried	322	45.0	295	45.7	27	38.6
Married	394	55.0	351	54.3	43	61.4
Age at graduation[1]	722	100.0	653	100.0	69	100.0
Less than 35 years	408	56.5	360	55.1	48	69.6
35-44	192	26.6	178	27.3	14	20.3
45 or more	122	16.9	115	17.6	7	10.1
Region[1,3]	717	100.0	649	100.0	68	100.0
Northeast	194	27.1	176	27.1	18	26.5
South	197	27.5	180	27.7	17	25.0
Midwest	132	18.4	118	18.2	14	20.6
West	194	27.1	175	27.0	19	27.9

[1]Includes only those graduates who responded to item.
[2]Includes Hispanics, American Indians, and Asians.
[3]Refers to location of graduates when they completed questionnaire for Phase II of project, which was mailed a minimum of 6 months following graduation. For states in each region, see Table I-C-3.
SOURCE: U.S. Department of Health, Education, and Welfare, Public Health Service, Health Resources Administration, Division of Nursing, *Longitudinal Study of Nurse Practitioners, Phase II*, DHEW Publication No. 78-92, September, 1978, p. 40.

Table I-C-6. Selected Demographic Characteristics of Nurse Practitioner Graduates, by Employment Status, Phase III

Demographic characteristics	Total		Employment status			
			Employed		Not employed	
	Number	Percent	Number	Percent	Number	Percent
Sex[1]	398	100.0	357	100.0	41	100.0
Male	13	3.3	13	3.6	...	...
Female	385	96.7	344	96.4	41	100.0
Racial/ethnic background[1]	396	100.0	355	100.0	41	100.0
White	363	91.7	326	91.8	37	90.2
Black	21	5.3	17	4.8	4	9.8
Other[2]	12	3.0	12	3.4	...	...
Marital status[1] ...	391	100.0	351	100.0	40	100.0
Unmarried	151	38.6	132	37.6	19	47.5
Married	240	61.4	219	62.4	21	52.5
Age at graduation[1]	398	100.0	357	100.0	41	100.0
Less than 35 years	218	54.8	194	54.3	24	58.5
35-44	111	27.9	101	28.3	10	24.4
45 or more	69	17.3	62	17.4	7	17.1
Region[1,3]	395	100.0	355	100.0	40	100.0
Northeast	114	28.9	101	28.5	13	32.5
South	133	33.7	115	32.4	18	45.0
Midwest	58	14.7	53	14.9	5	12.5
West	90	22.8	86	24.2	4	10.0

[1]Includes only those graduates who responded to item.
[2]Includes Hispanics, American Indians, and Asians.
[3]Refers to location of graduate. For states in each region, see Table I-C-3.

SOURCE: U.S. Department of Health, Education, and Welfare, Public Health Service, Health Resources Administration, Division of Nursing, *Longitudinal Study of Nurse Practitioners, Phase III*, DHEW Publication No. HRA 80-2, May, 1980, p. 88.

Table I-C-7. Selected Professional Characteristics of Nurse Practitioner Graduates, by Employment Status, Phase II

Professional characteristics	Total		Employment status			
			Employed		Not employed	
	Number	Percent	Number	Percent	Number	Percent
ANA membership[1]...	721	100.0	651	100.0	70	100.0
Member	347	48.1	316	48.5	31	44.3
Nonmember	374	51.9	335	51.5	39	55.7
Years in professional nursing[1]	716	100.0	647	100.0	69	100.0
Less than one year	16	2.2	12	1.9	4	5.8
1-5	259	36.2	233	36.0	26	37.7
6-10	194	27.1	167	25.8	27	39.1
11-15	114	15.9	105	16.2	9	13.0
16-20	70	9.8	69	10.7	1	1.4
21 or more	63	8.8	61	9.4	2	2.9
Previous employment setting[1] ...	705	100.0	641	100.0	64	100.0
Hospital outpatient service	74	10.5	68	10.6	6	9.4
Hospital inpatient service	259	36.7	232	36.2	27	42.2
Health center ...	101	14.3	96	15.0	5	7.8
Extended care facility	12	1.7	11	1.7	1	1.6
Fee-for-service physician	33	4.7	30	4.7	3	4.7
Prepaid group practice	7	1.0	6	0.9	1	1.6
Community/home health agency ..	110	15.6	100	15.6	10	15.6
School	47	6.7	45	7.0	2	3.1
Teaching	47	6.7	42	6.6	5	7.8
Other[2]	15	2.1	11	1.7	4	6.3
Prior nursing preparation[1]	724	100.0	654	100.0	70	100.0
Diploma	244	33.7	223	34.1	21	30.0
Associate degree	40	5.5	33	5.0	7	10.0
Baccalaureate ...	392	54.1	353	54.0	39	55.7
Master's	48	6.6	45	6.9	3	4.3
Employment changes after graduation[1]	709	100.0	644	100.0	65	100.0
None	531	74.9	515	80.0	16	24.6
One or more	178	25.1	129	20.0	49	75.4

[1]Includes only those graduates who responded to item.
[2]Includes settings within state and federal agencies, including the armed services, inservice education, and social agencies as well as combined inpatient/outpatient settings.

SOURCE: U.S. Department of Health, Education, and Welfare, Public Health Service, Health Resources Administration, Division of Nursing, *Longitudinal Study of Nurse Practitioners, Phase II*, DHEW Publication No. 78-92, September, 1978, p. 43.

Table I-C-8. Selected Professional Characteristics of Nurse Practitioner Graduates, by Employment Status, Phase III

Professional characteristics	Total		Employment status			
			Employed		Not employed	
	Number	Percent	Number	Percent	Number	Percent
ANA membership[1]...	397	100.0	356	100.0	41	100.0
Member	146	36.8	128	36.0	18	43.9
Nonmember	251	63.2	228	64.0	23	56.1
Years in professional nursing[1]	396	100.0	355	100.0	41	100.0
Less than one ...	4	1.0	3	0.8	1	2.4
1-5	140	35.4	123	34.6	17	41.5
6-10	123	31.1	110	31.0	13	31.7
11-15	51	12.9	47	13.2	4	9.8
16-20	43	10.9	41	11.5	2	4.9
21 or more	35	8.8	31	8.7	4	9.8
Previous employment setting[1] ...	394	100.0	354	100.0	40	100.0
Hospital outpatient service	36	9.1	32	9.0	4	10.0
Hospital inpatient service	156	39.6	136	38.4	20	50.0
Health center ...	64	16.2	62	17.5	2	5.0
Extended care facility	25	6.3	24	6.8	1	2.5
Fee-for-service physician	21	5.3	20	5.6	1	2.5
Prepaid group practice	1	0.3	...	...	1	2.5
Community/home health agency ..	54	13.7	49	13.8	5	12.5
School	8	2.0	7	2.0	1	2.5
Teaching	20	5.1	16	4.5	4	10.0
Other[2]	9	2.3	8	2.3	1	2.5
Prior nursing preparation[1]	398	100.0	357	100.0	41	100.0
Diploma	148	37.2	135	37.8	13	31.7
Associate degree	47	11.8	43	12.0	4	9.8
Baccalaureate ...	186	46.7	164	45.9	22	53.7
Master's	17	4.3	15	4.2	2	4.9
Employment changes after graduation[1]	396	100.0	355	100.0	41	100.0
None	346	87.4	318	89.6	28	68.3
One or more	50	12.6	37	10.4	13	31.7

[1]Includes only those graduates who responded to item.
[2]Includes setting within state and federal agencies, including the armed services, inservice education, and social agencies as well as combined inpatient/outpatient settings.

SOURCE: U.S. Department of Health, Education, and Welfare, Public Health Service, Health Resources Administration, Division of Nursing, *Longitudinal Study of Nurse Practitioners, Phase III*, DHEW Publication No. HRA 80-2, May, 1980, p. 89.

Table I-C-9. Phase II Nurse Practitioner Graduates[1] Who Were Not Employed, by Reason of Unemployment, and Type of Nurse Practitioner Program

	Type of program					
	Total		Certificate		Master's	
Reasons not employed[2]	Number	Percent	Number	Percent	Number	Percent
	N=63		N=50		N=13	
Nursing leadership at the place of employment is not familiar with, or not accepting of, the role	4	6.3	4	8.0	...	...
Not seeking employment	24	38.1	18	36.0	6	46.2
Physicians are accepting of the role, but there are no jobs available	12	19.0	11	22.0	1	7.7
Physicians approached are not familiar with, or not accepting of, the role	6	9.5	5	10.0	1	7.7
No job classification exists for this role at the place of employment	6	9.5	6	12.0	...	...
Attending another nurse practitioner program	1	1.6	1	2.0	...	...
Other[3]	23	36.5	18	36.0	5	38.5

[1] Includes only those graduates who supplied information on reasons they were not employed.
[2] Graduates may have selected more than one reason.
[3] "Other" reasons were primarily personal or to continue their education.
SOURCE: U.S. Department of Health, Education, and Welfare, Public Health Service, Health Resources Administration, Division of Nursing, *Longitudinal Study of Nurse Practitioners, Phase II*, DHEW Publication No. 78-92, September, 1978, p. 55.

Table I-C-10. Phase III Nurse Practitioner Graduates[1] Who Were Not Employed, by Reasons of Unemployment, and Type of Nurse Practitioner Program

Reasons not employed[2]	Type of program					
	Total		Certificate		Master's	
	Number	Percent	Number	Percent	Number	Percent
	N=41		N=34		N=7	
Nursing leadership at the place of employment is not familiar with, or not accepting of, the role	4	9.8	4	11.8	...	...
Not seeking employment	20	48.8	16	47.1	4	57.1
Physicians are accepting of the role, but there are no jobs available	8	19.5	8	23.5	...	...
Physicians approached are not familiar with, or not accepting of, the role	12	29.3	11	32.5	1	14.3
No job classification exists for this role at the place of employment	9	22.0	8	23.5	1	14.3
Attending another nurse practitioner program	3	7.3	3	8.8	...	...
Other[3]	2	4.9	2	5.9	...	...

[1] Includes only those graduates who supplied information on reasons they were not employed.
[2] Graduates may have selected more than one reason.
[3] "Other" refers to graduates waiting to begin a new job.

SOURCE: U.S. Department of Health, Education, and Welfare, Public Health Service, Health Resources Administration, Division of Nursing, *Longitudinal Study of Nurse Practitioners, Phase III*, DHEW Publication No. HRA 80-2, May, 1980, p. 98.

Table I-C-11. Nurse Practitioner Graduates Providing Primary Care, by the Employment Setting in Which They Spend Most of Their Time as Nurse Practitioners, and Type of Nurse Practitioner Program, Phase II and Phase III

	Type of program											
	Phase II						Phase III					
	Total		Certificate		Master's		Total		Certificate		Master's	
Employment setting	Number	Percent	Number	Percent	Number	Percent	Number	Percent	Number	Percent	Number	Percent
Total	500	100.0	403	100.0	97	100.0	288	100.0	253	100.0	35	100.0
Inhospital practice	35	7.0	22	5.5	13	13.4	32	11.1	30	11.8	2	5.7
Patient unit	29	5.8	17	4.2	12	12.4	24	8.3	22	8.7	2	5.7
Emergency room	6	1.2	5	1.3	1	1.0	8	2.8	8	3.1	...	...
Ambulatory clinical practice	317	63.4	248	61.5	69	71.2	176	61.0	154	60.9	22	62.9
Private practice	71	14.2	59	14.6	12	12.4	50	17.3	46	18.2	4	11.4
Prepaid group practice	20	4.0	15	3.7	5	5.2	12	4.2	10	4.0	2	5.7
Hospital based clinic	102	20.4	75	18.6	27	27.8	40	13.9	35	13.8	5	14.3
Community based clinic or center	116	23.2	93	23.1	23	23.7	74	25.6	63	24.9	11	31.5
Other ambulatory practice	8	1.6	6	1.5	2	2.1	...	...	...	...	...	...
Nonhospital institutional setting	81	16.2	80	19.9	1	1.0	27	9.4	24	9.5	3	8.6

School for mentally or physically handicapped..	4	0.8	4	1.0	...	...	8	2.8	8	3.2	...	...
Grades 1-12, public school system	32	6.4	32	7.9	...	...	5	1.7	2	0.8	3	8.6
College health program	44	8.8	43	10.7	1	1.0	12	4.2	12	4.7	...	...
Other nonhospital institutional setting	1	0.2	1	0.3	...	...	2	0.7	2	0.8	...	...
Nonhospital community setting........	*50*	*10.0*	*42*	*10.4*	*8*	*8.2*	*31*	*10.8*	*27*	*10.7*	*4*	*11.4*
Health department or home health agency	46	9.2	40	9.9	6	6.2	30	10.4	26	10.3	4	11.4
Social services or agency ...	3	0.6	2	0.5	1	1.0	1	0.4	1	0.4	...	...
Other nonhospital community setting	1	0.2	...	...	1	1.0	1	1.0	...	...	...	...
School of nursing..	*2*	*0.4*	...	...	*2*	*2.1*	*2*	*0.7*	...	...	*2*	*5.7*
Extended care facility	*7*	*1.4*	*4*	*1.0*	*3*	*3.1*	*14*	*4.9*	*12*	*4.7*	*2*	*5.7*
Other[1]	*8*	*1.6*	*7*	*1.7*	*1*	*1.0*	*6*	*2.1*	*6*	*2.4*	...	...

Includes industry, airport clinics, faculty in an Air Force nurse midwifery program for Phase II. Includes only industry for Phase III

SOURCE: U.S. Department of Health, Education, and Welfare, Public Health Service, Health Resources Administration, Division of Nursing, *Longitudinal Study of Nurse Practitioners, Phase II,* DHEW Publication No. 78-92, September, 1978, p. 68, and *Longitudinal Study of Nurse Practitioners, Phase III,* DHEW Publication No. HRA 80-2, May, 1980, p. 104.

Table I-C-12. Practice Setting Location of Nurse Practitioner Graduates[1] Who Provide Primary Care, by Type of Program, Phase II and Phase III

Practice setting location	Type of program											
	Phase II						Phase III					
	Total		Certificate		Master's		Total		Certificate		Master's	
	Number	Percent	Number	Percent	Number	Percent	Number	Percent	Number	Percent	Number	Percent
Total	497	100.0	400	100.0	97	100.0	283	100.0	248	100.0	35	100.0
Inner city	167	33.6	126	31.4	41	42.4	64	22.6	57	23.0	7	20.0
Other urban	89	17.9	65	16.3	24	24.7	53	18.7	42	16.9	11	31.5
Suburban	46	9.3	35	8.8	11	11.3	42	14.8	36	14.5	6	17.1
Rural	84	16.9	77	19.3	7	7.2	61	21.6	57	23.0	4	11.4
Combination[2]	19	3.8	16	4.0	3	3.1	22	7.8	17	6.9	5	14.3
Other[3]	92	18.5	81	20.2	11	11.3	41	14.5	39	15.7	2	5.7

[1] Includes only those graduates who supplied information on practice setting locations.
[2] Includes two or more of the practice setting locations.
[3] Includes military installations, VA hospitals, industry, college/university campuses, Indian reservations, religious communities and construction sites for Phase II. Includes various institutional settings for Phase III.

SOURCE: U.S. Department of Health, Education, and Welfare, Public Health Service, Health Resources Administration, Division of Nursing, *Longitudinal Study of Nurse Practitioners, Phase II*, DHEW Publication No. 78-92, September, 1978, p. 70, and *Longitudinal Study of Nurse Practitioners, Phase III*, DHEW Publication No. HRA 80-2, May, 1980, p. 105.

Table I-C-13. Average Number of Hours Per Week Nurse Practitioner Graduates Providing Patient Care, Functioned as Nurse Practitioners in Specific Employment Settings, by Type of Nurse Practitioner Program, Phase II

| Employment setting[1] | Total | | Type of program | | | |
| | | | Certificate | | Master's | |
	Number of nurse practitioners	Average hours per week	Number of nurse practitioners	Average hours per week	Number of nurse practitioners	Average hours per week
Total	500	33.7	403	33.5	97	34.9
Inhospital practice	115	15.6	74	16.0	41	14.9
Patient unit	95	16.6	59	16.5	36	16.7
Emergency room	32	10.8	20	13.0	12	7.1
Other hospital practice	4	4.5	3	4.3	1	5.0
Ambulatory practice	346	28.4	265	(2)	81	24.0
Private practice	76	28.9	62	29.0	14	28.4
Prepaid group practice	20	37.6	15	38.4	5	35.2
Hospital based clinic	125	25.0	84	27.5	41	20.1
Community based clinic or center	141	27.0	112	28.6	29	20.6
Other ambulatory practice	10	27.8	6	37.0	4	14.0
Nonhospital institutional setting	96	25.5	93	(2)	3	15.3
School for mentally or physically handicapped	6	21.8	6	21.8	⋮	⋮
Grades 1-12, public school system	37	21.3	37	21.3	⋮	⋮
College health program	47	32.7	44	33.9	3	14.7
Other nonhospital institutional setting	3	16.7	2	21.0	1	8.0
Nonhospital community setting	72	21.3	60	(2)	12	25.5
Health department or home health agency	66	22.0	57	21.0	9	28.3
Social services or agency	4	13.0	3	8.7	1	26.0
Other nonhospital community setting	3	9.3	1	3.0	2	12.5
School of nursing	21	9.5	4	4.0	17	10.8
Extended care facility	19	13.2	13	11.5	6	16.7
Other[3]	18	17.9	13	21.7	5	8.2

[1] Graduates may have selected more than one employment setting.
[2] Information not available.
[3] Includes industry, school of medicine, family practice, airport clinics, and faculty in an Air Force nurse midwifery program.

SOURCE: U.S. Department of Health, Education, and Welfare, Public Health Service, Health Resources Administration, Division of Nursing, *Longitudinal Study of Nurse Practitioners, Phase II*, DHEW Publication No. 78-92, September, 1978, p. 69.

Table I-C-14. Nurse Practitioner Graduates[1] by Type of Program, Percent of Time Spent in Nurse Practitioner Functions, and Major Employment Setting,[2] Phase II

Type of program and percent of time in nurse practitioner functions	Total		Major employment setting												
			Inhospital practice		Ambulatory practice		Nonhospital institutional setting		Nonhospital community setting		School of nursing		Extended care facility		Other[3]	
	Number	Percent	Number	Percent	Number	Percent	Number	Percent	Number	Percent	Number	Percent	Number	Percent	Number	Percent
Total	528	100.0	40	100.0	317	100.0	81	100.0	53	100.0	17	100.0	8	100.0	12	100.0
1-50	97	18.4	7	17.5	45	14.2	18	22.2	12	22.6	9	52.9	4	50.0	2	16.7
51-99	109	20.6	9	22.5	59	18.6	24	29.7	15	28.3	...	...	...	...	2	16.7
100	322	61.0	24	60.0	213	67.2	39	48.1	26	49.1	8	47.1	4	50.0	8	66.6
Certificate ...	413	100.0	22	100.0	248	100.0	80	100.0	45	100.0	3	100.0	4	100.0	11	100.0
1-50	68	16.5	3	13.6	29	11.7	18	22.5	12	26.6	2	66.7	2	50.0	2	18.2
51-99	89	21.5	4	18.1	47	19.0	23	28.8	13	28.9	...	...	...	...	2	18.2
100	256	62.0	15	68.3	172	69.3	39	48.7	20	44.5	1	33.3	2	50.0	7	63.6
Master's	115	100.0	18	100.0	69	100.0	1	100.0	8	100.0	14	100.0	4	100.0	1	100.0
1-50	29	25.2	4	22.3	16	23.2	...	...	2	25.0	7	50.0	2	50.0	...	...
51-99	20	17.4	5	27.8	12	17.4	1	100.0	6	75.0	...	...	...	...	...	...
100	66	57.4	9	49.9	41	59.4	...	...	...	...	7	50.0	2	50.0	1	100.0

[1]Includes only those graduates who supplied information on number of hours they were engaged in nurse practitioner functions and employment setting.

[2]Major employment setting in which they spend most of their time in nurse practitioner functions.

[3]Includes industry, airport clinics, and faculty in an Air Force midwifery program.

SOURCE: U.S. Department of Health, Education, and Welfare, Public Health Service, Health Resources Administration, Division of Nursing, *Longitudinal Study of Nurse Practitioners, Phase II*, DHEW Publication No. 78-92, September, 1978, p. 89.

Table I-C-15. Nurse Practitioners[1] and Average Number of Patients Seen Per Day, by Type of Program and Employment Setting, 1977

Employment setting	Total		Type of program			
			Certificate		Master's	
	Number of nurse practitioners	Average number of patients	Number of nurse practitioners	Average number of patients	Number of nurse practitioners	Average number of patients
Total	118	15.1	106	15.4	12	12.9
Inhospital practice	13	17.7	12	17.8	1	17.0
Patient unit	8	17.4	7	17.4	1	17.0
Emergency room	5	18.4	5	18.4	...	...
Ambulatory practice	73	14.2	63	14.7	10	11.7
Private practice	19	15.2	17	15.5	2	13.0
Prepaid group practice	9	15.6	8	15.9	1	13.0
Hospital-based clinic	17	12.7	15	12.3	2	16.0
Community-based clinic or center	28	14.1	23	15.2	5	9.2
Nonhospital institutional setting	11	15.9	11	15.9	...	...
Nonhospital community setting	16	11.6	16	11.6	...	...
Extended care facility	5	13.8	4	12.2	1	20.0

[1]Those working full-time as nurse practitioners in the one employment setting in which they reported spending most of their time.

SOURCE: U.S. Department of Health, Education, and Welfare, Public Health Service, Health Resources Administration, Division of Nursing, *Longitudinal Study of Nurse Practitioners, Phase III*, DHEW Publication No. HRA 80-2, May, 1980, p. 129.

Table I-C-16. Number of Nurse Practitioners[1] Providing Patient
Care and Average Percent of Patients in Selected Income Categories,
by Type of Program and Specialty, 1977

Type of program and specialty	Number of nurse practitioners	Patients' income		
		Less than $4,000 Average percent	$4,000-15,000 Average percent	More than $15,000 Average percent
Total	258	46	43	11
Pediatric	25	49	43	8
Midwifery	10	45	39	16
Maternity	41	54	36	10
Family	111	43	46	11
Adult	62	48	39	13
Psychiatric	2	23	74	3
Emergency	7	34	52	14
Certificate	227	46	43	11
Pediatric	15	51	42	7
Midwifery	10	45	39	16
Maternity	39	55	37	8
Family	100	41	48	11
Adult	55	49	38	13
Psychiatric	1	1	98	1
Emergency	7	34	52	14
Master's	31	49	40	11
Pediatric	10	45	45	10
Midwifery	...	...	...	...
Maternity	2	37	18	45
Family	11	59	32	9
Adult	7	44	47	9
Psychiatric	1	45	50	5
Emergency	...	...	...	...

[1]Includes only those graduates who supplied information on income of patients served and specialty.
SOURCE: U.S. Department of Health, Education, and Welfare, Public Health Service, Health Resources
Administration, Division of Nursing, *Longitudinal Study of Nurse Practitioners, Phase III,*
DHEW Publication No. HRA 80-2, May, 1980, p. 106.

Table I-C-17. Number of Active Anesthesiologists (M.D.)[1] and Nurse Anesthetists in the United States, and Ratio of Nurse Anesthetists per Anesthesiologist, by State, 1972

State	Anesthesiologist	Nurse anesthetist	Nurse anesthetist per anesthesiologist
United States, total	11,106	12,162	1.1
Alabama	92	304	3.3
Alaska	10	15	1.5
Arizona	100	100	1.2
Arkansas	47	121	2.6
California	1,597	685	0.4
Colorado	138	110	1.8
Connecticut	208	147	0.7
Delaware	24	26	1.0
District of Columbia	88	33	0.4
Florida	380	492	1.3
Georgia	189	257	1.4
Hawaii	33	67	2.0
Idaho	25	61	2.4
Illinois	527	649	1.2
Indiana	271	92	0.3
Iowa	105	157	1.5
Kansas	84	141	1.7
Kentucky	120	137	1.1
Louisiana	106	343	3.2
Maine	58	55	0.9
Maryland	261	168	0.6
Massachusetts	539	304	0.6
Michigan	340	605	1.8
Minnesota	183	499	2.7
Mississippi	43	165	3.8
Missouri	150	334	2.2
Montana	25	66	2.6
Nebraska	41	154	3.8
Nevada	33	30	0.9
New Hampshire	45	30	0.7
New Jersey	405	227	0.6
New Mexico	29	74	2.6
New York	1,569	635	0.4
North Carolina	97	457	4.7
North Dakota	11	85	7.7
Ohio	623	455	0.7
Oklahoma	94	139	1.5
Oregon	142	146	1.0
Pennsylvania	606	1,171	1.9
Rhode Island	65	28	0.4
South Carolina	65	164	2.5
South Dakota	10	96	9.6
Tennessee	147	259	1.8
Texas	530	763	1.4
Utah	88	55	0.6
Vermont	33	18	0.5
Virginia	183	298	1.6
Washington	247	239	1.0
West Virginia	54	165	3.1
Wisconsin	232	315	1.4
Wyoming	14	26	1.9

[1] Excludes 685 federally employed anesthesiologists and 61 anesthesiologists employed in the U.S. possessions.

SOURCE: U.S. Department of Health, Education, and Welfare, Public Health Service, Health Resources Administration, Bureau of Health Manpower, *Supply, Need and Distribution of Anesthesiologists and Nurse Anesthetists in the U.S., 1972 and 1980.* DHEW Publication No. (HRA) 77-31, 1976, p. 24.

Table I-C-18. Nurse Anesthetists Supply and Needs, 1972 and 1980

	Supply		Need	
Method	1972	1980	1972	1980
Method I[1]	12,162	15,835	23,480	25,530
Method II[2]	12,162	16,080	20,467	22,267

[1]Method I need estimates are based on the national total (actual for 1972 and projected for 1980) of operations and deliveries. It is assumed that nurse anesthetists deliver all services, that each nurse administers 800 anesthetics, and that one anesthesiologist supervises two anesthetists. See report for explanation of Method I supply projections.
[2]Method II need estimates, which are based on state supplies of hospitals, modify Method I assumptions so that all hospitals with less than 100 beds need one anesthesiologist and no anesthetists. Needs for larger hospitals would be determined in the same way as in Method I. See report for explanation of Method II supply projections.

SOURCE: U.S. Department of Health, Education, and Welfare, Public Health Service, Health Resources Administration, Bureau of Health Manpower, *Supply, Need and Distribution of Anesthesiologists and Nurse Anesthetists in the U.S., 1972 and 1980*, DHEW Publication No. (HRA) 77-31, 1976, p. 25.

Table I-C-19. U.S. Resident ACNM[1] Study Participants in Clinical Practice, by Number of Nurse-Midwifery Positions Concurrently Held and Number of Paid Work Hours Per Week, 1976-1977

	Positions concurrently held[2]		
	Total	One	Two or more
Number of weekly paid work hours	Percent	Percent	Percent
Total	100	85	15
Less than 35	13	8	5
35-44	63	56	7
45 or more	24	21	3

[1]American College of Nurse-Midwives.
[2]Includes only those responding to number of positions concurrently held.

SOURCE: American College of Nurse-Midwives, *Nurse-Midwifery in the United States: 1976-1977*, p. 17.

Table I-C-20. Percent of Work Time Spent in Various Activities by ACNM[1] Study Participants[2] in Clinical Practice, 1976-1977

Work activity	Percent distribution[3] by percent of work time				
	Total	0-24	25-49	50-74	75-100
Direct patient management and care	100.0	16	10	30	44
Education of health-care providers	100.0	77	11	5	7
Clinical instruction associated with patient care	100.0	81	11	5	3
Classroom instruction	100.0	95	4	(4)	(4)
Patient, client, or public education	100.0	86	12	2	(4)
Supervision and/or administration	100.0	89	7	3	1
Consultation	100.0	99	(4)	(4)	...
Research	100.0	100	(4)	...	...

[1] American College of Nurse-Midwives.
[2] N=623.
[3] Includes only those who responded to percent of time spent in work activity.
[4] Less than one percent.
SOURCE: American College of Nurse-Midwives, *Nurse-Midwifery in the United States: 1976-1977*, p. 17.

Table I-C-21. Mean Percent of Work Time Spent in Various Activities by ACNM[1] Study Participants[2] in Clinical Practice, 1976-1977

Work activity	Mean percent
Total	100.0
Direct patient management and care	60.6
Education of health-care providers	16.6
Clinical instruction associated with patient care	[3]11.3
Classroom instruction	[3]3.6
Patient, client, or public education	11.5
Supervision and/or administration	7.8
Consultation	1.8
Research	0.9
Other	0.8

[1] American Academy of Nurse-Midwives.
[2] N=623.
[3] Included in education of health-care providers.
SOURCE: American College of Nurse-Midwives, *Nurse-Midwifery in the United States: 1976-1977*, p. 17.

Table I-C-22. U.S. Resident ACNM[1] Study Participants[2] in Clinical Practice, by Size of Community and Field of Employment, 1976-1977

Field of employment	Nurse-midwives		Total	Size of community				
				Less than 10,000	10,000- 49,000	50,000- 199,999	200,000- 499,999	500,000 or more
	Number	Percent	Percent	Percent	Percent	Percent	Percent	Percent
Total	621	100.0	100.0	10	19	19	11	41
Hospital	283	45.6	100.0	5	11	20	9	55
Public health agency	86	13.8	100.0	20	25	13	16	26
Private practice with M.D.	80	12.9	100.0	14	40	20	9	17
U.S. military	51	8.2	100.0	14	29	37	6	14
Nurse-midwife maternity service[3]	47	7.6	100.0	21	19	9	7	44
University health service	31	5.0	100.0	...	10	20	30	40
Prepaid health plan	21	3.4	100.0	...	...	26	5	69
Private nurse-midwife practice	15	2.4	100.0	8	8	15	8	61
Other	7	1.1	100.0	13	29	29	29	...

[1] American College of Nurse-Midwives.
[2] Includes only those responding to size of community and field of employment.
[3] With medical backup.
SOURCE: American College of Nurse-Midwives, *Nurse-Midwifery in the United States: 1976-1977*, p. 18.

Table I-C-23. U.S. Resident ACNM[1] Study Participants Who Manage Deliveries and Number of Deliveries[2] by Field of Employment, 1976-1977

Field of employment	Nurse-midwives		Deliveries		
	Number	Percent	Number	Percent	Average per year
Total	521	100.0	33,613	100.0	65
Hospital	264	50.6	15,596	46.3	59
Public health agency	41	7.9	3,249	9.7	79
Private practice with M.D.	66	12.7	4,901	14.6	74
U.S. military	50	9.6	4,402	13.1	88
Nurse-midwife maternity service[3]	45	8.6	3,121	9.3	69
University health service	25	4.8	964	2.9	39
Prepaid health plan	13	2.5	623	1.9	48
Private nurse-midwife practice	15	2.9	601	1.8	40
Other	1	0.2	145	0.4	145
Unknown	1	0.2	11	(4)	11

[1] American College of Nurse-Midwives.
[2] Number of deliveries they managed during 12 months prior to filling out study questionnaire.
[3] With medical back-up.
[4] Less than 0.1 percent.
SOURCE: American College of Nurse-Midwives, *Nurse-Midwifery in the United States: 1976-1977*, p. 29.

Chapter I, Section D
NURSES FUNCTIONING IN INSTITUTIONS

A necessary adjunct to studies of individual nurses, such as the ANA inventories and the 1977 national sample survey of registered nurses, are statistics gathered from the employers of nurses. Detailed and diversified information on nurses functioning in employment settings are important for assessing significant changes in the utilization of nursing personnel. For example, data on the number of nurses-to-patients and staffing patterns are used as proxies for utilization. Obviously, these data on the characteristics of nurses within their work settings are essential for a more explicit understanding of the total nurse supply picture.

Hospitals remain the predominant employers of nurses. One important source of information on nurses within this sector is the American Hospital Association. All AHA data presented in this section are based on full-time equivalents (FTEs). An FTE was calculated by adding one-half of the number of part-time nurses to the number of full-time personnel. This statistic more accurately measures nursing staffing levels than does a total enumeration, and it thus provides a better indicator of utilization than mere totals. In 1978, the AHA reported there were 859,792 full-time equivalent licensed nurses, of whom 602,660 FTEs were registered nurses located in all U.S. hospitals. This reflected a 4.9 percent net gain in the number of FTE registered nurses employed in hospitals since 1977. However, there was wide variation in the amount of change in the number of FTE nurses according to the bed-size designation of the hospital, ranging from a decline of 2.1 percent in facilities with 25-49 beds to a 10.0 percent gain in those with 300-399 beds.

Short-term general and other special hospitals constituted the largest group of hospitals. In 1978, 84 percent of all hospitals were in this category, accounting for 534,857 FTE nurses (88.7 percent of all FTE hospital nurses). These hospitals provided a significant number of outpatient services as well as inpatient care. Therefore, the "adjusted" average daily census, a figure representing the average number of inpatients plus an equivalent figure for outpatients, is a better measure of utilization than the average daily census (average number of inpatients receiving care each day) for this group of facilities. For technical definitions the reader is referred to the AHA source documents indicated in the tables in this section. Ratios of the number of nurses per 100 adjusted average daily census in all U.S. short-term general and other special hospitals were calculated. There were 64.3 FTE registered nurses per 100 patients in 1978, up 4.6 percent over the previous year. Increases in the ratios of nurses to 100 patients were observed in each bed-size category, with the larger proportionate gains in the largest hospitals.

The nurse-to-patient population ratios varied by state and region. Excluded from the statistics are a small number of hospitals not registered with the AHA. In addition, special adjustments were made to estimate the state and regional adjusted average daily census for the 5,935 short-term general and other special hospitals registered with the AHA. This group consisted of two categories: 5,851 community hospitals and 84 hospital units of institutions. For the community hospitals the adjusted average daily census was reported by the AHA on a state and regional basis; however, for the hospital units of institutions it was not. The U.S. total adjusted average daily census for hospital units of institutions was 4,631. This number was proportionally allocated by state and region according to the distribution of the average daily census of the hospital units. The estimated total adjusted average daily census for AHA registered nonfederal short-term general and other special hospitals was then formed by adding the value provided by AHA for the community hospitals and the estimate for hospital units of institutions.

The 1978 FTE nurse-to-100 adjusted average daily census in non-federal short-term hospitals ranged from 48.1 in the East South Central states to 81.2 in the Pacific region. All regions exhibited growth in the nurse-to-patient ratios from 1977 to 1978. The largest gains were marked in the West South Central (7.0 percent) and the East South Central (6.9 percent), while the lowest was in the West North Central region (0.7 percent).

Nurse-to-100 average inpatient censuses were computed for all other categories of AHA registered nonfederal hospitals, resulting in ratios of 10.5 for psychiatric facilities, 24.6 for tuberculosis, and 18.4 for long-term general and other special hospitals in 1978. Increases of 9.4 percent, 5.6 percent, and 5.1 percent, respectively, were observed in the ratios of registered nurses to 100 inpatients since 1977. The ratio for federal hospitals was 41.7 nurses to 100 inpatient population in 1978.

The National Center for Health Statistics also supplied data on nursing personnel by employment setting, through its Master Facility Inventory. According to the latest (1976) survey, there were a total of 622,287 registered nurses working in hospitals; of the total, 460,954, or 74.1 percent, were considered full-time employees. The proportion of nurses employed part-time in hospitals has been on the decline since 1968. In 1968, about 30 percent of the nurses in hospitals held part-time positions; in 1970, 29 percent; in 1972, 27 percent; and 1976, 26 percent held part-time positions. Nonfederal hospitals had a larger porportion of part-time staff than federal hospitals. Within the nonfederal group, short-term general and other special hospitals accounted for the largest part-time complement.

Registered nurses constituted the largest proportion (26 percent) of professional patient care staff in mental health facilities. The Division of Biometry and Epidemiology of the National Institute of Mental Health reported 45,163 registered nurses employed in mental health facilities (excluding federally funded community mental health centers) as of January 1976. This figure represented a 15.1 percent increase in registered nurse staff from 1974. A breakdown by employment status revealed 77.8 percent of the nurses were working in full-time positions, indicating a continued growth in the proportion of full-time workers. About 13 percent of the nurses were employed on a part-time basis, and 9 percent were in trainee positions.

The National Center for Health Statistics also collected data on registered nurses working in nursing homes and related facilities. Data on the characteristics of nurses and of the nursing homes for 1977 are detailed in the tables. In 1977, there were 66,900 FTE registered nurses in nursing homes, accounting for 4.8 nurses per 100 beds. In 1976, 80,195 nurses worked in these facilities, of whom 57 percent were working full-time. The part-time complement in nursing and personal care homes increased slightly, from 41.4 percent in 1973 to 42.9 percent in 1976. Nationally, there were 32.4 full-time registered nurses and 24.3 part-time nurses per 1,000 beds. The number of nurses in relation to the number of beds varied by state and region. The Middle Atlantic region showed the highest ratio of full-time nurses, while the West South Central states had the lowest ratios. Nursing and personal care homes operating on a for-profit basis employed the majority (62.8 percent) of the nurses; 25.6 percent were working in church-related or other non-profit agencies; and 11.6 percent were employed in homes operated by government agencies. Calculations of the 1976 distribution of full-time equivalent nurses by the certification status of the home indicated the majority of FTE nurses were in combined skilled nursing and intermediate care facilities.

Table I-D-1. Full-time Equivalent Nursing Personnel¹ in Hospitals,² by Size of Hospital, 1977 and 1978

Number of beds	Full-time equivalent nursing personnel					
	1977			1978		
	Total	Registered nurse	Licensed practical nurse	Total	Registered nurse	Licensed practical nurse
Total	830,356	574,583	255,773	859,792	602,660	257,132
6-24 beds	4,384	3,038	1,346	4,422	3,040	1,382
25-49	23,944	15,144	8,800	23,653	14,820	8,833
50-99	66,919	41,640	25,279	68,292	42,262	26,030
100-199	146,352	96,937	49,415	151,722	101,491	50,231
200-299	143,920	100,890	43,030	146,359	103,119	43,240
300-399	112,681	80,854	31,827	121,969	88,882	33,087
400-499	98,079	70,005	28,074	98,982	72,122	26,860
500 or more	234,077	166,075	68,002	244,393	176,924	67,469

¹Data reflects the number of full-time equivalent (FTE) nursing personnel. The FTE is computed by adding one-half of the number of part-time nurses to the number of full-time nurses.
²Includes all U.S. hospitals, AHA registered and non-AHA registered hospitals.

SOURCE: American Hospital Association, *Hospital Statistics 1978*, pp. 13 and 213. *Hospital Statistics 1979*, pp. 13 and 213.

Table I-D-2. Nursing Personnel[1] per 100 Adjusted Average Daily Census[2] in All Nonfederal Short-term General and Other Special Hospitals,[3] by Size of Hospital, 1977 and 1978

| Number of beds | 1978 | | Full-time equivalent nursing personnel per 100 patients | | | 1977 | | Full-time equivalent nursing personnel per 100 patients | | |
	Number of hospitals	Adjusted average daily census	Total[4]	Registered nurse	Licensed practical nurse	Number of hospitals	Adjusted average daily census	Total[4]	Registered nurse	Licensed practical nurse
Total	6,076	831,726	91.0	64.3	26.6	6,120	826,905	88.0	61.4	26.6
6-24 beds	334	3,680	92.9	62.6	30.3	349	3,890	88.3	59.8	28.5
25-49	1,153	26,071	78.3	47.5	30.7	1,197	27,872	74.5	45.7	28.8
50-99	1,487	76,856	80.2	48.7	31.5	1,479	77,080	77.4	47.4	30.4
100-199	1,424	157,709	88.7	59.1	29.7	1,437	158,081	86.2	56.9	29.3
200-299	724	151,516	91.6	64.7	26.9	720	150,466	89.8	63.1	26.7
300-399	395	119,245	95.0	69.7	25.4	383	115,303	91.0	65.9	25.1
400-499	242	97,503	92.5	68.1	24.4	244	98,599	90.0	64.6	25.4
500 or more	317	199,146	94.8	71.4	23.4	311	195,614	91.3	67.3	23.9

[1]Data reflects the number of full-time equivalent (FTE) nursing personnel. The FTE is computed by adding one-half of the number of part-time nurses to the number of full-time nurses.
[2]Nurse to patient ratios were calculated using the adjusted average daily census as the denominator. The adjusted census includes the average number of inpatients receiving care plus an equivalent figure for outpatients.
[3]Includes all U.S. hospitals, AHA registered and non-AHA registered hospitals.
[4]Detail may not add to totals due to rounding.
SOURCE: Ratios were computed by the American Nurses' Association, Research and Policy Analysis Department, Statistics Unit, based upon data from the American Hospital Association, Hospital Statistics 1978, pp. 12 and 212, Hospital Statistics 1979, p. 12 and 212.

Table I-D.3. Nursing Personnel[1] Per 100 Average Daily Census in Nonfederal Hospitals,[2] by Type of Hospital, 1978

Region and state	Short-term general and other special[a] Number of hospitals	Total[b]	Registered nurse	Licensed practical nurse	Psychiatric[a] Number of hospitals	Total[b]	Registered nurse	Licensed practical nurse	Tuberculosis[a] Number of hospitals	Total[b]	Registered nurse	Licensed practical nurse	Long-term general and other special[a] Number of hospitals	Total[b]	Registered nurse	Licensed practical nurse
Total	5,935	91.0	64.3	26.6	526	18.7	10.5	8.2	15	51.2	24.6	26.6	169	31.2	18.4	12.8
New England	272	103.9	79.1	24.8	48	22.6	14.1	8.5	1	57.8	30.1	27.7	40	39.8	24.6	15.2
Connecticut	40	97.6	74.6	23.0	11	21.4	15.2	6.2	…	…	…	…	8	41.6	29.3	12.4
Maine	49	96.1	68.3	27.8	3	12.8	7.6	5.1	…	…	…	…	…	…	…	…
Massachusetts	124	107.8	84.7	23.0	27	28.2	15.2	13.0	1	57.8	30.1	27.7	30	42.9	26.1	16.8
New Hampshire	29	106.8	80.5	26.3	2	16.9	15.1	1.8	…	…	…	…	…	…	…	…
Rhode Island	14	103.3	71.4	31.9	3	12.9	10.7	2.2	…	…	…	…	2	20.9	11.4	9.5
Vermont	16	102.3	67.2	35.1	2	15.4	11.1	4.3	…	…	…	…	…	…	…	…
Middle Atlantic	647	88.2	67.3	20.9	100	16.5	11.7	4.7	1	87.5	68.8	18.8	41	28.9	16.4	12.5
New Jersey	108	84.7	62.2	22.5	13	19.6	10.4	9.2	…	…	…	…	14	49.7	33.9	15.9
New York	290	86.2	67.9	18.3	47	14.0	11.1	3.0	1	87.5	68.8	18.8	14	31.2	17.2	14.0
Pennsylvania	249	93.2	69.3	23.9	40	20.2	13.8	6.4	…	…	…	…	13	21.4	11.2	10.2
South Atlantic	822	89.0	61.5	27.5	90	14.1	8.7	5.4	7	41.9	22.6	19.3	25	27.4	15.4	12.1
Delaware	8	104.5	74.7	29.8	2	17.8	9.9	8.0	…	…	…	…	3	18.3	11.8	6.5
District of Columbia	13	104.5	83.4	21.2	1	60.6	60.0	0.6	…	…	…	…	1	132.3	33.8	98.5
Florida	211	93.1	65.5	27.6	18	9.3	6.7	2.5	1	29.5	17.1	12.4	1	32.4	13.9	18.5
Georgia	163	92.5	59.1	33.4	17	22.4	11.3	11.1	…	…	…	…	…	…	…	…
Maryland	53	88.7	70.4	18.3	13	16.8	9.6	7.1	1	33.5	12.4	21.1	8	31.5	18.2	13.3
North Carolina	129	86.4	58.7	27.6	13	12.4	9.6	2.8	3	46.9	27.2	19.6	4	33.8	23.9	9.9
South Carolina	74	76.7	48.2	28.5	5	11.0	7.0	4.0	1	53.1	33.3	19.8	1	83.3	61.1	22.2
Virginia	103	88.0	59.1	28.9	17	13.9	7.4	6.4	1	41.3	18.8	22.5	4	27.2	15.6	11.6
West Virginia	68	76.5	48.1	28.4	4	8.3	5.7	2.6	…	…	…	…	3	14.6	4.8	9.8
East North Central	925	88.1	62.9	25.1	103	17.2	10.3	6.8	…	…	…	…	18	28.5	16.2	12.3
Illinois	245	88.4	68.9	19.4	25	15.7	9.5	6.2	…	…	…	…	5	27.5	17.3	10.2
Indiana	116	78.0	57.3	20.7	13	10.5	6.4	4.1	…	…	…	…	2	27.0	15.1	11.9
Michigan	210	88.8	58.6	30.2	21	18.9	11.7	7.2	…	…	…	…	5	25.0	11.9	13.1
Ohio	209	92.3	63.6	29.7	23	17.9	9.5	8.4	…	…	…	…	4	34.4	18.4	15.9
Wisconsin	145	84.6	60.9	23.7	21	32.6	22.6	10.0	…	…	…	…	2	62.1	37.1	25.0

East South Central	*487*	*80.2*	*48.1*	*32.1*	*25*	*12.0*	*6.8*	*5.3*	…	…	…	…	*8*	*26.9*	*14.1*	*12.8*
Alabama	133	87.2	50.5	36.7	6	6.5	3.8	2.7	…	…	…	…	1	89.3	39.3	50.0
Kentucky	108	76.9	53.5	23.3	6	25.9	14.7	11.1	…	…	…	…	2	88.1	42.7	25.4
Mississippi	104	76.2	40.7	35.5	3	9.6	4.8	4.8	…	…	…	…	2	65.3	…	22.7
Tennessee	142	78.9	46.1	32.8	10	13.3	7.6	5.7	…	…	…	…	3	16.6	6.9	9.7
West North Central	*808*	*82.8*	*58.3*	*24.5*	*39*	*19.7*	*9.2*	*10.5*	*1*	*54.9*	*15.2*	*39.7*	*8*	*23.8*	*14.5*	*9.3*
Iowa	131	88.6	63.8	24.8	7	10.4	5.8	4.7	…	…	…	…	…	…	…	…
Kansas	147	77.4	54.9	22.6	10	40.3	11.5	28.8	…	…	…	…	…	…	…	…
Minnesota	173	87.0	62.2	24.8	8	15.7	7.1	8.6	…	…	…	…	2	17.9	7.4	10.5
Missouri	149	76.3	52.4	23.9	9	17.7	11.7	5.9	1	54.9	15.2	39.7	1	16.0	9.7	6.3
Nebraska	97	81.0	57.3	23.7	3	30.7	20.9	9.8	…	…	…	…	3	36.9	26.9	9.9
North Dakota	54	90.5	59.8	30.7	1	11.6	6.8	4.8	…	…	…	…	…	…	…	…
South Dakota	57	98.5	69.2	29.3	…	12.7	8.3	4.3	…	…	…	…	2	25.8	14.0	11.8
West South Central	*858*	*90.0*	*53.3*	*36.8*	*40*	*17.0*	*8.3*	*8.7*	*2*	*43.5*	*19.4*	*24.1*	*12*	*29.5*	*16.1*	*13.4*
Arkansas	91	88.0	45.9	43.0	1	80.1	10.1	69.9	…	…	…	…	…	…	…	…
Louisiana	140	81.0	47.6	33.4	7	15.0	8.1	6.9	…	…	…	…	3	14.3	7.6	6.7
Oklahoma	121	86.6	53.2	33.4	7	9.1	6.3	2.8	…	…	…	…	1	15.0	3.3	11.7
Texas	506	93.7	56.3	37.4	25	18.2	9.1	9.2	2	43.5	19.4	24.1	8	45.0	25.7	19.3
Mountain	*366*	*97.8*	*70.9*	*26.9*	*23*	*31.8*	*17.9*	*13.9*	…	…	…	…	*6*	*36.9*	*26.4*	*10.5*
Arizona	58	101.8	77.8	24.0	4	20.8	17.1	3.6	…	…	…	…	…	…	…	…
Colorado	86	100.5	75.8	24.7	6	53.5	26.1	27.4	…	…	…	…	2	88.0	76.1	12.0
Idaho	47	100.2	60.9	39.3	2	36.6	16.8	19.9	…	…	…	…	…	…	…	…
Montana	57	78.8	57.7	21.1	2	28.7	12.7	16.0	…	…	…	…	…	…	…	…
Nevada	19	94.8	62.8	32.0	2	45.9	36.7	9.2	…	…	…	…	…	…	…	…
New Mexico	37	91.7	60.9	30.8	4	23.1	14.9	8.2	…	…	…	…	2	19.0	9.1	10.0
Utah	35	104.2	76.7	27.5	2	17.8	11.7	6.2	…	…	…	…	2	33.3	23.0	10.3
Wyoming	27	101.6	74.3	27.3	1	8.3	5.1	3.2	…	…	…	…	…	…	…	…
Pacific	*750*	*110.4*	*81.2*	*29.1*	*58*	*34.3*	*10.4*	*23.9*	*3*	*74.6*	*34.4*	*40.2*	*11*	*31.4*	*21.0*	*10.4*
Alaska	16	102.0	75.2	26.8	1	27.3	17.5	9.8	…	…	…	…	…	…	…	…
California	526	109.6	80.8	28.8	45	35.2	9.5	25.7	2	113.8	57.5	56.3	7	23.0	19.3	3.7
Hawaii	20	101.1	68.0	33.1	7	73.9	35.2	38.7	1	56.8	23.9	33.0	4	87.9	31.9	56.0
Oregon	78	112.0	88.2	23.8	5	18.4	15.7	2.7	…	…	…	…	…	…	…	…
Washington	110	117.8	83.0	34.7	6	32.5	12.0	20.5	…	…	…	…	…	…	…	…

[1] Data reflects the number of full-time equivalent (FTE) nursing personnel. The FTE is computed by adding one-half the number of part-time nurses to the number of full-time nurses.

[2] Excludes 215 U.S. hospitals not registered with the American Hospital Association.

[3] Nurse-to-patient ratios based on the adjusted average daily census, which includes both the average number of inpatients plus an equivalent figure for outpatients.

[4] Nurse-to-patient ratios based on the average daily census, which includes only the number of inpatients receiving care each day.

[5] Detail may not add to totals due to rounding.

SOURCE: Ratios were computed by the American Nurses' Association, Research and Policy Analysis Department, Statistics Unit, based upon data from the American Hospital Association, *Hospital Statistics 1979*, pp. 20-141.

Table I-D-4. Nursing Personnel[1] Per 100 Average Daily Census in Nonfederal Hospitals,[2] by Type of Hospital, 1977

Region and state	Short-term general and other special[3]				Psychiatric[4]				Tuberculosis[4]				Long-term general and other special[4]			
	Number of hospitals	Full-time equivalent nursing personnel per 100 patients			Number of hospitals	Full-time equivalent nursing personnel per 100 patients			Number of hospitals	Full-time equivalent nursing personnel per 100 patients			Number of hospitals	Full-time equivalent nursing personnel per 100 patients		
		Total[5]	Registered nurse	Licensed practical nurse		Total[5]	Registered nurse	Licensed practical nurse		Total[5]	Registered nurse	Licensed practical nurse		Total[5]	Registered nurse	Licensed practical nurse
Total	5,973	88.0	61.5	26.6	541	17.9	9.6	8.3	19	46.4	23.3	23.1	189	29.7	17.5	12.2
New England	275	101.3	76.5	24.8	49	21.5	13.1	8.3	1	51.2	27.4	23.8	40	36.9	22.6	14.3
Connecticut	40	98.0	72.9	25.1	11	19.9	14.0	5.9	…	…	…	…	8	41.9	30.1	11.8
Maine	49	94.3	65.2	29.1	3	12.1	6.8	5.2	…	…	…	…	…	…	…	…
Massachusetts	127	103.5	81.5	22.0	28	26.0	13.9	12.1	1	51.2	27.4	23.8	30	39.3	23.3	16.0
New Hampshire	29	103.6	77.5	26.0	2	18.4	15.9	2.4	…	…	…	…	…	…	…	…
Rhode Island	14	103.9	70.7	33.2	3	11.4	9.7	1.7	…	…	…	…	2	19.7	11.2	8.5
Vermont	16	98.1	64.6	33.4	2	16.3	11.4	4.9	…	…	…	…	…	…	…	…
Middle Atlantic	662	84.9	63.9	21.0	100	14.9	10.9	4.1	1	59.7	45.5	14.3	47	27.8	15.8	12.0
New Jersey	108	83.3	60.9	22.5	13	18.8	10.2	8.6	…	…	…	…	15	49.1	30.2	18.9
New York	303	81.9	63.3	18.6	48	13.0	10.4	2.6	1	59.7	45.5	14.3	15	30.4	17.2	13.2
Pennsylvania	251	90.6	66.6	24.0	39	17.3	12.1	5.2	…	…	…	…	17	20.6	11.3	9.3
South Atlantic	820	86.8	59.3	27.5	91	13.2	7.7	5.5	7	37.4	20.5	16.9	29	24.6	13.9	10.7
Delaware	8	95.3	66.1	29.3	3	11.4	7.4	4.0	…	…	…	…	3	13.2	8.5	4.6
District of Columbia	13	97.8	75.7	22.2	1	46.2	45.6	0.6	…	…	…	…	2	16.8	10.7	6.2
Florida	212	90.5	62.2	28.3	19	8.9	6.5	2.4	1	25.9	14.7	11.2	1	24.8	12.8	11.9
Georgia	160	90.1	57.3	32.8	17	20.5	9.7	10.8	…	…	…	…	1	54.5	34.8	19.7
Maryland	51	85.7	67.2	18.5	12	18.7	8.6	10.1	1	32.7	13.6	19.1	8	32.8	19.3	13.6
North Carolina	130	83.7	57.5	26.2	12	9.9	7.7	2.2	3	44.0	24.7	19.3	6	30.7	18.8	11.9
South Carolina	75	77.3	48.1	29.2	5	9.8	6.8	3.0	1	41.3	24.8	16.5	1	55.2	34.5	20.7
Virginia	103	87.2	58.4	28.8	16	13.4	6.8	6.6	1	30.4	19.6	10.7	4	28.5	15.8	12.7
West Virginia	68	77.5	48.4	29.1	6	9.0	5.4	3.6	…	…	…	…	3	12.8	2.6	10.2
East North Central	933	84.5	59.6	24.9	109	15.3	9.1	6.2	…	…	…	…	20	28.4	15.7	12.7
Illinois	246	83.9	63.9	20.0	25	17.4	10.3	7.1	…	…	…	…	5	25.0	14.9	10.2
Indiana	116	77.5	56.6	20.8	13	9.2	5.6	3.7	…	…	…	…	2	22.7	12.6	10.1
Michigan	215	85.8	56.2	29.6	24	15.2	9.8	5.5	…	…	…	…	5	25.4	12.0	13.4
Ohio	211	88.6	59.5	29.1	26	14.0	7.4	6.6	…	…	…	…	5	41.6	23.1	18.6
Wisconsin	145	81.4	58.2	23.2	21	25.7	17.0	8.7	…	…	…	…	3	60.2	36.7	23.4

Region and State															
East South Central	488	77.0	45.0	32.0	25	10.9	6.1	4.8	3	42.9	24.8	18.0	10	29.0	15.6	13.4
Alabama	133	84.9	47.0	37.9	6	5.7	3.5	2.2	…	…	…	…	2	52.3	30.8	21.5
Kentucky	107	72.0	48.8	23.1	6	25.5	13.7	11.8	2	51.4	29.7	21.6	2	48.1	37.3	10.8
Mississippi	104	75.7	39.5	36.2	3	6.9	3.6	3.3	…	…	…	…	4	111.0	52.1	58.9
Tennessee	144	75.0	43.4	31.6	10	12.9	7.3	5.6	1	35.6	20.7	14.9	4	15.8	7.3	8.5
West North Central	808	82.5	57.9	24.7	42	16.1	9.4	6.7	1	58.2	16.4	41.8	7	24.0	13.8	10.2
Iowa	131	88.6	63.5	25.2	7	11.1	6.2	4.9	…	…	…	…	…	…	…	…
Kansas	146	74.3	52.9	21.4	9	23.4	10.9	12.4	…	…	…	…	2	15.0	7.4	7.6
Minnesota	173	90.3	64.2	26.2	9	14.7	6.5	8.2	…	…	…	…	1	15.3	8.4	7.0
Missouri	150	74.8	51.2	23.6	10	14.8	11.7	3.0	1	58.2	16.4	41.8	2	67.2	42.6	24.6
Nebraska	97	84.7	60.7	24.0	4	33.5	24.5	9.0	…	…	…	…	…	…	…	…
North Dakota	54	86.8	56.6	30.2	2	12.6	7.1	5.5	…	…	…	…	2	22.6	14.0	8.6
South Dakota	57	86.1	57.2	28.9	1	12.8	9.0	3.8	…	…	…	…	…	…	…	…
West South Central	860	88.1	49.8	38.3	43	16.5	8.3	8.3	2	35.5	15.2	20.4	13	29.3	15.4	13.9
Arkansas	91	88.8	45.0	43.8	2	30.8	8.2	22.5	…	…	…	…	2	14.0	6.7	7.3
Louisiana	142	83.0	44.9	38.1	7	15.3	8.7	6.6	…	…	…	…	1	13.6	4.0	9.7
Oklahoma	122	84.3	50.3	34.0	7	8.7	6.2	2.5	…	…	…	…	…	…	…	…
Texas	505	90.4	52.0	38.3	27	17.6	8.9	8.7	2	35.5	15.2	20.4	10	45.7	25.3	20.5
Mountain	365	96.3	69.6	26.7	23	29.7	16.1	13.6	…	…	…	…	8	45.5	33.1	12.4
Arizona	59	96.2	74.2	21.9	4	17.1	13.9	3.2	…	…	…	…	…	…	…	…
Colorado	87	95.2	72.7	22.4	6	57.7	27.6	30.2	…	…	…	…	3	65.0	57.0	8.0
Idaho	46	102.5	63.0	39.5	2	26.3	10.1	16.2	…	…	…	…	1	146.2	69.2	76.9
Montana	57	92.1	65.6	26.5	2	24.0	9.7	14.3	…	…	…	…	…	…	…	…
Nevada	19	91.7	60.3	31.4	2	23.0	14.3	8.7	…	…	…	…	…	…	…	…
New Mexico	37	98.9	62.4	36.5	4	19.4	12.5	6.9	…	…	…	…	2	21.4	9.8	11.6
Utah	34	99.7	71.6	28.1	2	27.2	17.7	9.5	…	…	…	…	2	45.5	32.0	13.5
Wyoming	26	93.7	68.8	24.7	1	8.0	5.3	2.7	…	…	…	…	…	…	…	…
Pacific	762	104.4	76.8	27.7	59	41.5	9.2	32.3	4	71.0	36.4	34.6	15	28.9	20.7	8.2
Alaska	16	110.1	82.1	27.9	1	25.5	17.2	8.3	…	…	…	…	…	…	…	…
California	535	102.8	76.0	26.7	46	44.5	8.7	35.9	2	105.3	76.3	28.9	10	23.6	19.9	3.7
Hawaii	20	97.5	67.3	30.2	1	54.4	26.4	28.0	1	59.5	21.1	38.4	5	71.6	27.3	44.4
Oregon	81	103.1	79.0	24.1	5	13.7	9.6	4.1	…	…	…	…	…	…	…	…
Washington	110	118.7	82.3	36.3	6	36.5	12.1	24.4	1	50.0	27.3	22.7	…	…	…	…

[1] Data reflects the number of full-time equivalent (FTE) nursing personnel. The FTE is computed by adding one-half of the number of part-time nurses to the number of full-time nurses.

[2] Excludes 208 U.S. hospitals not registered with the American Hospital Association.

[3] Nurse-to-patient ratios based on the adjusted average daily census, which includes both the average number of inpatients plus an equivalent figure for outpatients.

[4] Nurse-to-patient ratios based on the average daily census, which includes only the number of inpatients receiving care each day.

[5] Detail may not add to totals due to rounding.

SOURCE: Ratios were computed by the American Nurses' Association, Research and Policy Analysis Department, Statistics Unit, based upon data from the American Hospital Association, *Hospital Statistics 1978*, pp. 20-141.

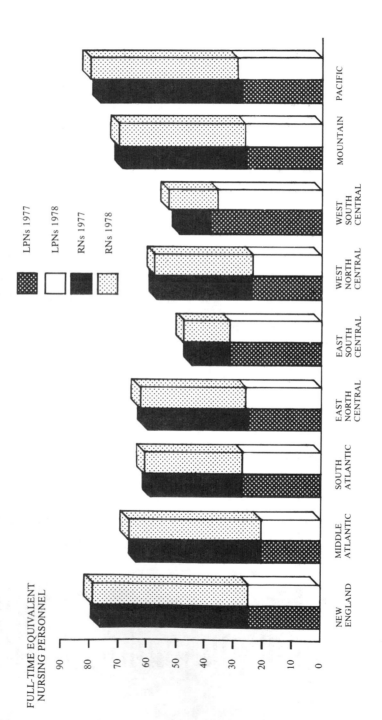

CHART 4. RATIO OF FULL-TIME EQUIVALENT NURSING PERSONNEL TO 100 ADJUSTED AVERAGE DAILY CENSUS IN SHORT-TERM GENERAL AND OTHER SPECIAL HOSPITALS, BY REGION, 1977 and 1978

FULL-TIME EQUIVALENT NURSING PERSONNEL

LPNs 1977
LPNs 1978
RNs 1977
RNs 1978

NEW ENGLAND MIDDLE ATLANTIC SOUTH ATLANTIC EAST NORTH CENTRAL EAST SOUTH CENTRAL WEST NORTH CENTRAL WEST SOUTH CENTRAL MOUNTAIN PACIFIC

SOURCE: Ratios were computed by the American Nurses' Association, Research and Policy Analysis Department, Statistics Unit, based upon data from the American Hospital Association, *Hospital Statistics 1978*, and *Hospital Statistics 1979*.

Table I-D-5. Nursing Personnel[1] Per 100 Average Daily Census[2] in Federal Hospitals,[3] 1978

Region and state	Number of hospitals	Average daily census	Full-time equivalent nursing personnel per 100 patients		
			Total[4]	Registered nurse	Licensed practical nurse
Total	370	95,585	55.8	41.7	14.1
New England	18	5,115	48.7	38.7	10.0
Connecticut	5	690	67.7	58.3	9.4
Maine	1	586	34.1	29.0	5.1
Massachusetts ...	7	3,044	40.1	31.3	8.8
New Hampshire ..	2	286	58.7	47.2	11.5
Rhode Island	2	317	83.6	67.5	16.1
Vermont	1	192	88.5	53.6	34.9
Middle Atlantic	31	15,602	41.7	32.2	9.4
New Jersey	4	2,147	40.8	33.2	7.6
New York	16	8,442	45.4	35.1	10.3
Pennsylvania	11	5,013	35.8	27.1	8.7
South Atlantic	70	18,821	59.4	43.9	15.5
Delaware	2	261	72.4	62.5	10.0
District of Columbia	4	3,639	44.8	31.7	13.2
Florida	14	3,300	61.7	46.9	14.8
Georgia	9	2,164	64.4	45.1	19.3
Maryland	10	2,369	63.5	52.0	11.5
North Carolina ...	9	2,473	50.5	38.5	12.0
South Carolina ...	7	1,112	83.6	54.1	29.5
Virginia	10	2,531	68.6	49.9	18.7
West Virginia .	5	972	53.1	39.2	13.9
East North Central	30	13,534	43.9	30.9	12.9
Illinois	10	4,892	39.1	31.3	7.8
Indiana	4	1,616	32.5	26.4	6.1
Michigan	8	1,945	51.8	32.6	19.1
Ohio	5	3,375	42.3	32.3	10.9
Wisconsin	3	1,706	60.7	29.7	31.0
East South Central	23	7,505	46.1	36.0	10.1
Alabama	8	2,101	46.1	33.8	12.3
Kentucky	5	1,479	59.6	45.1	14.5
Mississippi	5	1,499	42.4	32.9	9.5
Tennessee	5	2,426	40.1	34.3	5.8
West North Central	42	8,105	53.0	40.6	12.4
Iowa	3	1,203	43.9	32.4	11.5
Kansas	7	1,452	45.9	35.7	10.3
Minnesota	5	1,381	51.3	41.5	9.8
Missouri	7	2,255	50.3	39.2	11.0
Nebraska	5	663	74.2	57.0	17.2
North Dakota	5	286	79.0	61.9	17.1
South Dakota	10	865	62.7	42.5	20.1
West South Central	49	11,284	59.9	44.6	15.3
Arkansas	4	1,591	45.9	32.9	13.0
Louisiana	9	1,756	57.1	43.4	13.7
Oklahoma	12	835	106.6	71.1	35.4
Texas	24	7,102	58.3	44.4	13.9
Mountain	51	4,828	82.9	60.9	22.0
Arizona	16	1,313	102.6	72.0	30.5
Colorado	7	1,447	70.4	50.7	19.7
Idaho	2	116	128.4	100.9	27.6
Montana	6	241	93.8	68.5	25.3
Nevada	4	199	82.9	68.8	14.1
New Mexico	11	659	95.6	72.4	23.2
Utah	2	405	67.7	51.9	15.8
Wyoming........	3	448	42.4	34.2	8.3
Pacific	56	10,791	80.4	59.2	21.2
Alaska	9	352	122.2	91.8	30.4
California	33	7,437	79.7	61.0	18.8
Hawaii	1	429	103.5	56.6	46.9
Oregon	2	737	52.4	41.0	11.4
Washington	11	1,836	81.0	53.8	27.3

[1] Data reflects the number of full-time equivalent (FTE) nursing personnel. The FTE is computed by adding one half of the number of part-time nurses to the number of full-time nurses.

[2] Nurse-to-patient ratios based upon the average number of inpatients receiving care each day.

[3] Excludes one federal hospital not registered with the American Hospital Association.

[4] Detail may not add to totals due to rounding.

SOURCE: Ratios were computed by the American Nurses' Association, Research and Policy Analysis Department, Statistics Unit, based upon data from the American Hospital Association, *Hospital Statistics 1979*, pp. 20-141.

Table I-D-6. Registered Nurses Employed in Hospitals, by Hospital Control and Service, 1976

Hospital control and service	Total hospitals			Number of registered nurses		
	Number	Beds	Average daily census	Total	Full-time	Part-time
Total	7,271	1,381,267	1,053,317	622,287	460,954	161,333
Federal	380	126,916	102,502	38,197	36,314	1,883
Long-term	48	41,684	36,039	6,820	6,286	534
Short-term	332	85,232	66,463	31,377	30,028	1,349
Nonfederal	6,891	1,254,351	950,815	584,090	424,640	159,450
Psychiatric	477	219,590	180,959	18,779	16,820	1,959
Tuberculosis	21	3,546	2,081	468	422	46
Long-term other	216	51,061	42,798	7,460	5,951	1,509
Short-term other	6,177	980,154	724,977	557,383	401,447	155,936

SOURCE: U.S. Department of Health, Education, and Welfare, Public Health Service, Health Resources Administration, National Center for Health Statistics, Division of Health Manpower and Facilities Statistics, 1976 Master Facility Inventory. Unpublished data.

Table I-D-7. Distribution of Registered Nurses Employed in Hospitals, by State and Region, 1976

Region and state	Number of beds	Total	Registered nurses Full-time Number	Registered nurses Full-time Number per 1,000 beds	Registered nurses Part-time Number	Registered nurses Part-time Number per 1,000 beds
Total	1,381,267	622,287	460,954	333.7	161,333	116.8
New England	84,700	47,943	32,095	378.9	15,848	187.1
Connecticut	17,941	9,930	6,574	366.4	3,356	187.1
Maine	6,699	3,510	2,312	345.1	1,198	178.8
Massachusetts	44,827	26,710	18,311	408.5	8,399	187.4
New Hampshire	5,082	2,735	1,823	358.7	912	179.5
Rhode Island	7,017	3,437	2,011	286.6	1,426	203.2
Vermont	3,134	1,621	1,064	339.5	557	177.7
Middle Atlantic	272,174	127,554	98,218	360.9	29,336	107.8
New Jersey	45,041	22,332	16,072	356.8	6,260	139.0
New York	137,488	64,235	51,645	375.6	12,590	91.6
Pennsylvania	89,645	40,987	30,501	340.2	10,486	117.0
South Atlantic	225,406	87,659	70,564	313.1	17,095	75.8
Delaware	4,073	1,764	1,253	307.6	511	125.5
District of Columbia	10,541	4,383	3,758	356.5	625	59.3
Florida	54,798	22,572	18,873	344.4	3,699	67.5
Georgia	32,391	11,822	9,724	300.2	2,098	64.8
Maryland	25,322	11,717	8,555	337.8	3,162	124.9
North Carolina	32,438	12,196	10,284	317.0	1,912	58.9
South Carolina	17,405	5,581	4,441	255.2	1,140	65.5
Virginia	32,409	12,690	9,750	300.8	2,940	90.7
West Virginia	16,029	4,934	3,926	244.9	1,008	62.9
East North Central ...	250,480	121,822	83,751	334.4	38,071	152.0
Illinois	71,776	36,407	26,426	368.2	9,981	139.1
Indiana	32,610	13,661	9,685	297.0	3,976	121.9
Michigan	50,581	25,036	17,228	340.6	7,808	154.4
Ohio	65,432	32,472	21,811	333.3	10,661	162.9
Wisconsin	30,081	14,246	8,601	285.9	5,645	187.7
East South Central ...	93,017	29,643	24,495	263.3	5,148	55.3
Alabama	23,482	7,971	6,709	285.7	1,262	53.7
Kentucky	19,473	7,762	6,166	316.6	1,596	82.0
Mississippi	17,660	4,435	3,631	205.6	804	45.5
Tennessee	32,402	9,475	7,989	246.6	1,486	45.9
West North Central....	125,125	55,763	36,996	295.7	18,767	150.0
Iowa	19,892	9,765	6,279	315.7	3,486	175.2
Kansas	17,003	6,898	4,728	278.1	2,170	127.6
Minnesota	29,468	15,336	8,883	301.4	6,453	219.0
Missouri	35,869	13,800	10,461	291.6	3,339	93.1
Nebraska	11,539	5,501	3,643	315.7	1,858	161.0
North Dakota	5,470	2,282	1,514	276.8	768	140.4
South Dakota	5,884	2,181	1,488	252.9	693	117.8
West South Central....	132,619	43,880	35,872	270.5	8,008	60.4
Arkansas	13,625	4,088	3,399	249.5	689	50.6
Louisiana	25,128	7,521	6,168	245.5	1,353	53.8
Oklahoma	17,005	5,543	4,257	250.3	1,286	75.6
Texas	76,861	26,728	22,048	286.9	4,680	60.9
Mountain	52,698	27,152	19,843	376.5	7,309	138.7
Arizona	11,198	6,471	5,155	460.4	1,316	117.5
Colorado	15,123	8,865	6,543	432.7	2,322	153.5
Idaho	3,610	1,802	1,207	334.3	595	164.8
Montana	5,426	2,156	1,335	246.0	821	151.3
Nevada	3,358	1,392	1,162	346.0	230	68.5
New Mexico	6,239	2,510	1,932	309.7	578	92.6
Utah	5,105	2,947	1,826	357.7	1,121	219.6
Wyoming	2,639	1,009	683	258.8	326	123.5
Pacific	145,048	80,871	59,120	407.6	21,751	150.0
Alaska	1,629	909	715	438.9	194	119.1
California	111,176	60,653	45,382	408.2	15,271	137.4
Hawaii	3,877	2,029	1,704	439.5	325	83.8
Oregon	12,076	6,796	4,194	347.3	2,602	215.5
Washington	16,290	10,484	7,125	437.4	3,359	206.2

SOURCE: U.S. Department of Health and Human Services, Public Health Service, Health Resources Administration, National Center for Health Statistics, Division of Health Manpower and Facilities Statistics, 1976 Master Facility Inventory. Unpublished data.

Table I-D-8. Number of Registered Nurses Employed in Mental Health Facilities, January 1976

	Number of facilities		Number of registered nurses employed			
Type of facility	Total	Reporting	Total	Full-time	Part-time	Trainee
Total	3,791	3,231	45,163	35,147	6,013	4,003
Psychiatric hospital	487	464	20,280	16,780	1,959	1,541
State and county mental hospitals	304	297	16,022	14,020	907	1,095
Private mental hospitals	183	167	4,258	2,760	1,052	446
VA psychiatric services	198	189	5,726	4,992	438	296
Neuropsychiatric hospitals	24	24	3,124	2,777	330	17
General hospital inpatient psychiatric unit	89	85	2,422	2,066	84	272
General hospital outpatient psychiatric unit	85	80	180	149	24	7
Non-federal general hospital psychiatric service	1,094	849	11,403	8,062	2,279	1,062
Inpatient psychiatric service	791	612	10,940	7,737	2,200	1,003
Outpatient psychiatric service	303	237	463	325	79	59
Residential treatment center for emotionally disturbed children	331	278	399	248	118	33
Freestanding outpatient clinics	1,076	904	1,097	717	254	126
Community mental health centers	528	486	5,761	3,973	923	865
Other	77	61	497	375	42	80
Freestanding day/night facilities	38	29	24	12	8	4
Other multi-service facilities	39	32	473	363	34	76

SOURCE: U.S. Department of Health, Education, and Welfare, Public Health Service, Alcohol, Drug Abuse, and Mental Health Administration, *Staffing of Mental Health Facilities, United States, 1976*, National Institute of Mental Health, Series B, No. 14, DHEW Publication No. (ADM) 78-522, p. 2 and p. 45.

Table I-D-9. Estimated Number and Percent of Registered Nurses Employed in Nursing Homes, by Selected Employee Characteristics, 1977

Employee characteristics[1]	Registered nurse					
	Total		Full-time		Part-time	
	Number	Percent	Number	Percent	Number	Percent
Total	84,500	100.0	43,800	100.0	40,700	100.0
Racial/ethnic background						
White (not Hispanic) ...	77,800	92.1	39,400	90.0	38,400	94.3
Black (not Hispanic)	3,500	4.1	2,200	5.0	1,300	3.2
Hispanic	(2)	(2)	(2)	(2)	(2)	(2)
Other	2,700	3.2	1,900	4.3	800	2.0
Sex						
Male	1,000	1.2	1,000	2.3	(2)	(2)
Female	83,100	98.3	42,900	97.9	40,200	98.8
Age group						
Under 35 years of age	23,900	28.3	12,900	29.5	11,000	27.0
35-44	21,400	25.3	8,900	20.3	12,500	30.7
45-54	21,200	25.1	12,100	27.6	9,100	22.4
55 years and over	18,000	21.3	9,900	22.6	8,100	19.9
Years of education						
Less than 12 years	(2)	(2)	(2)	(2)	(2)	(2)
12	1,800	2.1	900	2.1	900	2.2
13-14	10,300	12.2	6,100	13.9	4,200	10.3
15-16	63,700	75.4	31,800	72.6	31,900	78.4
17 years or more	8,600	10.2	5,000	11.4	3,600	8.8
Years of current employment						
Less than 2 years	39,100	46.3	20,100	45.9	19,000	46.7
2-4	24,600	29.1	12,100	27.6	12,500	30.7
5-9	14,200	16.8	7,200	16.4	7,000	17.2
10-14	4,400	5.2	3,000	6.8	1,400	3.4
15 years or more	2,300	2.7	1,500	3.4	800	2.0
Years of total experience						
Less than 5 years	28,100	33.3	15,000	34.2	13,100	32.2
5-9	20,500	24.3	9,300	21.2	11,200	27.5
10-14	12,500	14.8	6,100	13.9	6,400	15.7
15 years or more	23,400	27.7	13,400	30.6	10,000	24.6

[1]Detail in each employee characteristic may not add to total due to rounding.
[2]Figure does not meet standards of reliability or precision (more than 30 percent relative standard error).

SOURCE: U.S. Department of Health, Education, and Welfare, Public Health Service, Office of Health Research, Statistics, and Technology, National Center for Health Statistics, *The National Nursing Home Survey: 1977 Summary for the United States*, Vital and Health Statistics, Series 13, No. 43, DHEW Publication No. (PHS) 79-1794, 1979, p. 20.

Table I-D-10. Estimated Number and Percent of Registered Nurses Employed in Nursing Homes, by Selected Nursing Home Characteristics, 1977

| Nursing home characteristics[1] | Registered nurse | | | | | |
| | Total | | Full-time | | Part-time | |
	Number	Percent	Number	Percent	Number	Percent
Total	84,500	100.0	43,800	100.0	40,700	100.0
Ownership						
Proprietary	52,400	62.0	25,100	57.3	27,300	67.1
Voluntary nonprofit	23,200	27.5	12,300	28.1	10,900	26.8
Government	8,900	10.5	6,400	14.6	2,500	6.1
Certification						
Skilled nursing facility ...	26,200	31.0	13,300	30.4	12,900	31.7
Skilled nursing facility and intermediate care facility	40,000	47.3	20,800	47.5	19,200	47.2
Intermediate care facility	12,300	14.6	6,700	15.3	5,600	13.8
Not certified	6,000	7.1	3,100	7.1	2,900	7.1
Bed size						
Less than 50 beds	11,400	13.5	4,600	10.5	6,800	16.7
50-99	25,800	30.5	12,000	27.4	13,800	33.9
100-199	31,600	37.4	17,000	38.8	14,600	35.9
200 beds or more	15,600	18.5	10,200	23.3	5,400	13.3
Location						
Region						
Northeast	31,900	37.8	14,800	33.8	17,100	42.0
North Central	25,400	30.1	12,800	29.2	12,600	31.0
South	13,500	16.0	8,800	20.1	4,700	11.5
West	13,700	16.2	7,400	16.9	6,300	15.5
Standard federal administrative region						
Region I	10,200	12.1	3,400	7.8	6,800	16.7
Region II	13,300	15.7	7,400	16.9	5,900	14.5
Region III	11,000	13.0	5,500	12.6	5,500	13.5
Region IV	8,100	9.6	5,300	12.1	2,800	6.9
Region V	20,300	24.0	10,000	22.8	10,300	25.3
Region VI	2,900	3.4	2,100	4.8	800	2.0
Region VII	4,000	4.7	2,300	5.3	1,700	4.2
Region VIII	3,800	4.5	1,900	4.3	1,900	4.7
Region IX	8,200	9.7	4,500	10.3	3,700	9.1
Region X	2,700	3.2	1,400	3.2	1,300	3.2
Type of facility						
Nursing care	77,500	91.7	40,700	92.9	36,800	90.4
Other	7,000	8.3	3,100	7.1	3,900	9.6

[1]Detail in each nursing home characteristic may not add to total due to rounding.

SOURCE: U.S. Department of Health, Education, and Welfare, Public Health Service, Office of Health Research, Statistics, and Technology, National Center for Health Statistics, *The National Nursing Home Survey: 1977 Summary for the United States*, Vital and Health Statistics, Series 13, No. 43, DHEW Publication No. (PHS) 79-1794, 1979, p. 17.

Table I-D-11. Distribution of Registered Nurses Employed in Nursing and Personal Care Homes, by State, 1976

Region and state	Number of beds	Registered nurses				
		Total	Full-time		Part-time	
			Number	Number per 1,000 beds	Number	Number per 1,000 beds
Total	1,414,865	80,195	45,817	32.4	34,378	24.3
New England	103,371	9,673	4,448	43.0	5,225	50.5
Connecticut	24,573	3,018	1,283	52.2	1,735	70.6
Maine	9,020	558	337	37.4	221	24.5
Massachusetts	50,940	4,388	1,879	36.9	2,509	49.3
New Hampshire	6,378	753	431	67.6	322	50.5
Rhode Island	7,330	616	318	43.4	298	40.7
Vermont	5,130	340	200	39.0	140	27.3
Middle Atlantic	200,390	18,097	10,801	53.9	7,296	36.4
New Jersey	33,976	3,548	1,963	57.8	1,585	46.7
New York	104,523	8,789	5,543	53.0	3,246	31.1
Pennsylvania	61,891	5,760	3,295	53.2	2,465	39.8
South Atlantic	151,142	7,799	5,060	33.5	2,739	18.1
Delaware	2,228	205	92	41.3	113	50.7
District of Columbia	2,873	145	109	37.9	36	12.5
Florida	33,097	2,001	1,395	42.1	606	18.3
Georgia	29,455	1,119	765	26.0	354	12.0
Maryland	19,154	1,222	705	36.8	517	27.0
North Carolina	24,614	1,103	729	29.6	374	15.2
South Carolina	8,701	492	333	38.3	159	18.3
Virginia	25,435	1,194	741	29.1	453	17.8
West Virginia	5,585	318	191	34.2	127	22.7
East North Central ...	310,152	17,622	9,452	30.5	8,170	26.3
Illinois	88,311	4,823	2,850	32.3	1,973	22.3
Indiana	37,611	1,768	1,063	28.3	705	18.7
Michigan	66,750	3,457	1,819	27.3	1,638	24.5
Ohio	64,903	4,144	2,281	35.1	1,863	28.7
Wisconsin	52,577	3,430	1,439	27.4	1,991	37.9
East South Central ...	69,554	2,224	1,485	21.4	739	10.6
Alabama	19,489	605	400	20.5	205	10.5
Kentucky	20,950	632	387	18.5	245	11.7
Mississippi	9,023	421	307	34.0	114	12.6
Tennessee	20,092	566	391	19.5	175	8.7
West North Central....	172,464	7,682	3,887	22.5	3,795	22.0
Iowa	33,874	1,483	836	24.7	647	19.1
Kansas	23,195	831	462	19.9	369	15.9
Minnesota	43,036	2,615	1,138	26.4	1,477	34.3
Missouri	33,746	1,009	631	18.7	378	11.2
Nebraska	23,349	905	433	18.5	472	20.2
North Dakota	6,878	380	170	24.7	210	30.5
South Dakota	8,386	459	217	25.9	242	28.9
West South Central....	167,727	3,477	2,284	13.6	1,193	7.1
Arkansas	19,803	464	367	18.5	97	4.9
Louisiana	19,135	497	356	18.6	141	7.4
Oklahoma	26,650	566	360	13.5	206	7.7
Texas	102,139	1,950	1,201	11.8	749	7.3
Mountain	50,343	3,529	2,116	42.0	1,413	28.1
Arizona	5,914	602	435	73.6	167	28.2
Colorado	22,731	1,549	834	36.7	715	31.5
Idaho	4,823	322	193	40.0	129	26.7
Montana	5,335	432	230	43.1	202	37.9
Nevada	1,638	159	116	70.8	43	26.3
New Mexico	3,366	128	98	29.1	30	8.9
Utah	4,613	233	139	30.1	94	20.4
Wyoming	1,923	104	71	36.9	33	17.2
Pacific	189,722	10,092	6,284	33.1	3,808	20.1
Alaska	782	103	75	95.9	28	35.8
California	138,219	6,693	4,145	30.0	2,548	18.4
Hawaii	3,188	345	260	81.6	85	26.7
Oregon	17,189	932	573	33.3	359	20.9
Washington	30,344	2,019	1,231	40.6	788	26.0

SOURCE: U.S. Department of Health and Human Services, Public Health Service, Health Resources Administration, National Center for Health Statistics, Division of Health Manpower and Facilities Statistics, 1976 Master Facility Inventory. Unpublished data.

Chapter I, Section E
REGISTERED NURSES EMPLOYED BY
COMMUNITY HEALTH AGENCIES

The Division of Nursing of the Public Health Service periodically collects data on nurses employed in public health agencies. As of January 1, 1974, there were 61,036 registered nurses working in 11,516 national, university, state and local (including boards of education) community health agencies, as printed in *Facts About Nursing 76-77*.

The Annual Inventory of Community Mental Health Centers conducted by the Division of Biometry and Epidemiology, National Institute of Mental Health contains information on registered nurses in federally funded agencies. The 1977 survey data estimated 6,117 registered nurses were working in these facilities, representing a 6.2 percent increase from the previous year. Of the total nurses employed, 69.0 percent were full-time staff; 16.6 percent, part-time; 12.8 percent, trainees; and 1.6 percent, volunteers. The total nurse count in 1977 was translated into a full-time equivalency of 4,898 nurses. The number of FTE nurses per community mental health center averaged 8.9 that year. The aggregate number of registered nurse positions in community mental health centers varied by the number of years the center had been in operation. The general trend is toward increased numbers of nursing positions in the older facilities.

The volunteer nurse enrollments in the American Red Cross chapters and the number of nurses providing direct services in chapter activities decreased between fiscal years 1978 and 1979, 14.0 percent and 4.4 percent, respectively. In fiscal year 1979, the American Red Cross served in 14 major national disaster operations. A total of 1,369 nurse assignments were made, totaling 5,182 days of service. In fiscal 1978, there were 2,307 nurses functioning in staff positions for the Red Cross Blood Program, up 6.4 percent from the previous year. Additionally, 42,033 nurse volunteers participated in blood service programs in fiscal 1978.

Table I-E-1. Registered Nurse Positions in Federally Funded Community Mental Health Centers, by Employment Status and Number of Years Facility has been in Operation, February 1977

Number of years in operation	Total	Employment status			
		Full-time	Part-time	Trainee	Volunteer
Total	195,903	166,514	19,741	8,836	812
1-2 years ...	26,227	21,845	3,243	1,093	46
3-5	58,487	49,439	5,684	3,064	300
6-7	47,322	40,726	4,804	1,513	279
8 years or more	63,867	54,504	6,010	3,166	187

SOURCE: U.S. Department of Health, Education, and Welfare, Public Health Service, National Institute of Mental Health, Division of Biometry and Epidemiology, Survey and Reports Branch, *Provisional Data on Federally Funded Community Mental Health Centers, 1976-77*, May 1978, pp. 12-14.

Table I-E-2. Registered Nurses in Federally Funded Community Mental Health Centers, 1973-1977

Year	Registered nurse		
	Total	Full-time equivalent	Average FTE per CMHC
1977	6,117	4,898	8.9
1976	5,761	4,588	8.7
1975	4,764	3,682	8.9
1974	4,148	3,459	8.7
1973	3,532	2,791	8.5

SOURCE: U.S. Department of Health, Education, and Welfare, Public Health Service, National Institute of Mental Health, Division of Biometry and Epidemiology, Survey and Reports Branch, *Provisional Data on Federally Funded Community Mental Health Centers, 1976-77*, May 1978, p. 30.

Table I-E-3. Percentage Distribution of Registered Nurses by Employment Status in Federally Funded Community Mental Health Centers, 1973-1977

Year	Total	Employment status			
		Full-time	Part-time	Trainee	Volunteer
1977	100.0	69.0	16.6	12.8	1.6
1976	100.0	69.0	14.5	15.0	1.5
1975	100.0	71.5	18.3	8.9	1.3
1974	100.0	71.9	17.0	9.4	1.7
1973	100.0	67.7	17.1	14.2	1.0

SOURCE: U.S. Department of Health, Education, and Welfare, Public Health Service, National Institute of Mental Health, Division of Biometry and Epidemiology, Survey and Reports Branch, *Provisional Data on Federally Funded Community Mental Health Centers, 1976-77*, May 1978, p. 29.

Table I-E-4. Nurse Enrollment in American Red Cross Chapters, Nurses Providing Direct Service in Chapter Activities, and Paid Nursing Staff, 1977-78 and 1978-79

Item	1978-79	1977-78
Volunteer staff		
Nurses enrolled during the year	5,594	6,502
Nurses providing direct services in chapter activities		
Registered nurses	58,698	61,404
Licensed practical nurses	11,136	12,308
Nursing students	12,451	11,217
Paid staff		
National headquarters nurses	7	7
Registered nurses on staff in Red Cross chapters	137	...
Licensed practical nurses on staff in Red Cross chapters	2	...
Number of people served through chapter activities	9,286,451	10,018,368

SOURCE: American Red Cross, 1980.

Table I-E-5. Disaster Health Services, American Red Cross, 1977-78 and 1978-79

Item	1978-79	1977-78
Major disaster operations during which Red Cross nurses served	[1]14	[1]13
Nursing assignments on operations	1,369	1,109
Days served by nurses assigned	5,182	3,441
Persons attending Red Cross disaster nursing courses	12,996	13,609

[1] Represents national assignments only.
SOURCE: American Red Cross, 1980.

Table I-E-6. Blood Service Nursing, American Red Cross, 1977-78 and 1978-79

Item	1978-79	1977-78
National headquarter's nurses—administrative, educational, supervisory	(1)	5
Registered nurses on staff in blood centers	(1)	2,307
Licensed practical nurses on staff in blood centers	(1)	160
Volunteers participating in blood services		
Registered nurses	46,605	42,033
Licensed practical nurses	10,015	8,537
Nursing students	7,288	6,226

[1] Information not available.
SOURCE: American Red Cross, 1980.

Chapter I, Section F
NURSE FACULTY MEMBERS

Survey results from the National League for Nursing biennial study showed there were 33,633 nurse faculty members employed in all nursing educational programs as of January 1978. Excluded from this count are 2,343 program administrators. Data were collected by mail questionnaires sent to all state-approved schools of nursing in the country. About 91 percent of the 2,730 nursing programs surveyed responded. Estimates of the total employed nurse faculty were derived for nonresponding programs by assessing that the average number of faculty members in the nonresponding programs was the same as in responding programs.

The relative proportion of nurse faculty members employed in RN programs has been steadily increasing over the past decade. These programs accounted for about 78 percent of the total nurse faculty in 1968 and for about 81 percent in 1978. Among the 27,333 nurses employed in RN programs in 1978, 24.8 percent were in diploma programs; 29.5 percent were in associate degree programs; and 45.7 percent, in basic and graduate baccalaureate and higher degree programs. Approximately 18.1 percent of the nurse faculty in both initial and graduate programs preparing registered nurses work on a part-time basis. The associate degree programs continued to have a larger proportion of part-time faculty than either the diploma or baccalaureate and higher degree programs. Practical nursing educational programs were the locus of the employment for about 19 percent of the nurse faculty. Twenty percent of the 6,300 nurse faculty in programs preparing for practical nurse licensure were part-timers.

In the 1978 nurse faculty census, NLN estimated there were 1,008 budgeted unfilled positions in nursing educational programs as of January, 909 in programs preparing registered nurses, and 99 in programs preparing licensed practical nurses. Since the total nurse faculty in these programs includes both full-time and part-time employees, the data presented on the number of budgeted positions (both filled and unfilled) reflect full-time equivalent positions. Each part-time position was counted as one-half of a full-time position in order to make comparison of needs for nurse faculty. With respect to the total budgeted positions in schools of nursing, there was a 5.6 percent increase between January 1976 and January 1978. In 1976, there were 29,871 full-time equivalent positions available, as contrasted to 31,534 in 1978. Budgeted vacancies amounted to 925 in 1976 and 1,008 in 1978. While the number of unfilled positions has increased, their relative proportion in relation to the total budgeted positions in 1976 and 1978 has remained fairly constant (3.1 percent and 3.2 percent, respectively). There were no exaggerated shifts from previous trends when the various programs were viewed separately. Associate degree and practical nursing programs continued a general decline in the percentage of vacant positions from 1976 to 1978. Baccalaureate programs, after having a marked decrease in vacant positions from 1974 to 1976, appeared to change direction in 1978. There was no change in the proportion of vacant positions in diploma programs over the biennium.

Looking at the data on the highest earned credentials of full-time nurse faculty members (exclusive of administrators) in programs preparing registered nurses, it could be observed that more than two-thirds (67.8 percent) held at least a master's degree. Slightly over 5 percent of the full-time faculty members had doctorates. These data reflected an increase of almost 9 percent in the number of full-time nurse faculty holding a master's or doctoral degree and a 20 percent gain in the number of nurse faculty with earned doctorates over the interval 1976 to 1978. In 1978, 91.7 percent of the full-time nurse faculty in baccalaureate and higher degree programs, 64.8 percent in associate degree programs, and 32.6 percent in diploma programs held at least a master's degree. Similar statistics on full-time nurse faculty in LPN programs showed 16.9 percent to hold graduate degrees. Examination on the basis of NLN accreditation of the program indicated higher percentages of the full-time nurse faculty in the accredited programs had earned master's or doctoral degrees than in nonaccredited programs, regardless of the type of program. Relatively smaller proportions of the part-time nurse faculty held advanced degrees. Overall, 47.2 percent of those in RN programs and 12.9 percent in the LPN programs had earned at least a master's degree.

Registered nurses holding administrative positions in nursing educational programs in 1978 numbered 2,343. The preponderance (97.3 percent) of the administrators in RN programs held at least a master's degree. In contrast, less than half (44.8 percent) of the administrators in practical nursing programs held master's degrees. While the baccalaureate programs had the largest proportion of administrators with at least a master's degree (99.4 percent), their counterparts in associate degree and diploma programs did not lag far behind in graduate preparation. Almost 95 percent of those in diploma programs and 97.6 percent in associate degree programs held at least a master's degree. The gap among the various nursing programs in terms of the educational preparation of the nurse administrator widened markedly when earned doctorates were taken into consideration, however. Here almost 70 percent of the administrators in baccalaureate and higher degree programs had a doctorate, while only 2.4 percent of those in diploma programs and 8.5 percent in associate degree programs held a doctoral degree.

Data collected by the Association of Schools of Public Health reported 21 nurses on the faculty of the public health nursing programs in schools of public health. There have been decreases each year since 1974-75 in the number of nurse faculty in public health nursing programs. These data excluded nurse faculty in other public health programs, such as epidemiology or maternal-child health.

Table I-F-1. Estimated Total Number of Nurse Faculty Members in Nursing Educational Programs,[1] Janaury 1976 and 1978

			Nurse faculty members			
	Total		Full-time		Part-time	
Type of program	1976	1978	1976	1978	1976	1978
Total programs ...	31,648	33,633	26,242	27,419	5,406	6,214
Nursing programs-RN	25,445	27,333	21,197	22,395	4,248	4,938
Diploma	7,407	6,769	6,448	5,800	959	969
Associate degree	7,288	8,065	5,831	6,335	1,457	1,730
Baccalaureate and higher degree	10,750	12,499	8,918	10,260	1,832	2,239
Practical nursing programs...	6,203	6,300	5,045	5,024	1,158	1,276

[1] Excludes administrators employed by various programs.

SOURCE: National League for Nursing, *NLN Nursing Data Book*, 1978, p. 57, and unpublished data, 1979.

Table I-F-2. Estimated Number of Full-time Nurse Faculty Positions¹ in Nursing Educational Programs, January 1978

Type of program	Estimated total budgeted positions²		Estimated total filled positions²		Estimated budgeted unfilled positions	
	Number	Percent	Number	Percent	Number	Percent
Total programs	31,534	100.0	30,526	96.8	1,008	3.2
Nursing programs-RN	25,773	100.0	24,864	96.5	909	3.5
Diploma	6,432	100.0	6,285	97.7	147	2.3
Associate degree	7,407	100.0	7,200	97.2	207	2.8
Baccalaureate and higher degree	11,934	100.0	11,379	95.3	555	4.7
Practical nursing programs	5,761	100.0	5,662	98.3	99	1.7

¹Excludes administrators employed by the various programs.
²Includes full-time equivalency of part-time faculty.
SOURCE: National League for Nursing, *NLN Nursing Data Book*, 1978, p. 57, and unpublished data, 1979.

Table I-F-3. Highest Earned Credential of Administrators in Nursing Educational Programs, January 1978¹

Type of program	Total		Highest earned credential									
			Diploma		Associate degree		Baccalaureate		Master's degree		Doctorate	
	Number	Percent²	Number	Percent	Number	Percent	Number	Percent	Number	Percent	Number	Percent
Total programs	2,343	100.0	149	6.4	24	1.0	454	19.4	1,398	59.7	318	13.6
Nursing programs-RN	1,270	100.0	...	...	...	...	34	2.7	939	73.9	297	23.4
Diploma	337	100.0	...	...	...	...	18	5.3	311	92.3	8	2.4
Associate degree	590	100.0	...	...	...	...	14	2.4	526	89.1	50	8.5
Baccalaureate and higher degree	343	100.0	...	...	...	...	2	0.6	102	29.7	239	69.7
Practical nursing programs	1,073	100.0	149	13.9	24	2.2	420	39.1	459	42.8	21	2.0

¹Replies were received from 2,480 of the 2,730 nursing programs surveyed; nurses included are those for whom information on highest earned credential was reported.
²Percentages may not add to 100.0 due to rounding.
SOURCE: National League for Nursing, *NLN Nursing Data Book*, 1978, p. 64, and unpublished data, 1979.

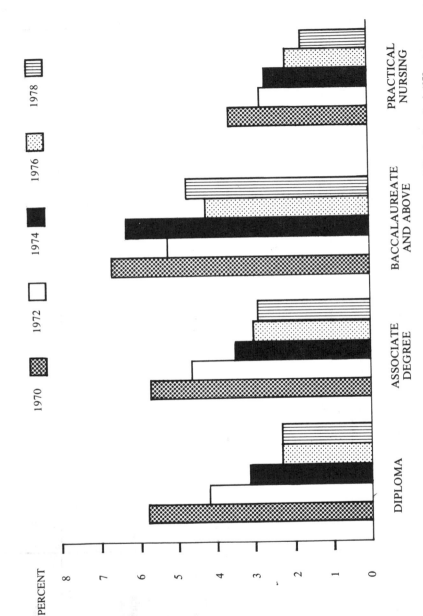

CHART 5. PERCENT OF VACANT POSITIONS FOR R.N.
FACULTY IN NURSING EDUCATIONAL PROGRAMS, 1970-1978

SOURCE: National League for Nursing, *Nurse-Faculty Census, 1970 to 1976*, NLN *Nursing Data Book*, 1978.
Prepared by American Nurses' Association, Research and Policy Analysis Department, Statistics Unit, 1980.

Table I-F-4. Highest Earned Credential of Full-time Nurse Faculty Members in Nursing Educational Programs, January 1978[1]

| Type of program | Total | | Highest earned credential | | | | | | | | | |
| | | | Diploma | | Associate degree | | Baccalaureate | | Master's degree | | Doctorate | |
	Number	Percent[2]	Number	Percent	Number	Percent	Number	Percent	Number	Percent	Number	Percent
Total programs	24,741	100.0	1,916	7.7	320	1.3	8,040	32.5	13,401	54.2	1,064	4.3
Nursing programs-RN	20,217	100.0	570	2.8	83	0.4	5,865	29.0	12,637	62.5	1,062	5.3
Diploma	5,484	100.0	456	8.3	23	0.4	3,221	58.7	1,770	32.3	14	0.3
Associate degree	5,939	100.0	105	1.8	56	0.9	1,927	32.5	3,795	63.9	56	0.9
Baccalaureate and higher degree	8,794	100.0	9	0.1	4	(3)	717	8.2	7,072	80.4	992	11.3
Practical nursing programs	4,524	100.0	1,346	29.8	237	5.2	2,175	48.1	764	16.9	2	(3)

[1] Replies were received from 2,480 of the 2,730 nursing programs surveyed; nurses included are those for whom information on highest earned credential was reported.
[2] Percentages may not add to 100.0 due to rounding.
[3] Less than 0.1 percent.
SOURCE: National League for Nursing, NLN Nursing Data Book, 1978, p. 58, and unpublished data, 1979.

Table I-F-5. Highest Earned Credential of Part-time Nurse Faculty Members in Nursing Educational Programs, January 1978[1]

| Type of program | Total | | Highest earned credential | | | | | | | | | |
| | | | Diploma | | Associate degree | | Baccalaureate | | Master's degree | | Doctorate | |
	Number	Percent	Number	Percent	Number	Percent	Number	Percent	Number	Percent	Number	Percent
Total programs	5,606	100.0	657	11.7	112	2.0	2,583	46.1	2,120	37.8	134	2.4
Nursing programs-RN	4,457	100.0	259	5.8	49	1.1	2,043	45.9	1,975	44.3	131	2.9
Diploma	916	100.0	153	16.7	6	0.7	532	58.1	211	23.0	14	1.5
Associate degree	1,622	100.0	96	5.9	43	2.6	989	61.0	486	30.0	8	0.5
Baccalaureate and higher degree	1,919	100.0	10	0.5	...	...	522	27.2	1,278	66.6	109	5.7
Practical nursing programs	1,149	100.0	398	34.6	63	5.5	540	47.0	145	12.6	3	0.3

[1] Replies were received from 2,480 of the 2,730 nursing programs surveyed; nurses included are those for whom information on highest earned credential was reported.
SOURCE: National League for Nursing, NLN Nursing Data Book, 1978, p. 62, and unpublished data, 1979.

Table I-F-6. Percentage Distribution of Full-time Nurse Faculty Members in Programs of Nursing Education-RN, by Highest Earned Credential and NLN Accreditation, January 1978[1]

Type of program	Total		Highest earned credential				
	Number	Percent	Diploma Percent	Associate degree Percent	Baccalaureate Percent	Master's degree Percent	Doctorate Percent
Total RN programs							
Accredited	16,483	100.0	2.7	0.3	27.9	63.2	5.9
Nonaccredited	3,734	100.0	3.4	1.1	34.1	59.3	2.1
Diploma							
Accredited	5,177	100.0	8.0	0.3	58.5	32.9	0.3
Nonaccredited...	307	100.0	13.4	2.9	62.5	21.2	...
Associate degree							
Accredited	3,464	100.0	0.7	0.8	29.3	68.2	1.0
Nonaccredited...	2,475	100.0	3.3	1.1	36.8	58.0	0.8
Baccalaureate and higher degree							
Accredited	7,842	100.0	...	...	7.0	81.1	11.9
Nonaccredited...	952	100.0	0.5	0.4	17.9	75.1	6.1

[1]Replies were received from 1,340 of the 1,464 programs surveyed; nurses included are those for whom information on highest earned credential was reported.

SOURCE: National League for Nursing, NLN Nursing Data Book, 1978, p. 59.

Table I-F-7. Faculty in Schools of Public Health and Public Health Nursing Programs, 1974-75 to 1978-79

		Schools of public health	
		Public health nursing programs	
		Nurse faculty	
Year	Total faculty	Number	Percent
1978-79	1,763	21	1.2
1977-78	1,751	26	1.5
1976-77	1,752	35	2.0
1975-76	2,268	65	2.9
1974-75	2,066	74	3.6

SOURCE: Association of Schools of Public Health. Unpublished data, 1980.

Chapter I, Section G
FEDERAL GOVERNMENT SERVICES

The military nurse corps employed 10,333 registered nurses in 1979, an increase of 4.2 percent in the total number serving in the Army, the Navy, and the Air Force from the previous year. The 1979 figure reflects the largest number of registered nurses in the nurse corps since 1975. In 1979, there were 3,876 nurses in the army, 2,600 nurses in the Navy, and 3,857 nurses in the Air Force, accounting for a 8.7 percent, a 1.6 percent, and 1.8 percent change respectively since 1978. While each of the three branches of the corps in 1979 exhibited growth over 1978, the Army Nurse Corps increased the greatest in both size and percent.

The U.S. Office of Personnel Management reported 34,438 registered nurses were employed full-time by selected federal government departments and agencies in 1978, an increase of 4.6 percent over 1977. The largest numerical increases in registered nurses were observed in the Veterans Administration and in the Department of Health, Education, and Welfare (Department of Health and Human Services as of May 1980), up 1,261 and 463 nurses, respectively. The largest proportionate gains in the employment of full-time civilian registered nurses were in the Department of Justice and the Department of Health, Education, and Welfare.

Registered nurse volunteers in the Peace Corps totaled 153 in 1976 and 137 in 1977, representing a 10.5 percent decline. The 1977 percentage distribution of Peace Corps nurses by geographic area is as follows: 70.1 percent in Latin American countries; 15.3 percent in Africa; and the remaining 14.6 percent in North Africa, the Near East, Asia, and the Pacific countries.

Table I-G-1. Registered Nurses Serving in the Military Nurse Corps, as of June 30, 1959-1979

Year	Army	Navy	Air Force
1979	3,876	2,600	3,857
1978	3,567	2,560	3,788
1977	3,646	2,560	3,732
1976	3,535	2,550	3,771
1975	3,706	2,560	4,060
1974	3,731	2,624	3,750
1973	3,769	2,436	3,785
1972	4,173	2,336	3,817
1971	4,752	2,231	3,811
1970	4,825	2,242	3,818
1969	4,829	2,382	3,961
1968	4,734	2,374	3,928
1967	4,545	2,322	4,102
1966	3,704	2,038	3,757
1965	3,121	1,874	3,488
1964	2,969	1,968	3,412
1963	2,981	2,038	3,409
1962	3,402	2,145	3,438
1961	3,283	2,200	3,113
1960	3,310	2,198	2,977
1959	3,364	2,168	2,880

SOURCE: Army Nurse Corps, Office of the Surgeon General; Air Force Nurse Corps, Office of the Surgeon General; Navy Nurse Corps, Bureau of Medicine and Surgery, 1980 and previous years. Unpublished data.

Table I-G-2. Full-time Civilian Registered Nurses Employed by Selected Federal Government Departments and Agencies, as of October 31, 1976-1978[1]

Department or agency	1976	1977	1978
Total	31,850	32,918	34,438
Executive Department	6,944	6,896	7,376
Department of Agriculture	19	19	18
Department of Commerce	22	23	21
Department of Defense	3,636	3,701	3,714
Department of the Air Force	861	858	775
Department of the Army	1,948	2,003	2,040
Department of the Navy	809	826	868
Defense Supply Agency[2]	10	6	7
Other Defense Activities	8	8	24
Department of Energy	(3)	7	7
Department of Health, Education, and Welfare	3,049	2,912	3,375
Department of the Interior	16	17	16
Department of Justice	54	59	69
Department of Labor	2	3	3
Department of State	44	48	47
Agency of International Development	...	...	...
Other Department of State	44	48	47
Department of Transportation	61	63	60
Department of the Treasury	41	44	46
Legislative Branch	22	22	26
Architect of the Capitol	15	16	16
Government Printing Office	2	2	7
Library of Congress	5	4	3
Independent Agencies	24,884	26,000	27,036
Action	4	14	12
Canal Zone Government	205	112	105
Civil Service Commission	4	1	3
Energy Research and Development Administration	8	(3)	(3)
Environmental Protection Agency	1	2	2
Federal Deposit Insurance Corporation	1	1	1
General Services Administration	5	4	2
National Aeronautics and Space Administration	7	7	8
National Science Foundation	1	1	1
Panama Canal Company	4	4	5
Railroad Retirement Board	1	1	1
Smithsonian Institution	4	2	5
Soldiers' and Airmen's Home	40	43	44
United States Postal Service	308	299	77
Veterans Administration	24,291	25,509	26,770

[1]Data as of October 31, 1976 includes all federal departments and agencies with the following exceptions: Congress, the Congressional Budget Office, most of the Judicial Branch, Board of Governors of the Federal Reserve System, Central Intelligence Agency, National Security Agency, and foreign nationals employed overseas. The 1977 data also excludes the following: Copyright Royalty Tribunal, Office of Technology Assessment, Office of Special Representative for Trade Negotiations, National Commission on the Observance of International Women's Year; judicial branch reports cover only employees of the administrative office of the U.S. courts, employees of the individual courts are not reported.
[2]Renamed Defense Logistics Agency in 1977.
[3]The Energy Research and Development Administration is now part of a new executive branch agency, the Department of Energy, established October 1, 1977 by Public Law 95-91.
SOURCE: U.S. Office of Personnel Management, Agency Compliance and Evaluation Work Force Information Division, 1978 and 1980.

Table I-G-3. Peace Corps Volunteer Nurses, by Country of Assignment, 1976-1977

Country or area	1976	1977
Total	153	137
Africa	32	21
Botswana	3	....
Cameroon	...	1
Ivory Coast	1	...
Kenya	6	2
Lesotho	3	...
Liberia	14	10
Mauritania	...	4
Niger	2	...
Sierra Leone	1	1
Upper Volta	...	2
Zaire	2	1
North Africa, Near East, Asia and Pacific	20	20
Afghanistan	...	2
Bahrain	4	1
Korea (South)	...	1
Micronesia	1	1
Nepal	1	...
Oman	6	2
Philippines	1	1
Thailand	...	1
Tunisia	1	...
Western Samoa	1	1
Yemen	5	10
Latin America	101	96
Belize	2	1
Brazil	23	30
Colombia	27	14
Costa Rica	16	17
Dominican Republic	...	1
Eastern Caribbean Islands	4	1
Ecuador	7	7
El Salvador	...	2
Guatemala	...	8
Honduras	10	7
Jamaica	1	2
Nicaragua	8	4
Paraguay	3	2

SOURCE: Peace Corps Volunteer System, Office of Management/PC, 1978. Unpublished data.

Chapter I, Section H
LICENSURE FOR PRACTICE AND CREDENTIALLING

One function of state government is the legal regulation of nursing practice through licensure. The requirements for licensure are mandated by each state's nursing practice act. It is the prerogative of the state board of nursing to administer the nursing practice act either on an independent basis or within a department of state government. Additionally, the state boards are responsible for establishing minimum standards for and approving basic nursing educational programs, determining by examination the applicant's competence to practice nursing, and issuing licenses.

It is estimated there are over 1.6 million licenses to practice as a registered nurse in existence at any one time; however, neither the total number of licenses nationally nor the number of licenses issued by each state can be used as an estimate of the actual number of nurses. Since a substantial number of nurses hold licenses in more than one state, the total number of licenses reflects the duplicate licenses some nurses hold. Moreover, with regard to the number of licenses issued by the state, some nurses holding state licenses are not located within the state in which they are licensed. For this reason, ANA periodically conducts national inventories of nurses, which provides unduplicated counts of the nurse population. The inventory includes the nurse in the state of employment, if employed in nursing or in the state of residence, if not employed in nursing. Selected data from the 1977-78 study are presented in Section A of this chapter.

The ANA periodically canvasses the state boards of nursing to update licensure statistics. In 1979, 47 state boards responded to the survey, and the analysis in this section reflects the responses of the participating state boards. In 1979, 46 states reported a total of 1,290,812 license renewals. Since some states have 2-year renewal periods, renewal figures may not be comparable from year to year. For this group, licensure renewal covers a 2-year span; therefore, the annual totals should not be compared unless appropriate adjustments are made. The license expiration dates are shown on a separate table in the following section.

Students graduating from schools of nursing must take the licensing examination administered by the state board of nursing. The examination is uniform throughout the nation. In 1979, 47 states reported that 65,112 state graduates wrote the examination for the first time. Overall, 84.8 percent of these candidates passed. There were 17,168 in-state graduates retaking the exam, of whom 58.2 percent passed. Of the 5,137 out-of-state graduates and 9,368 foreign nurse graduates taking the licensing exam for the first time, 83.2 percent and 21.9 percent passed, respectively. About 49.7 percent of the out-of-state and 19.3 percent of the foreign nurse graduates repeating the exam passed.

In 1979, a total of 73,938 licenses were issued to registered nurses for the first time in the United States by the responding states. Of these, 591 were reported as "first" licenses issued on the basis of endorsement of a license or certificate from a foreign country. In some instances, nurses from foreign countries are required to take the licensing examination. The count of those passing is included in the column denoting first license issued by "examination" on the table.

As nursing practice acts have undergone revisions, the trend has been to remove minimum age and citizenship requirements. In 1979, only six states reported minimum age requirements and four required citizenship or "registered resident alien" status.

A fee is established either by law or by board regulation in order to obtain a license in a state or to renew an already existing license. Fees for examination in states varied from $10.00 in Pennsylvania and the Virgin Islands to $75.00 in New Mexico. Endorsement fees also ranged from $10.00 to $65.00; and license renewal fees, from $1.00 to $20.00. A table providing the citation and the dates of enactment and amendment of each state's nursing practice act is included in this section.

The Commission on Graduates of Foreign Nursing Schools (CGFNS) administers a testing and evaluation program for graduates of foreign nursing schools to determine the probability of successfully passing the state licensing examination. A total of 7,124 foreign nurse graduates submitted application or reapplication for the CGFNS examination from October 1978 through October 1980. Of that number, 5,256 were eligible and scheduled to take the examination; about 91.8 percent of these nurses actually took the examination. More detailed statistics were presented for 4,417 foreign nurse graduates in 56 countries tested by CGFNS in the period. Almost three-fourths (72.2 percent) did not pass the examination. Looking at the results of those taking the examination for the first time, failure to pass the nursing portion was the most predominant category (39.6 percent), followed by 32.6 percent who failed both the nursing portion and the English tests. The examination also revealed that the major areas of weakness for foreign nurse graduates were psychiatric nursing and the nursing of children, with passing rates of 38.6 percent and 47.7 percent, respectively. Data on the personal characteristics of foreign nurse graduates tested is also presented.

Recent years have marked trends among professions to establish certification programs to identify members who practice on a level higher than that determined by state licensure examinations. The American Nurses' Association has been responsive to this trend by establishing a program of certification in nursing. The principal and central focus of ANA certification is one of quality assurance. The formal definition of ANA certification was made in 1977. "Certification is the documented validation of specific qualifications demonstrated by the individual registered nurse in the provision of professional nursing care in a defined area of practice." In prior years, the definition appeared in a slightly simpler form. As of August 1980 a total of 4,734 nurses had been certified by ANA since 1975. The program has been marked by steady growth since its initiation. The number of nurses certified in 1980 was greater than the total number certified in the three previous years.

Table I-H-1. Licenses Renewed for Registered Nurses, 1976-1979

State or territory	Type of renewal and licensing period	Number of licenses renewed during			
		1976	1977	1978	1979
Total		*1,386,764*	*1,138,220*	*1,099,183*	*1,290,812*
Alabama	Annual (calendar)	13,991	...	...	...
	Biennial (1/1/odd year-12/31/even year)	...	482	[1]192	[1]16,837
Alaska	Biennial (7/1/even year-6/30/even year)	1,805	...	2,596	4
Arizona	Annual (calendar)	16,700	16,467	17,699	19,044
Arkansas	Biennial (5/1/even year-4/30/even year)	7,510	...	(2)	(2)
California	Biennial (birthdate)	80,752	87,767	79,570	86,576
Colorado	Biennial (1/1/even year-12/31/odd year)	18,495	[2]22,400	(3)	(3)
Connecticut	Annual (birthdate)	[4]23,327	[4]23,427	[4]26,099	[4]33,283
Delaware	Biennial (1/1/even year-12/31/odd year)	66	5,762	...	5,421
District of Columbia	Annual (fiscal)	(3)	(3)	(3)	(3)
Florida	Annual	49,626	53,631	57,645	58,551
Georgia	Biennial (1/1/odd year-12/31/even year)	[5]31,600	...	23,283	5,228
Guam	Annual (fiscal)	337	343	343	348
Hawaii	Annual (fiscal)	[5]5,897	...	...	...
	Biennial (7/1/odd year-6/30/odd year)	...	6,397	...	[6]7,651
Idaho	Annual (fiscal)	4,608	[5]5,055	[5]5,364	...
	Biennial (7/1/odd year-6/30/odd year)				
Illinois	Annual	82,689	(3)	...	...
	Biennial (5/1/even year-4/30/even year)	...	...	[1]91,420	[1]9,515
Indiana	Biennial (1/1/even year-12/31/odd year)	3,764	26,301	[2]30,295	[1]31,090
Iowa	Annual (fiscal)	[2]22,674	[2]23,584	[2]24,449	[2]25,288
Kansas	Biennial (birthdate even or odd year)	[6]18,179	[6]19,692	[2]20,896	[2]20,502
Kentucky	Annual	19,112	20,621	21,868	22,812
Louisiana	Annual (calendar)	14,683	15,285	16,302	17,499
Maine	Annual (calendar)	9,947	9,797	10,092	10,404
Maryland	Biennial (1/1/even or odd year-12/31/odd or even year)ᴺ	[2]12,222	[2]24,125	[2]17,417	[1]19,392
Massachusetts	Biennial (birthdate-even year)	[1]76,466	(3)	(3)	(3)
Michigan	Annual	[1]63,352	(3)	[2]73,724	[1]76,350
Minnesota	Annual (calendar)	30,930	32,643	(3)	(3)
Mississippi	Annual (calendar)	9,474	...	9,756	...
	Biennial (1/1/odd year-12/31/even year)				

State	Registration				
Missouri	Annual (fiscal)	[1]26,883	[1]28,668	(2)	[1]30,178
Montana	Annual (calendar)	[4]5,672	[4]6,507	[4]6,555	[4]6,635
Nebraska	Annual (calendar)	[11]16,772	[11]16,989	[11]17,138	[11]17,185
Nevada	Biennial (3/1/even year-2/28/even year)	3,143		3,710	
New Hampshire	Biennial (birthdate-odd year)	[1]9,253	2,448	8,748	2,075
New Jersey	Biennial (1/1/even or odd year-12/31/odd or even year)	[1]41,921	[1]43,566	[1]30,146	[4]45,266
New Mexico	Biennial (birthdate-odd year)	273	5,927	181	5,797
New York	Biennial (9/1/odd year-8/31/odd year)	[4]201,799	[4]172,298	[4]186,975	[1]180,894
North Carolina	Biennial (1/1/even or odd year-12/31/odd or even year)	15,691	[1]16,963	[1]18,453	[1]15,982
North Dakota	Annual (calendar)	4,834	5,117	5,035	5,220
Ohio	Annual	[4]75,013	[8]81,821	[8]82,477	[8]85,952
Oklahoma	Annual (fiscal)	11,809	12,675	13,508	14,401
Oregon	Biennial (4/1/odd year-3/31/odd year)		15,939		18,078
Pennsylvania	Biennial (11/1/odd year-10/31/odd year)	[1,9]137,875	[1]135,946	[1]143,074	[1]145,313
Rhode Island	Annual	[10]9,388	[10]9,706	[11]9,762	[11]10,125
South Carolina	Annual (calendar)	[4]13,452	12,711	[4]15,480	[4]16,882
South Dakota	Annual (calendar)	5,189	(3)	564	5,466
Tennessee	Biennial (birthdate-even or odd year)	[1]21,976	[12]24,609	[4]24,827	[4]26,998
Texas	Biennial (1/1/odd year-12/31/even year)	57,228	61,935	62,578	67,966
Utah	Annual	[1]9,154	[4]9,838	(3)	(3)
Vermont	Annual (calendar)		5,241		[4]5,432
Virgin Islands	Biennial (5/1/odd year-4/30/odd year)	441	456	468	515
Virginia	Annual (fiscal)	[1]30,600	[13]32,102	[13]33,700	[13]37,568
Washington	Annual (birthdate)	[1]28,870	(3)	[13]35,054	[13]37,442
West Virginia	Annual (birthdate)	[1]10,142	[1]11,303	[1]11,740	[1]12,439
Wisconsin	Annual (calendar)	[1]29,075	[1]29,347	(3)	[1]31,208
Wyoming	Biennial (2/1/even year-1/31/even year) / Annual (fiscal)	2,105	2,329	(3)	(3)

[1] Includes reinstatements.
[2] Información not available.
[3] Not reported.
[4] Current registration as of December 31.
[5] Estimated.
[6] Current registration as of June 30.
[7] Current registration as of April 30.
[8] Even or odd year based on last digit of registration number.
[9] One year registration in order to change licensing period to biennial beginning in odd year.
[10] Current registration as of July 1.
[11] Number of licenses renewed as of June 30.
[12] Current registration as of June 1.
[13] Current registration as of January 1.
[14] Current registration as of May, 1978.

SOURCE: American Nurses' Association, Research and Policy Analysis Department, Statistics Unit, special tabulations from licensure table update sheets, 1980.

Table I-H-2. Licenses Issued to Registered Nurses Previously Licensed in the U.S.,[1] by Method of Licensure and State Issuing License, 1978 and 1979

	1978			1979		
State or territory	Endorse-ment	Exam-ination	Rein-statement	Endorse-ment	Exam-ination	Rein-statement
Total	53,050	1,551	2,599	54,813	1,453	4,137
Alabama	863	...	(2)	865	...	(2)
Alaska	409	...	...	352	...	63
Arizona	1,616	...	...	1,782	...	...
Arkansas	(3)	(3)	(3)	(3)	(3)	(3)
California	5,302	...	12	5,417	..	18
Colorado	(4)	(4)	(4)	(4)	(4)	(4)
Connecticut	1,217	...	4	1,214	...	6
Delaware	234	...	155	210	...	42
District of Columbia	(4)	(4)	(4)	(4)	(4)	(4)
Florida	5,210	...	...	5,326	...	...
Georgia	⁵1,500	...	...	1,600	...	...
Guam	39	...	8	53	1	4
Hawaii	667	12	...	...	15	(2)
Idaho	484	...	...	450	...	(2)
Illinois	2,863	...	(2)	2,218	...	(2)
Indiana	1,046	...	(2)	1,099	1	(2)
Iowa	872	...	(2)	749	...	(2)
Kansas	769	...	(2)	910	...	(2)
Kentucky	852	...	228	876	...	408
Louisiana	952	...	596	898	3	596
Maine	575	...	374	474	...	403
Maryland	1,711	...	(2)	1,743	...	(2)
Massachusetts	(4)	(4)	(4)	(4)	(4)	(4)
Michigan	1,122	13	(2)	1,194	2	(2)
Minnesota	(4)	(4)	(4)	(4)	(4)	(4)
Mississippi	449	...	140	504	...	1,078
Missouri	(3)	(3)	(3)	1,381	36	(2)
Montana	390	...	(2)	373	...	(2)
Nebraska	454	...	(2)	497	...	(2)
Nevada	584	...	196	452	...	50
New Hampshire	774	...	298	730	...	196
New Jersey	1,754	...	(2)	2,149	...	(2)
New Mexico	586	...	108	528	...	...
New York	...	1,515	(2)	...	1,389	(2)
North Carolina	1,414	...	(2)	1,762	...	(2)
North Dakota	207	...	1	192	...	1
Ohio	1,532	...	(2)	1,582	...	(2)
Oklahoma	775	2	240	779	2	225
Oregon	1,283	...	230	1,328	...	809
Pennsylvania	1,739	8	(2)	2,030	3	(2)
Rhode Island	300	...	(2)	343	...	(2)
South Carolina	775	...	(2)	918	...	(2)
South Dakota	226	...	...	236	...	...
Tennessee	1,141	...	(2)	1,096	...	(2)
Texas	4,378	...	9	4,200	...	12
Utah	(4)	(4)	(4)	(4)	(4)	(4)
Vermont	362	1	...	370	1	226
Virgin Islands	71	...	...	83	...	...
Virginia	2,043	...	(2)	2,166	...	(2)
Washington	1,808	...	(2)	2,085	...	(2)
West Virginia	482	...	(2)	560	...	(2)
Wisconsin	1,220	...	(2)	1,039	...	(2)
Wyoming	(4)	(4)	(4)	(4)	(4)	(4)

[1]Includes foreign nurses previously licensed in the U.S. and territories.
[2]Reinstatements included with renewals, see Table I-H-1.
[3]Information not available.
[4]Not reported.
[5]Estimated.

SOURCE: American Nurses' Association, Research and Policy Analysis Department, Statistics Unit, special tabulations from licensure table update sheets, 1980.

Table I-H-3. Licenses Issued to Registered Nurses for the First Time in the U.S., by Method of Licensure and State Issuing License, 1978 and 1979

State or territory	1978				1979			
	Total	Waiver	Exami-nation[1]	Endorse-ment[2]	Total	Waiver	Exami-nation[1]	Endorse-ment[2]
Total	67,760	...	67,245	515	73,938	...	73,347	591
Alabama	1,422	...	1,381	41	1,519	...	1,506	13
Alaska	70	...	70	...	65	...	65	...
Arizona	741	...	741	...	740	...	740	...
Arkansas	(3)	(3)	(3)	(3)	(3)	(3)	(3)	(3)
California	5,220	...	5,220	...	5,483	...	5,483	...
Colorado	(4)	(4)	(4)	(4)	(4)	(4)	(4)	(4)
Connecticut	1,036	...	1,036	...	1,117	...	1,117	...
Delaware	290	...	290	...	300	...	300	...
District of Columbia	(4)	(4)	(4)	(4)	(4)	(4)	(4)	(4)
Florida	2,909	...	2,909	...	3,237	...	3,237	...
Georgia	(3)	(3)	(3)	(3)	1,682	...	1,682	...
Guam	23	...	23	...	25	...	25	...
Hawaii	166	...	166	...	167	...	167	...
Idaho	209	...	209	...	238	...	238	...
Illinois	4,893	...	4,893	...	5,185	...	5,185	...
Indiana	1,883	...	1,883	...	2,184	...	2,184	...
Iowa	1,338	...	1,336	2	1,358	...	1,356	2
Kansas	(3)	(3)	(3)	(3)	(3)	(3)	(3)	(3)
Kentucky	1,209	...	1,209	...	1,294	...	1,294	...
Louisiana	1,186	...	1,089	97	1,269	...	1,160	109
Maine	440	...	401	39	449	...	420	29
Maryland	1,490	...	1,490	...	1,282	...	1,282	...
Massachusetts	(4)	(4)	(4)	(4)	(4)	(4)	(4)	(4)
Michigan	3,185	...	3,185	...	3,355	...	3,355	...
Minnesota	(4)	(4)	(4)	(4)	(4)	(4)	(4)	(4)
Mississippi	712	...	700	12	717	...	710	7
Missouri	(3)	(3)	(3)	(3)	2,006	...	2,006	...
Montana	295	...	295	...	329	...	329	...
Nebraska	689	...	689	...	690	...	689	1
Nevada	331	...	135	196	439	...	152	287
New Hampshire	283	...	283	...	272	...	272	...
New Jersey	2,693	...	2,690	3	2,688	...	2,681	7
New Mexico	367	...	362	5	349	...	346	3
New York	8,853	...	8,853	...	9,081	...	9,081	...
North Carolina	1,792	...	1,748	44	1,917	...	1,853	64
North Dakota	336	...	334	2	354	...	346	8
Ohio	4,164	...	4,164	...	4,330	...	4,330	...
Oklahoma	763	...	759	4	737	...	731	6
Oregon	957	...	957	...	942	...	942	...
Pennsylvania	4,804	...	4,777	27	5,127	...	5,090	37
Rhode Island	447	...	447	...	424	...	424	...
South Carolina	791	...	791	...	732	...	732	...
South Dakota	464	...	464	...	361	...	361	...
Tennessee	1,509	...	1,509	...	1,615	...	1,615	...
Texas	4,279	...	4,279	...	4,123	...	4,123	...
Utah	(4)	(4)	(4)	(4)	(4)	(4)	(4)	(4)
Vermont	167	...	167	...	171	...	171	...
Virgin Islands	6	...	6	...	15	...	15	...
Virginia	1,635	...	1,635	...	1,796	...	1,796	...
Washington	1,288	...	1,264	24	1,334	...	1,329	5
West Virginia	662	...	662	...	683	...	683	...
Wisconsin	1,763	...	1,744	19	1,757	...	1,744	13
Wyoming	(4)	(4)	(4)	(4)	(4)	(4)	(4)	(4)

[1] Includes some foreign nurses required to write the SBTP examination but licensed through the endorsement procedure.
[2] License issued on the basis of license or certificate from foreign country.
[3] Information not available.
[4] Not reported.

SOURCE: American Nurses' Association, Research and Policy Analysis Department, Statistics Unit, special tabulations from licensure table update sheets, 1980.

Table I-H-4. Registered Nurse Licensing Examination

State or territory	State graduates						Out-of-state		
	First time candidates			Retakes			First time candidates		
	Number written	Number passed	Percent passed	Number written	Number passed	Percent passed	Number written	Number passed	Percent passed
Alabama	1,405	1,101	78.4	515	324	62.9	58	49	84.5
Alaska	41	33	80.5	6	4	66.7	27	23	85.2
Arizona	632	564	89.2	123	72	58.5	81	67	82.7
Arkansas	(1)	(1)	(1)	(1)	(1)	(1)	(1)	(1)	(1)
California	5,192	4,556	87.8	1,329	461	34.7	490	422	86.1
Colorado	(2)	(2)	(2)	(2)	(2)	(2)	(2)	(2)	(2)
Connecticut	971	845	87.0	145	108	74.5	137	115	83.9
Delaware	301	243	80.7	73	38	52.1	13	11	84.6
District of Columbia	(2)	(2)	(2)	(2)	(2)	(2)	(2)	(2)	(2)
Florida	2,545	2,172	85.3	720	345	47.9	244	218	89.3
Georgia	1,373	1,132	82.4	506	279	55.1	187	143	76.5
Guam	29	11	37.9	29	8	27.6	2	2	100.0
Hawaii	139	119	85.6	18	14	77.8	29	25	86.2
Idaho	190	170	89.5	47	32	68.1	28	26	92.9
Illinois	4,247	3,534	83.2	1,040	682	65.6	392	328	83.7
Indiana	1,794	1,678	93.5	527	430	81.6	89	64	71.9
Iowa	1,295	1,155	89.2	137	99	72.3	89	81	91.0
Kansas	⁴1,005	⁴859	⁴85.5	⁴205	⁴132	⁴64.4	...	...	...
Kentucky	1,161	977	84.2	332	213	64.2	82	74	90.2
Louisiana	1,050	866	82.5	359	190	52.9	115	81	70.4
Maine	376	317	84.3	53	42	79.2	59	56	94.9
Maryland	1,375	1,196	87.0	305	189	62.0	92	77	83.7
Massachusetts ...	(2)	(2)	(2)	(2)	(2)	(2)	(2)	(2)	(2)
Michigan	3,028	2,730	90.2	393	277	70.5	100	85	85.0
Minnesota	(2)	(2)	(2)	(2)	(2)	(2)	(2)	(2)	(2)
Mississippi	734	512	69.8	281	173	61.6	18	16	88.9
Missouri	2,465	2,006	81.4	274	141	51.5	106	96	90.6
Montana	229	199	86.9	41	34	82.9	22	18	81.8
Nebraska	648	600	92.6	75	60	80.0	34	29	85.3
Nevada	119	110	92.4	28	19	67.9	18	17	94.4
New Hampshire...	206	185	89.8	31	21	67.7	63	49	77.8
New Jersey	2,157	1,731	80.3	720	433	60.1	254	178	70.1
New Mexico	291	231	79.4	107	55	51.4	52	45	86.5
New York	7,524	5,631	74.8	3,856	1,847	47.9	456	348	76.3
North Carolina ...	1,718	1,310	76.3	721	426	59.1	117	99	84.6
North Dakota	326	276	84.7	72	50	69.4	16	13	81.3
Ohio	3,948	3,534	89.5	519	392	75.5	387	321	82.9
Oklahoma	(5)	(5)	(5)	(5)	(5)	(5)	(5)	(5)	(5)
Oregon	786	712	90.6	56	38	67.9	173	149	86.1
Pennsylvania	4,398	4,161	94.6	778	664	85.3	204	161	78.9
Rhode Island	401	319	79.6	125	83	66.4	22	22	100.0
South Carolina ...	625	495	79.2	247	113	45.7	75	60	80.0
South Dakota	310	270	87.1	57	31	54.4	23	21	91.3
Tennessee	1,519	1,340	88.2	305	185	60.7	33	26	78.8
Texas	3,501	2,868	81.9	⁶1,129	⁶694	⁶61.5	242	206	85.1
Utah	(2)	(2)	(2)	(2)	(2)	(2)	(2)	(2)	(2)
Vermont	146	108	74.0	36	26	72.2	29	26	89.7
Virgin Islands	17	5	29.4	30	7	23.3	2	...	...
Virginia	1,504	1,298	86.3	324	206	63.6	242	219	90.5
Washington	1,168	1,075	92.0	141	90	63.8	74	63	85.1
West Virginia	613	515	84.0	185	136	73.5	25	22	88.0
Wisconsin	1,610	1,479	91.9	168	130	77.4	136	123	90.4
Wyoming	(2)	(2)	(2)	(2)	(2)	(2)	(2)	(2)	(2)

¹Information not available.
²Not reported.
³Includes foreign nurse graduates who repeated the examination.

SOURCE: American Nurses' Association, Research and Policy Analysis Department, Statistics Unit, special

Given by State and Territorial Boards, 1979

graduates			Foreign nurse graduates					
Retakes			First time candidates			Retakes		
Number written	Number passed	Percent passed	Number written	Number passed	Percent passed	Number written	Number passed	Percent passed
23	14	60.9	17	5	29.4	32	13	40.6
4	3	75.0	2	1	50.0	4	...	...
28	11	39.3	88	15	17.0	37	11	29.7
(1)	(1)	(1)	(1)	(1)	(1)	(1)	(1)	(1)
125	44	35.2	1,163	159	13.7	2,739	218	8.0
(2)	(2)	(2)	(2)	(2)	(2)	(2)	(2)	(2)
31	25	80.6	40	14	35.0	29	10	34.5
3	3	100.0	...	...	...	8	3	37.5
(2)	(2)	(2)	(2)	(2)	(2)	(2)	(2)	(2)
124	46	37.1	977	324	33.2	1,283	318	24.8
66	42	63.1	80	24	30.0	198	67	33.8
4	1	25.0	15	1	6.7	8	2	25.0
15	7	46.7	58	10	17.2	44	7	15.9
5	5	100.0	2	1	50.0	4	1	25.0
71	46	64.8	[3]3,171	[3]628	[3]19.8	...	...	...
19	12	63.2	17	7	41.2	16	6	37.5
16	9	56.3	22	3	13.6	31	9	29.0
...	...	...	...	...	...	...	...	...
36	20	55.6	...	...	...	19	4	21.1
52	23	44.2	12	5	41.7	35	7	20.0
6	6	100.0	46	4	8.7	38	8	21.1
46	33	71.7	75	9	12.0	185	52	28.1
(2)	(2)	(2)	(2)	(2)	(2)	(2)	(2)	(2)
16	12	75.0	465	172	37.0	272	81	29.8
(2)	(2)	(2)	(2)	(2)	(2)	(2)	(2)	(2)
8	6	75.0	10	1	10.0	6	2	33.3
12	8	66.7	111	40	36.0	172	77	44.8
5	4	80.0	18	10	55.6	3	1	33.3
2	1	50.0	...	...	...	...	...	...
1	1	100.0	4	1	25.0	13	4	30.8
13	9	69.2	6	5	83.3	6	3	50.0
226	63	27.9	282	60	21.3	854	218	25.5
13	5	38.5	17	2	11.8	22	8	36.4
186	79	42.5	1,849	275	14.9	5,962	1,037	17.4
...	...	...	23	7	30.4	31	12	38.7
8	6	75.0	8	1	12.5	5	...	...
52	36	69.2	63	28	44.4	59	19	32.2
(5)	(5)	(5)	(5)	(5)	(5)	(5)	(5)	(5)
31	21	67.7	40	8	20.0	25	6	24.0
46	25	54.3	56	11	19.6	246	71	28.9
5	4	80.0	10	1	10.0	11	3	27.3
29	16	55.2	18	5	27.8	9	1	11.1
1	1	100.0	2	...	...	2	...	...
29	20	69.0	51	8	15.7	133	36	27.1
...	...	...	374	144	38.5	504	202	40.1
(2)	(2)	(2)	(2)	(2)	(2)	(2)	(2)	(2)
3	2	66.7	11	8	72.7	4	2	50.0
1	1	100.0	8	1	12.5	17	5	29.4
48	27	56.3	53	24	45.3	83	22	26.5
24	13	54.2	82	24	29.3	178	30	16.9
7	4	57.1	10	3	30.0	9	2	22.2
5	4	80.0	12	4	33.3	21	4	19.0
(2)	(2)	(2)	(2)	(2)	(2)	(2)	(2)	(2)

[4]Includes out-of-state and foreign nurse candidates.
[5]Permission to publish withheld.
[6]Includes out-of-state graduates who repeated the examination.

tabulations from licensure update sheets, 1980.

Table I-H-5. Registered Nurse Licensing Examinations Given

	State graduates						Out-of-state		
	First time candidates			Retakes			First time candidates		
State or territory	Number written	Number passed	Percent passed	Number written	Number passed	Percent passed	Number written	Number passed	Percent passed
Alabama	1,367	1,073	78.5	425	239	56.2	41	29	70.7
Alaska	39	33	84.6	6	4	66.7	29	29	100.0
Arizona	665	581	87.4	128	80	62.5	56	48	85.7
Arkansas	(1)	(1)	(1)	(1)	(1)	(1)	(1)	(1)	(1)
California	4,951	4,353	87.9	1,092	418	38.3	462	409	88.5
Colorado	(2)	(2)	(2)	(2)	(2)	(2)	(2)	(2)	(2)
Connecticut	868	765	88.1	146	109	74.7	122	96	78.7
Delaware	269	230	85.5	57	31	54.4	24	21	87.5
District of Columbia	(2)	(2)	(2)	(2)	(2)	(2)	(2)	(2)	(2)
Florida	2,460	2,126	86.4	575	262	45.6	259	215	83.0
Georgia	1,390	1,098	79.0	676	358	53.0	153	121	79.1
Guam	43	18	41.9	11	1	9.1	...	...	...
Hawaii	135	117	86.7	24	17	70.8	24	16	66.7
Idaho	197	162	82.2	33	25	75.8	16	16	100.0
Illinois	4,267	3,796	89.0	847	520	61.4	393	348	88.5
Indiana	1,863	1,620	87.0	311	220	70.7	49	38	77.6
Iowa	1,217	1,143	93.9	98	72	73.5	110	103	93.6
Kansas	³963	³858	³89.1	³175	³104	³59.4	...	...	...
Kentucky	1,170	964	82.4	271	171	63.1	88	76	86.4
Louisiana	1,042	850	81.6	249	138	55.4	103	77	74.8
Maine	408	361	88.5	53	34	64.2	7	6	85.7
Maryland	1,441	1,211	84.0	279	168	60.2	53	52	98.1
Massachusetts	(2)	(2)	(2)	(2)	(2)	(2)	(2)	(2)	(2)
Michigan	2,930	2,632	89.8	387	257	66.4	99	85	85.9
Minnesota	(2)	(2)	(2)	(2)	(2)	(2)	(2)	(2)	(2)
Mississippi	679	483	71.1	338	184	54.4	27	20	74.1
Missouri	(1)	(1)	(1)	(1)	(1)	(1)	(1)	(1)	(1)
Montana	287	248	86.4	16	14	87.5	37	33	89.2
Nebraska	640	582	90.0	32	24	75.0	42	41	97.6
Nevada	115	99	86.1	27	17	63.0	11	10	90.9
New Hampshire	223	203	91.0	22	16	72.7	64	57	89.1
New Jersey	2,318	1,880	81.1	634	325	51.3	269	208	77.3
New Mexico	319	264	82.8	74	37	50.0	45	38	84.4
New York	7,889	6,039	76.5	3,604	1,500	41.6	461	374	81.1
North Carolina	1,762	1,340	76.0	614	307	50.0	98	85	86.7
North Dakota	328	280	85.4	59	36	61.0	18	13	72.2
Ohio	3,942	3,542	89.9	449	337	75.1	232	204	87.9
Oklahoma	(5)	(5)	(5)	(5)	(5)	(5)	(5)	(5)	(5)
Oregon	724	683	94.3	92	56	60.9	190	173	91.1
Pennsylvania	4,646	3,984	85.8	826	553	66.9	169	139	82.2
Rhode Island	418	320	76.6	80	57	71.3	23	18	78.3
South Carolina	752	585	77.8	225	140	62.2	57	44	77.2
South Dakota	352	303	86.1	65	46	70.8	10	8	80.0
Tennessee	1,425	1,242	87.2	277	147	53.1	71	61	85.9
Texas	3,764	3,053	81.1	⁶1,257	⁶665	⁶52.9	182	161	88.5
Utah	(2)	(2)	(2)	(2)	(2)	(2)	(2)	(2)	(2)
Vermont	156	125	80.1	25	20	80.0	18	16	88.9
Virgin Islands	13	1	7.7	17	3	17.6	1	1	100.0
Virginia	1,450	1,249	86.1	307	176	57.3	185	164	88.6
Washington	1,225	1,123	91.7	119	74	62.2	75	71	94.7
West Virginia	670	523	78.1	144	108	75.0	23	22	95.7
Wisconsin	1,664	1,521	91.4	140	109	77.9	101	97	96.0
Wyoming	(2)	(2)	(2)	(2)	(2)	(2)	(2)	(2)	(2)

¹ Information not available.
² Not reported.
³ Includes foreign nurse graduates who repeated the examination.

SOURCE: American Nurses' Association, Research and Policy Analysis Department, Statistics Unit, special

by State and Territorial Boards, 1978

graduates			Foreign nurse graduates					
Retakes			First time candidates			Retakes		
Number written	Number passed	Percent passed	Number written	Number passed	Percent passed	Number written	Number passed	Percent passed
8	6	75.0	37	8	21.6	80	26	32.5
5	2	40.0	8	1	12.5	4	...	...
17	8	47.1	33	14	42.4	27	10	37.0
(1)	(1)	(1)	(1)	(1)	(1)	(1)	(1)	(1)
108	40	37.0	1,051	179	17.0	2,161	167	7.7
(2)	(2)	(2)	(2)	(2)	(2)	(2)	(2)	(2)
40	30	75.0	54	22	40.7	45	12	26.7
4	2	50.0	4	2	50.0	11	1	9.1
(2)	(2)	(2)	(2)	(2)	(2)	(2)	(2)	(2)
89	30	33.7	833	299	35.9	1,018	222	21.8
68	38	55.9	138	21	15.2	304	86	28.3
6	2	33.3	8	1	12.5	28	1	3.6
17	12	70.6	14	12	85.7	21	4	19.0
6	1	16.7	2	...	...	7	3	42.9
48	29	60.4	[1]2,098	[1]468	[1]22.3	...	...	...
9	5	55.6	20	12	60.0	32	13	40.6
10	6	60.0	35	8	22.9	26	4	15.4
...	...	...	...	...	...	...	...	...
28	12	42.9	...	...	...	27	5	18.5
39	24	61.5	16	2	12.5	35	5	14.3
...	...	...	22	4	18.2	22	6	27.3
26	12	46.2	80	11	13.8	205	36	17.6
(2)	(2)	(2)	(2)	(2)	(2)	(2)	(2)	(2)
17	10	58.8	367	169	46.0	153	45	29.4
(2)	(2)	(2)	(2)	(2)	(2)	(2)	(2)	(2)
8	1	12.5	17	4	23.5	20	8	40.0
(1)	(1)	(1)	(1)	(1)	(1)	(1)	(1)	(1)
2	2	100.0	21	12	57.1	4	2	50.0
7	7	100.0	3	3	100.0	...	...	...
...	...	...	...	...	...	12	9	75.0
7	1	14.3	7	4	57.1	7	2	28.6
146	32	21.9	248	42	16.9	845	203	24.0
14	9	64.3	13	1	7.7	33	7	21.2
151	58	38.4	1,754	215	12.3	5,986	808	13.5
...	...	...	19	5	26.3	43	12	27.9
2	...	...	8	2	25.0	12	3	25.0
60	36	60.0	50	15	30.0	74	30	40.5
(5)	(5)	(5)	(5)	(5)	(5)	(5)	(5)	(5)
33	19	57.6	52	11	21.2	31	14	45.2
34	22	64.7	101	8	7.9	359	78	21.7
...	...	...	4	1	25.0	12	2	16.7
20	12	60.0	16	4	25.0	15	6	40.0
2	1	50.0	...	...	...	...	...	...
34	14	41.2	84	18	21.4	123	27	22.0
...	...	...	427	137	32.1	911	251	27.6
(2)	(2)	(2)	(2)	(2)	(2)	(2)	(2)	(2)
2	2	100.0	12	4	33.3	3	1	33.3
...	...	...	8	1	12.5	6	2	33.3
42	15	35.7	30	13	43.3	109	18	16.5
14	8	57.1	124	24	19.4	162	21	13.0
3	2	66.7	15	6	40.0	7	1	14.3
8	8	100.0	14	6	42.9	16	3	18.8
(2)	(2)	(2)	(2)	(2)	(2)	(2)	(2)	(2)

[a]Includes out-of-state and foreign nurse candidates.
[s]Permission to publish withheld.
[h]Includes out-of-state graduates who repeated the examination.

tabulations from licensure table update sheets, 1980.

Table I-H-6. Licenses Issued to Registered Nurses from Foreign Countries[1] by Method of Licensure and State Issuing License, 1978 and 1979

State or territory	1978			1979		
	Total	Exam-ination[2]	Endorse-ment	Total	Exam-ination[2]	Endorse-ment
Total	5,943	3,612	2,331	5,834	3,325	2,509
Alabama	75	34	41	31	18	13
Alaska	1	1	...	1	1	...
Arizona	50	24	26	65	26	39
Arkansas	(3)	(3)	(3)	(3)	(3)	(3)
California	1,925	346	1,579	1,876	377	1,499
Colorado	(4)	(4)	(4)	(4)	(4)	(4)
Connecticut	34	34	...	24	24	...
Delaware	5	5	...	...	...	...
District of Columbia	(4)	(4)	(4)	(4)	(4)	(4)
Florida	521	521	...	280	280	...
Georgia	(3)	(3)	(3)	(3)	(3)	(3)
Guam	7	2	5	18	3	15
Hawaii	16	16	...	17	17	...
Idaho	3	3	...	2	2	...
Illinois	468	468	...	628	628	...
Indiana	54	25	29	43	13	30
Iowa	20	12	8	22	12	10
Kansas	(3)	(3)	(3)	(3)	(3)	(3)
Kentucky	11	3	8	10	3	7
Louisiana	127	7	120	142	12	130
Maine	39	10	29	29	12	17
Maryland	56	46	10	71	61	10
Massachusetts	(4)	(4)	(4)	(4)	(4)	(4)
Michigan	214	214	...	...	..	...
Minnesota	(4)	(4)	(4)	(4)	(4)	(4)
Mississippi	24	12	12	10	3	7
Missouri	(3)	(3)	(3)	153	117	36
Montana	14	14	...	11	11	...
Nebraska	8	3	5	8	7	1
Nevada	205	9	196	294	7	287
New Hampshire	7	6	1	9	8	1
New Jersey	...	...	...	...	...	...
New Mexico	16	8	8	19	10	9
New York	1,044	1,044	...	[5]977	[5]977	...
North Carolina	61	17	44	83	19	64
North Dakota	7	5	2	9	1	8
Ohio	70	45	25	104	47	57
Oklahoma	11	5	6	22	8	14
Oregon	25	25	...	14	14	...
Pennsylvania	106	79	27	116	79	37
Rhode Island	1	1	...	1	1	...
South Carolina	10	10	...	6	6	...
South Dakota	2	1	.1	3	3	...
Tennessee	46	45	1	50	44	6
Texas	388	388	...	346	346	...
Utah	(4)	(4)	(4)	(4)	(4)	(4)
Vermont	8	5	3	13	10	3
Virgin Islands	...	...	...	5	5	...
Virginia	136	31	105	155	46	109
Washington	96	72	24	136	54	82
West Virginia	7	7	..	5	5	...
Wisconsin	25	9	16	26	8	18
Wyoming	(4)	(4)	(4)	(4)	(4)	(4)

[1]Includes those being licensed for the first time and those previously licensed in another state or territory of the U.S.
[2]Includes some foreign nurses required to write the SBTP examination but licensed through the endorsement procedure.
[3]Information not available.
[4]Not reported.
[5]Incomplete count.

SOURCE: American Nurses' Association, Research and Policy Analysis Department, Statistics Unit, special tabulations from licensure table update sheets, 1980.

Table I-H-7. Minimum Age and Citizenship Requirement of Nursing Practice Acts for Registered Nurses, 1979

State or territory	Minimum age	Citizenship	State or territory	Minimum age	Citizenship
Alabama	…	…	Montana	…	…
Alaska	…	…	Nebraska	…	…
Arizona	…	…	Nevada	…	…
Arkansas	…	…	New Hampshire	…	…
California	…	…	New Jersey	18	…
Colorado	…	…	New Mexico	…	…
Connecticut	…	…	New York	18	…
Delaware	19	…	North Carolina	…	…
District of Columbia	…	…	North Dakota	…	…
Florida	…	…	Ohio	…	…
Georgia	…	…	Oklahoma	…	…
Guam	…	…	Oregon	…	…
Hawaii	…	…	Pennsylvania	…	…
Idaho	18	…	Rhode Island	…	…
Illinois	…	Yes[1]	South Carolina	18	…
Indiana	…	…	South Dakota	…	Yes[2]
Iowa	…	…	Tennessee	…	…
Kansas	…	…	Texas	…	…
Kentucky	…	…	Utah	…	…
Louisiana	…	…	Vermont	…	…
Maine	…	…	Virgin Islands	…	…
Maryland	…	…	Virginia	…	…
Massachusetts	…	…	Washington	…	…
Michigan	…	…	West Virginia	…	…
Minnesota	…	…	Wisconsin	…	Yes[1]
Mississippi	19	Yes	Wyoming	…	…
Missouri	19	…			

[1]Citizenship requirement still included in Act but not enforced based on Supreme Court ruling.
[2]Or registered "resident alien."
SOURCE: American Nurses' Association, Research and Policy Analysis Department, Statistics Unit, special tabulations from licensure table update sheets, 1980:

Table I-H-8. Expiration Dates[1] for Renewal of License or Registration for Registered Nurses, 1980

State or territory	Expiration date	State or territory	Expiration date
Alabama	December 31[2]	Montana	December 31
Alaska	June 30[2]	Nebraska	December 31
Arizona	December 31	Nevada	February 28[2]
Arkansas	Birthdate[2]	New Hampshire	Birthdate[2]
California	Last day of month following birthday month of registrant[2]	New Jersey	December 31[2]
Colorado	December 31[2]	New Mexico	Birthdate[2]
Connecticut	Birthdate	New York	August 31[2]
Delaware	December 31[2]	North Carolina	December 31[2]
District of Columbia	June 30	North Dakota	December 31
Florida	March 31	Ohio	February 28
Georgia	December 31[2]	Oklahoma	June 30
Guam	June 30	Oregon	March 31[2]
Hawaii	June 30[2]	Pennsylvania	October 31[2]
Idaho	June 30[2]	Rhode Island	March 1
Illinois	May 1[2]	South Carolina	December 31
Indiana	December 31[2]	South Dakota	Birthdate[2]
Iowa	June 30	Tennessee	December 31[2]
Kansas	Birthdate[2]	Texas	March 31
Kentucky	April 30	Utah	December 31
Louisiana	December 31	Vermont	April 30[2]
Maine	December 31	Virgin Islands	June 30
Maryland	December 31[2]	Virginia	Birthdate
Massachusetts	Birthdate[2]	Washington	Birthdate
Michigan	March 31	West Virginia	December 31
Minnesota	August 1[2]	Wisconsin	January 31[2]
Mississippi	December 31[2]	Wyoming	June 30
Missouri	June 30		

[1] Excludes grace period.
[2] Biennial renewal.

SOURCE: American Nurses' Association, Research and Policy Analysis Department, Statistics Unit, special tabulations from licensure table update sheets, 1980.

Table I-H-9. Responsibility for Selected Functions Relating to Registered Nurse Licensure, 1979

State or territory	Conducting examination		Approval of application		Approval of basic nursing programs	
	State board of nursing	Department of state government	State board of nursing	Department of state government	State board of nursing	Department of state government
Alabama	X	...	X	...	X	...
Alaska	X	...	X	...	X	...
Arizona	X	...	X	...	X	...
Arkansas	X	...	X	...	X	...
California	X	...	X	...	X	...
Colorado	X	...	X	...	X	...
Connecticut...............	X	...	X	...	X	...
Delaware	X	...	X	...	X	...
District of Columbia	X	...	X	...	X	...
Florida	X	...	X	...	X	...
Georgia	X	...	X	...	X	...
Guam	X	...	X	...	X	...
Hawaii	X	...	X	...	X	...
Idaho	X	...	X	...	X	...
Illinois	...	X	...	X	...	X
Indiana	X	...	X	...	X	...
Iowa	X	...	X	...	X	...
Kansas	X	...	X	...	X	...
Kentucky	X	...	X	...	X	...
Louisiana	X	...	X	...	X	...
Maine	X	...	X	...	X	...
Maryland.................	X	...	X	...	X	...
Massachusetts	X	...	X	...	X	...
Michigan	X	...	X	...	X	...
Minnesota	X	...	X	...	X	...
Mississippi	X	...	X	...	X	...
Missouri	X	...	X	...	X	...
Montana	X	...	X	...	X	...
Nebraska	X	...	X	...	X	...
Nevada	X	...	X	...	X	...
New Hampshire	X	...	X	...	X	...
New Jersey	X	...	X	...	X	...
New Mexico	X	...	X	...	X	...
New York	...	X	...	X	...	X
North Carolina	X	...	X	...	X	...
North Dakota	X	...	X	...	X	...
Ohio	X	...	X	...	X	...
Oklahoma	X	...	X	...	X	...
Oregon	X	...	X	...	X	...
Pennsylvania	X	...	X	...	X	...
Rhode Island	X	...	X	...	X	...
South Carolina	X	...	X	...	X	...
South Dakota	X	...	X	...	X	...
Tennessee	X	...	X	...	X	...
Texas	X	...	X	...	X	...
Utah	X	...	X	...	X	...
Vermont..................	X	...	X	...	X	...
Virgin Islands	X	...	X	...	X	...
Virginia	X	...	X	...	X	...
Washington	X	...	X	...	X	...
West Virginia	X	...	X	...	X	...
Wisconsin	X	...	X	...	X	...
Wyoming	X	...	X	...	X	...

SOURCE: American Nurses' Association, Research and Policy Analysis Department, Statistics Unit, special tabulations from licensure table update sheets, 1980.

Table I-H-10. Citation and Chronology of Nursing Practice Acts for Registered Nurses, 1980

State or territory	Citation	Year first law enacted	Amendments to first law	Year of repeal and enactment of new law	Amendments to new law
Alabama	Title 46, Code of Alabama of 1940, as amended.	1915	1927, '31, '35, '39, '40, '45, '55	1966	1976
Alaska	Chapter 68, Title 8, Alaska Statutes.	1941	1949	1953, '57, '67, '72	1960, '62, '66, '68, '69, '70, '73, '74, '76
Arizona	Arizona Revised Statutes Annotated 1956, Chapter 15, Section 32-1601 through 32-1667.	1921	1927, '28, '37	1941, '52	1958, '60, '62, '64, '70, '72, '73, '74, '77
Arkansas	Arkansas Statutes 1947 Annotated, Sections 72-701 through 72-725.	1913	1945, '47, '57	1967, '71	...
California	Chapter 6, Business and Professions Code, enacted 1939, last amended 1978.	1905	1913	1939	1941, '43, '45, '47, '49, '51, '53, '55, '57, '59, '61, '63, '65, '66, '67, '68, '69, '70, '71, '72, '73, '74, '75, '76, '77, '78
Colorado	Chapter 12, Article 38, Part 2 Colorado Revised Statutes, 1973, as amended.	1905	1933, '53	1957, '74	1962, '77
Connecticut	Chapter 378 of General Statutes of State of Connecticut.	1905	1915, '29, '30, '35, '39, '41, '43, '47, '49, '53, '55, '57, '59, '61, '69, '71, '75, '76, '77	...	...
Delaware	Delaware Code, Chapter 153, Vol. 54.	1909	1913, '21, '31, '43, '53, '55	1963	1970
District of Columbia	Code of Laws of D.C., 1973 edition, Title 2, Chapter 4.	1907	...	1929	1945, '46, '63

State	Citation				
Florida	Chapter 464, Florida Revised Statutes, 1975.	1913	1919, '47	1951, '75	1955, '57, '67, '76, '77
Georgia	Georgia Code Annotated, Title 84, Chapters 1001-1041, 9915.	1907	1916, '21	1927, '75	1931, '46, '56, '66, '74, '78
Guam	Government Code of Guam, Chapter 3, Public Law 7-34.	1952	...	1963	1964
Hawaii	Hawaii Revised Statutes, Chapter 457.	1917	1919, '25, '31, '47, '55	1959	1961, '70, '74
Idaho	Idaho Code, Sections 54-1401 through 54-1415.	1911	...	1947, '51, '77	1965, '71, '74
Illinois	Chapter 91, Illinois Revised Statutes.	1907	1910, '13, '17, '19, '31, '35, '39, '41, '43, '47, '49	1951	1959, '61, '63, '65, '73, '75, '80
Indiana	Indiana Code 1976, Title 25, Article 23, Chapter 1, Section 1-28. Amended by Acts 1977. Public Law 172 and Acts 1978. Public Law 2. Acts 1979. Public Law 17. (Burns Indiana Statutes Annotated 24-23-1-1 through 25-23-1-28 (Code Edition)).	1905	1911, '13, '21, '29, '31	1949	1951, '71, '74, '75, '76, '77, '78, '79
Iowa	Code of Iowa, Chapter 147, (general provisions-practice acts), Chapter 152 (Practice of nursing).	1907	1949	1963, '76	1975, '77
Kansas	K.S.A. Chapter 65, Article 11, Chapter 231, Laws of Kansas 1968.	1913	1915, '21, '33, '43, '45	1949	1963, '65, '68, '72, '73, '74, '75, '76
Kentucky	Kentucky Revised Statutes, Chapter 314.	1914	1942, '46	1950, '66, '78	...
Louisiana	Louisiana Revised Statutes 37:911 et seq as amended and reenacted by Act 351 and 200 of 1976 and Act 131 of 1977.	1912	1922, '26, '42, '50, '66, '76, '77	...	...
Maine	Title 32, Revised Statutes 1964, Chapter 31.	1915	1917, '23, '29, '35, '39, '45, '47, '55, '57	1959	1961, '63, '65, '67, '69, '70, '71, '72, '73, '74, '75, '76, '77
Maryland	(1971 Replacement Vol. 1974 Supplement) as amended by Chapter 591 of the General Assembly of Md., 1975.	1904	1917, '22, '46, '55, '62	1967, '75	1969, '70, '73, '74, '75
Massachusetts	Chapters 13 and 112 of G.L., as amended; Chapter 620 Acts of 1941; Chapter 693 Acts of 1960.	1910	1919, '41, '48, '51, '52, '53, '54, '56, '57	...	...

Table I-H-10. (continued)

State or territory	Citation	Year first law enacted	Amendments to first law	Year of repeal and enactment of new law	Amendments to new law
Massachusetts (continued)			'58, '59, '60, '61, '62, '63, '64, '66, '67, '68, '69, '70, '71, '75, '76, '79		
Michigan	Act 149, Public Acts of 1967, as amended.	1909	1913, '21, '39, '52, '54, '57, '65	1967	1973, '74, '75, '76
Minnesota	Minnesota Statutes, Sections 148.171-148.299 (1976 and 1977 Supplement).	1907	1923, '29	1945	1947, '55, '59, '61, '67, '69, '71, '73, '74, '75, '76, '77
Mississippi	Mississippi Code of 1942, Sections 8806-8831.	1914	1932, '48, '54	1954, '70	1968, '70, '74, '76, '77
Missouri	Chapter 335, Missouri Revised Statutes, Supplement 1976.	1909	1914, '21, '23	1953, '76	1971, '73
Montana	Title 37, 8101-8409, 82A-1602.18, RCM-1947.	1913	1919, '25, '33, '43	1947	1953, '63, '67, '74, '75, '77, '79
Nebraska	Compiled Statutes of Nebraska 71-1, 132.04-71-1, 132.42.	1909	1919, '27	1935, '53	1937, '41, '45, '47, '51, '55, '59, '61, '65, '75, '76, '78
Nevada	Nevada Revised Statutes, 1963, Chapter 632.	1923	1933	1945, '47, '63	1949, '55, '59, '61, '69, '73, '75, '77, '79
New Hampshire	Revised Statutes Annotated, 1955, Chapter 326, Chapter 281, Laws of 1975.	1907	1915, '19, '25, '39, '42, '43	1947, '75	1976, '77, '79
New Jersey	P.L. 1947, c.262, as amended; Revised Statutes of New Jersey, Title 45, Chapter 11; Revised Statutes Cumulative Supplement, amended 1958 and 1966.	1903	...	1912, '36, '47	1915, '17, '20, '23, '42, '49, '52, '53, '55, '58, '64, '66, '71, '74

State	Statute				
New Mexico	New Mexico Statutes, Annotated, Chapter 220, Law 1977.	1923	1925, '28	1937, '53	1947, '49, '59, '68, '73, '77
New York	Education Law-Title VIII Education Law 1971, Article 130 and Article 139.	1903	1920, '27	1938, '71	1940, '41, '42, '51, '53, '54, '55, '61, '69, '71, '73, '74, '75, '76
North Carolina	North Carolina General Statutes Chapter 90, Article 9, 158 to 171.18.	1903	1917, '19, '25, '31, '33, '47	1954, '65	1955, '61, '69, '71, '73, '74, '77, '78
North Dakota	Laws governing Professional Nursing N.D. Century Code 43-12.1.	1915	1927, '39, '53, '63, '71	1977	...
Ohio	Ohio Revised Code, Chapter 4723.	1915	1919, '23	1941, '56	1963, '67
Oklahoma	59 Oklahoma Statutes, 1971-567.51.	1909	1913, '21, '25, '35, '39, '43, '45, '49	1953	1963, '67, '76, '78
Oregon	Oregon Laws, Chapter 678, Sections 678.010 to 678.410.	1911	1917, '45, '47, '53, '57, '63, '65, '67, '69, '71	1973	1975, '77, '79
Pennsylvania	The Professional Nurse Law, 63 P.S. 211 et seq.	1909	1915, '19, '23, '27, '35, '45	1951	1959, '68, '70, '74
Rhode Island	Chapter 5-34 of the General Laws, 1956.	1912	1914, '18, '35, '48	1952	1956, '59, '62, '71, '73, '74
South Carolina	1962 Code of Laws of South Carolina, Volume 5, Chapter 17, Articles 1 through 6.	1910	...	1935	1947, '52, '59, '62, '66, '68, '69, '74, '75, '77
South Dakota	Chapter 36-9, Session Laws of 1976.	1917	1919, '31, '37, '39	1947, '49, '55, '67, '76	1969, '72, '74, '75, '77, '78, '79

Table I-H-10. (continued)

State or territory	Citation	Year first law enacted	Amendments to first law	Year of repeal and enactment of new law	Amendments to new law
Tennessee	Public Acts, Chapter No. 7, Title 63, Public Act Annotated 1967.	1911	...	1915, '35, '45, '51, '67	1939, '55, '59, '72, '76
Texas	Vernon's Civil Statutes, Articles 4513-4528.	1909	...	1923	1935, '49, '59, '61, '67, '69, '75, '77, '79
Utah	58-31-1 to 58-31-17 Utah Code Annotated, as amended to and including Session Laws 1963.	1917	1943, '45, '47, '49, '53, '55	1963	1965, '71, '75
Vermont	Title 26, V.S.A. Chapter 27, Section 1551-1552.	1911	1915, '17, '21, '33, '35, '39, '45, '47, '51, '53, '56, '57	1961	1967, '68, '73, '74, '75, '76
Virgin Islands	Virgin Islands Code Title 27.	1945	1945, '46	1952	1956, '60, '69
Virginia	Code of Virginia, Title 54, Chapter 13.1 (as amended at the 1975 session of the General Assembly).	1903	1916, '18, '22, '44, '46, '56, '60, '66, '70, '74, '75, '79	...	...
Washington	Chapter 18.88, Revised Code of Washington.	1909	1923, '33, '49, '55, '61, '71, '73	...	...
West Virginia	Chapter 30, Article 7, Code of West Virginia of 1931, as amended.	1907	1917, '25, '37	1945	1951, '57, '65, '71, '72, '73
Wisconsin	Chapter 441, Wisconsin Statutes.	1911	1913, '15, '18, '21, '41, '43, '45, '47, '49, '55, '59, '61, '63, '65, '67, '69, '71, '73, '75, '77, '79	...	...
Wyoming	Wyoming Statutes 33-279.1 through 33-279.18.	1909	1943, '47, '51, '53	1955, '75	1967

SOURCE: American Nurses' Association, Research and Policy Analysis Department, Statistics Unit, special tabulations from licensure table update sheets, 1980.

Table I-H-11. Selected Fees Charged for Licensure of Registered Nurses, 1980

State or territory	Examination	Endorsement	Renewal[1]	Verification of original license to other boards
Alabama	$55.00	$45.00	[2]$12.00	$5.00
Alaska	40.00	40.00	[2]15.00	...
Arizona	50.00	45.00	10.00	...
Arkansas	30.00	30.00	[2]10.00	15.00
California	35.00	35.00	[2]16.00	2.00
Colorado	40.00	30.00	[2]10.00	10.00
Connecticut	30.00	30.00	10.00	2.00
Delaware	30.00	30.00	[2]10.00	2.00
District of Columbia	(3)	(3)	(3)	(3)
Florida	50.00	30.00	6.00	6.00
Georgia	30.00	50.00	[2]20.00	...
Guam	50.00	50.00	10.00	10.00
Hawaii	30.00	30.00	[2]10.00	5.00
Idaho	65.00	50.00	[2]25.00	5.00
Illinois	25.00	25.00	[2]10.00	...
Indiana	40.00	25.00	[2]10.00	...
Iowa	40.00	25.00	6.00	5.00
Kansas	35.00	35.00	[2]12.00	5.00
Kentucky	50.00	35.00	10.00	4.00
Louisiana	55.00	25.00	10.00	10.00
Maine	40.00	40.00	10.00	2.00
Maryland	35.00	35.00	[2]2.00	2.00
Massachusetts	30.00	50.00	[2]6.00	2.00
Michigan	45.00	25.00	5.00	...
Minnesota	60.00	35.00	[2]15.00	5.00
Mississippi	50.00	50.00	[2]8.00	6.00
Missouri	25.00	25.00	5.00	...
Montana	35.00	35.00	10.00	...
Nebraska	50.00	50.00	7.00	5.00
Nevada	65.00	45.00	[2]15.00	...
New Hampshire	40.00	40.00	[2]10.00	5.00
New Jersey	35.00	25.00	[2]10.00	5.00
New Mexico	75.00	62.00	[2]15.00	5.00
New York	60.00	40.00	[2]10.00	10.00
North Carolina	27.00	30.00	[2]12.00	10.00
North Dakota	65.00	65.00	20.00	10.00
Ohio	30.00	30.00	3.00	...
Oklahoma	55.00	55.00	10.00	...
Oregon	45.00	35.00	[2]25.00	...
Pennsylvania	10.00	10.00	[2]4.00	...
Rhode Island	30.00	30.00	5.00	3.00
South Carolina	50.00	50.00	10.00	5.00
South Dakota	45.00	45.00	[2]15.00	5.00
Tennessee	50.00	50.00	[2]8.00	...
Texas	30.00	30.00	4.00	5.00
Utah	30.00	30.00	7.50	...
Vermont	46.00	25.00	[2]10.00	...
Virgin Islands	10.00	...	1.00	...
Virginia	50.00	30.00	5.00	5.00
Washington	25.00	25.00	8.00	3.00
West Virginia	40.00	30.00	5.00	5.00
Wisconsin	50.00	50.00	[2]25.00	10.00
Wyoming	50.00	50.00	8.00	5.00

[1] Renewal fee applies to annual registration unless otherwise indicated.
[2] Biennial renewal.
[3] Not reported.

SOURCE: American Nurses' Association, Research and Policy Analysis Department, Statistics Unit, special tabulations from licensure table update sheets, 1980.

**Table I-H-12. Applications and Re-applications of Foreign Nurse
Graduates Submitted for the First 5 CGFNS Examinations,
October 1978-October 1980**

Applications and re-applications	Number	Percent
Submitted to CGFNS	7,124	100.0
Eligible and scheduled for examination	5,256	73.8
Tested or re-tested	4,823	(91.8)
Did not appear	433	(8.2)
Ineligible for examination	459	6.4
Cancelled application	98	1.4
Deferred application	202	2.8
Incomplete application	1,109	15.6

SOURCE: Commission on Graduates of Foreign Nursing Schools, 1980. Unpublished data.

**Table I-H-13. Graduates of Nursing Schools in 56 Foreign Countries
Tested by CGFNS, October 1978-October 1980**

Foreign nurse graduates	Number	Percent
Tested by CGFNS	4,417	100.0
Received CGFNS Certificate (passed nursing and English)	1,230	27.8
On first examination	1,163	(94.6)
On repeat examination	67	(5.4)
Have not passed nursing and English	3,187	72.2

SOURCE: Commission on Graduates of Foreign Nursing Schools, 1980. Unpublished data.

Table I-H-14. Personal Characteristics of Foreign Nurse Graduates Tested by CGFNS, October 1978-October 1980

Personal characteristics	Applicants	
	Number	Percent
Total	4,417	100.0
Sex		
Female	4,160	94.2
Male	257	5.8
Age		
22 years or under	1,002	22.7
23-27	2,733	61.9
28-32	468	10.6
33-37	134	3.0
38 years or over	80	1.8
Marital status		
Single	3,811	86.3
Married	535	12.1
Divorced	32	0.7
Widowed	11	0.2
Not applicable	28	0.6
Type of nursing program		
Degree	2,116	47.9
Non-degree	2,301	52.1

SOURCE: Commission on Graduates of Foreign Nursing Schools, 1980. Unpublished data.

Table I-H-15. Examination Results of Foreign Nurse Graduates Taking CGFNS Examination for First Time, October 1978-October 1980

Nursing and English examination results	Number	Percent
Total	4,417	100.0
Nursing passed/English passed	1,163	26.3
Nursing passed/English failed	65	1.5
Nursing failed/English passed	1,748	39.6
Nursing failed/English failed	1,441	32.6

SOURCE: Commission on Graduates of Foreign Nursing Schools, 1980. Unpublished data.

Table I-H-16. Distribution of Nursing Subject Areas Passed by Foreign Nurse Graduates Taking CGFNS Examination for First Time, October 1978-October 1980

Nursing subject areas	Number passed	Percent passed
	N = 4,417	
Medical nursing	2,963	67.1
Psychiatric nursing	1,706	38.6
Obstetric nursing	2,853	64.6
Surgical nursing	2,376	53.8
Nursing of children	2,107	47.7

SOURCE: Commission on Graduates of Foreign Nursing Schools, 1980. Unpublished data.

Table I-H-17. Registered Nurses Certified by the American Nurses' Association, 1975-1980

Structural unit and certification program title	Total	1980	1979	1978	1977	1976	1975
Total	4,734	2,190	997	285	722	441	99
Commission on Nursing Services							
Nursing Administration	321	321	...	...	...	...	...
Nursing Administration, Advanced	164	164	...	...	...	...	...
Community Health Nursing Practice							
Adult Nurse Practitioner	1,248	635	340	...	273	...	...
Community Health Nurse	89	6	18	10	32	23	...
Family Nurse Practitioner	1,230	573	293	...	364	...	...
School Nurse Practitioner	130	130	...	...	...	...	...
Gerontological Nursing Practice							
Gerontological Nurse	307	69	55	27	53	68	35
Gerontological Nurse Practitioner	15	15	...	...	...	...	...
Maternal and Child Health Nursing Practice							
Maternal-Gynecological-Neonatal Nursing[1]	378	...	97	110	...	171	...
Pediatric Nurse Practitioner	208	74	44	32	...	43	15
Nursing of Child/Adolescent with Acute/Chronic Illness/Disabling Condition	11	11	...	...	...	...	...
Medical-Surgical Nursing Practice							
Medical-Surgical Nurse	105	40	22	...	...	43	...
Medical-Surgical Clinical Specialist	46	22	10	2	...	12	...
Psychiatric-Mental Health Nursing Practice							
Psychiatric and Mental Health Nurse	259	70	55	4	...	81	49
Psychiatric and Mental Health Clinical Specialist-Adult	209	55	62	92	...	...	...
Psychiatric and Mental Health Clinical Specialist-Child	14	5	1	8	...	...	...

[1]A joint certification program with NAACOG Certification Corporation.

SOURCE: American Nurses' Association, Credentialing Department, 1980. Unpublished data.

Chapter I, Section I
NURSING ASSOCIATIONS

The American Nurses' Association, the national professional organization for registered nurses, was first established in 1896. As enunciated in its bylaws, the purposes of the association are to foster high standards for nursing practice, promote the professional and educational advancement of nurses, and promote the welfare of nurses to the end that all people have better nursing care. The nursing profession has become an effective national force through the leadership and resources of ANA. By providing a forum for seeking solutions to the problems the profession encounters, ANA is instrumental in advancing the nursing profession in today's society.

As of December 31, 1979, ANA membership totalled 181,212. About 83.6 percent of the members were full members, and 16.4 percent paid reduced membership dues. Nurses eligible for reduced membership fees include those not employed, registered nurse students engaged in full-time study, new graduates for the first year of membership, and those 62 years of age or older who earn no more than social security allows without loss of payment.

Membership in ANA is tri-level: national, state, and district. The 50 states, the District of Columbia, Guam, and the Virgin Islands comprise ANA's 53 constituents. In turn, the state nurses' associations are composed of over 800 district nurses' associations. State nurses' association memberships as of December 31, 1979, ranged from 167 nurses in the Virgin Islands to 16,576 nurses in California.

Nurses belonging to ANA may affiliate at the national level with one or two of five divisions on practice: community health nursing, gerontological nursing, medical-surgical nursing, maternal and child health nursing, and psychiatric and mental health nursing. These ANA divisions establish standards for nursing practice, recognize professional achievement, conduct clinical conferences, promote research, and disseminate information to advance nursing practice.

Structural units based upon occupational and/or clinical interest groups at the state level are depicted in two tables in this section. In 1979, SNAs reported 143 conferences and special interest groups and 61 sections.

Participation in preprofessional organizational activities for undergraduate nursing students is provided by membership in the National Student Nurses' Association. As of August 1977, 31,893 nursing students enrolled in basic nursing educational programs belonged to the NSNA. California was the constituent with the largest membership (6,022 students), followed by Texas, with 2,800 members.

The national nurses' associations of 89 countries belong to the International Council of Nurses, headquartered in Geneva, Switzerland, as of December 31, 1979. Among the largest organizations in the ICN federation are Japan, the United States, Canada, and the United Kingdom.

Further information about the structures and programs of ANA, NSNA, ICN, and other nursing organizations appear in Chapter VI.

Table I-I-1. Membership in the American Nurses' Association, by Type of Membership, December 31, 1978 and 1979

State or territory	1979 Total	1979 Members	1979 Reduced membership dues group	1978 Total	1978 Members	1978 Reduced membership dues group
Total	181,212	151,560	29,652	186,573	155,689	30,884
Alabama	3,362	2,681	681	3,914	3,087	827
Alaska	360	286	74	403	320	83
Arizona	1,857	1,407	450	2,032	1,552	480
Arkansas	764	569	195	821	640	181
California	16,576	14,350	2,226	16,602	14,147	2,455
Colorado	2,681	2,094	587	2,958	2,263	695
Connecticut	1,720	1,401	319	1,715	1,392	323
Delaware	726	562	164	712	557	155
District of Columbia	1,522	1,279	243	1,685	1,432	253
Florida	3,489	3,019	470	3,142	2,669	473
Georgia	2,550	2,109	441	2,553	2,078	475
Guam	177	170	7	176	168	8
Hawaii	1,467	1,362	105	1,958	1,830	128
Idaho	817	689	128	815	689	126
Illinois	9,535	8,032	1,503	10,288	8,572	1,716
Indiana	2,779	2,260	519	2,804	2,276	528
Iowa	1,883	1,608	275	1,869	1,599	270
Kansas	1,858	1,555	303	1,934	1,602	332
Kentucky	1,694	1,393	301	1,857	1,565	292
Louisiana	2,467	2,067	400	2,388	2,038	350
Maine	796	644	152	845	687	158
Maryland	3,815	3,031	784	3,817	3,037	780
Massachusetts	9,807	8,536	1,271	9,911	8,617	1,294
Michigan	8,295	7,021	1,274	8,303	7,028	1,275
Minnesota	10,089	9,062	1,027	9,650	8,675	975
Mississippi	2,371	1,882	489	2,367	1,937	430
Missouri	3,797	2,850	947	4,108	3,094	1,014
Montana	1,272	1,108	164	1,273	1,108	165
Nebraska	1,269	1,006	263	1,354	1,091	263
Nevada	522	423	99	541	445	96
New Hampshire	878	712	166	889	713	176
New Jersey	6,819	5,602	1,217	5,785	4,629	1,156
New Mexico	825	617	208	806	613	193
New York	14,779	12,616	2,163	15,842	13,347	2,495
North Carolina	3,259	2,594	665	3,216	2,621	595
North Dakota	738	629	109	779	669	110
Ohio	9,649	7,592	2,057	9,852	7,566	2,286
Oklahoma	1,747	1,373	374	1,828	1,435	393
Oregon	4,332	3,973	359	4,350	3,916	434
Pennsylvania	9,989	8,476	1,513	9,861	8,519	1,342
Rhode Island	617	442	175	1,140	976	164
South Carolina	1,388	1,131	257	1,561	1,288	273
South Dakota	698	608	90	726	621	105
Tennessee	2,692	2,136	556	2,716	2,196	520
Texas	5,413	4,069	1,344	6,003	4,597	1,406
Utah	888	679	209	1,062	814	248
Vermont	515	426	89	492	407	85
Virginia	2,510	1,844	666	2,553	1,925	628
Virgin Islands	167	152	15	132	117	15
Washington	7,838	7,114	724	8,035	7,226	809
West Virginia	1,437	1,183	254	1,488	1,197	291
Wisconsin	2,330	1,985	345	3,334	2,989	345
Wyoming	387	322	65	448	378	70
Individual	1,000	829	171	880	735	145

SOURCE: American Nurses' Association, Research and Policy Analysis Department, Statistics Unit, 1980. Unpublished data.

Table I-1-2. Sections of State and Territorial Nurses' Associations, 1979

State or territory	Educational administrators, consultants, and teachers	General duty	Nursing service administration	Office	Private duty	Public health	School nurse	Community health	Psychiatric/ mental health practice	Geriatric nursing practice	Maternal and child health	Medical/ surgical	Other
Total	4	4	5	2	5	5	3	5	5	5	6	6	6
Alabama	(1)												
Alaska	(1)	(1)	(1)	(1)	(1)	(1)	(1)	(1)	(1)	(1)	(1)	(1)	(1)
Arizona													
Arkansas													
California													
Colorado													
Connecticut													
Delaware						X		[2]X	[2]X	[2]X	[2]X	[1]X	
District of Columbia													
Florida								[4]X	[4]X	[4]X	[4]X	[4]X	[5]X
Georgia													[6]X
Guam	(1)	(1)	(1)	(1)	(1)	(1)	(1)	(1)	(1)	(1)	(1)[2]X	(1)[3]X	(1)
Hawaii													
Idaho													
Illinois													
Indiana													
Iowa													
Kansas													
Kentucky				X	X	X							
Louisiana						X		X					
Maine													
Maryland								[7]X	[7]X	[7]X	[7]X	[7]X	
Massachusetts	X	X	X										
Michigan	X	X	X	X				X					[8]X
Minnesota								X					
Mississippi													
Missouri													
Montana													
Nebraska													
Nevada													

New Hampshire											
New Jersey											
New Mexico											
New York	X	X	X	X	X	X	X				
North Carolina					X						
North Dakota	X	X	X	X	X	X	[2]X	X	X	[2]X	[2]X	[9]X
Ohio	X	X	X	X	X	X	X	X	X	X	X	[10]X
Oklahoma								X	X	X	X	[5,10,11]X
Oregon												
Pennsylvania												
Rhode Island												
South Carolina												
South Dakota												
Tennessee												
Texas												
Utah												
Vermont												
Virginia												
Virgin Islands	(1)	(1)	(1)	(1)	(1)	(1)	(1)	(1)	(1)	(1)	(1)	(1)
Washington												
West Virginia												
Wisconsin												
Wyoming												

[1] Not reported.
[2] Includes both a clinical practice and an advanced practice section.
[3] Advanced practice section.
[4] Includes divisions.
[5] Advanced practice areas combined (community health, gerontological, maternal/child health, medical/surgical and psychiatric/mental health); includes divisions in Florida.
[6] Awards—annual, district honorees.
[7] Advanced practice clinical sections.
[8] Head nurse.
[9] Current and long-term goals.
[10] Occupational health nurse.
[11] Operating room nursing practice.

SOURCE: American Nurses' Association, Research and Policy Analysis Department, Statistics Unit. Special tabulation prepared by the American Nurses' Association in cooperation with the state nurses' associations, 1980. Unpublished data.

Table I-1.3. Conference and Special Interest Groups in State and Territorial Nurses' Associations, 1979

State or territory	Advanced practice areas combined	Community health	Gerontological	Maternal/child health	Medical/surgical	Psychiatric/mental health	Educational administrators, consultants, and teachers	Nursing service administration	Occupational health	Operating room nursing practice	Private duty	School nurse	Other
Total	3	14	16	17	12	15	9	9	4	4	7	10	23
Alabama													
Alaska	(1)	(1)	(1)	(1)	(1)	(1)	(1)	(1)	(1)	(1)	(1)	(1)	(1)
Arizona			X	X	X	X		[2]X				[2]X	[3]X
Arkansas													[4]X
California													
Colorado						X						X	[4,5]X
Connecticut												X	
Delaware													[6]X
District of Columbia													
Florida													
Georgia	(1)	[?]X	[?]X	[?]X	[?]X	[?]X	(1)	(1)	(1)	(1)	(1)	(1)	(1)
Guam	(1)	(1)	(1)	(1)	(1)	(1)		X				X	
Hawaii												X	
Idaho		X	X	X	X	X	X		X				
Illinois													
Indiana		[?]X	X	X	[10]X	X		X	X	X	X	X	[11]X
Iowa		X	X	[?]X	[?]X	[?]X	X	X					
Kansas		X	X	X	X	X							[12]X
Kentucky													
Louisiana													
Maine													
Maryland									X		X		[13,14]X
Massachusetts													[15]X
Michigan										X			[16]X
Minnesota				X		X				X			[17]X
Mississippi		[?]X	[?]X	[?]X	[?]X	[?]X	[?]X	[?]X	[?]X	[?]X	[?]X	[?]X	[18]X
Missouri		[?]X	[?]X	[?]X	[?]X	[?]X							
Montana													
Nebraska													
Nevada	[19]X												
New Hampshire													
New Jersey													
New Mexico	X	X	X	X								X	
New York							[20]X						[21]X
North Carolina						[?]X							[?]X

State										
North Dakota									X	[14,22] X
Ohio										
Oklahoma				X	X	X		X	X	[19,23] X
Oregon	X			X	X	X		X	X	[17] X
Pennsylvania					X	X				
Rhode Island	X			X	X	X			X	[4,25,24] X
South Carolina						X		X	X	[25] X
South Dakota	[1] X	[1] X	X	X	X	X		X	X	[25] X
Tennessee	X	X	X	X	X	X	X	X	X	[13,26] X
Texas	X		X	X	X	X		X	X	
Utah	[1] X	[1] X								[12,27] X
Vermont	X	X	X	X	[1] X					[28] X
Virginia	[1] X	[1] X	X	X	X	X		X	X	[4,29] X
Virgin Islands	[1] X	[1] X	[1]	[1]	[1]	[1]	[1]	[1]	[1]	[1]
Washington										
West Virginia										
Wisconsin										
Wyoming	X									

[1] Not reported.
[2] Occupational interest group.
[3] Gynecological nurse practitioner and primary care nurse practitioner occupational interest groups.
[4] Nurse practitioners.
[5] Inservice education.
[6] Current and long-term goals—board retreat, annual.
[7] Advanced practice.
[8] Includes both clinical and advanced practice.
[9] Includes occupational health nurse, office nurse and public health nurse.
[10] Includes nursing care of the adult.
[11] Nurses as change agents; emergency nursing, intensive and coronary care nursing.
[12] Public health nurse.
[13] Advanced practice (area not specified).
[14] Research and studies.
[15] Ambulatory care functional specialty group; nurse practitioner functional specialty group; staff development functional specialty group.
[16] Advocates for child psychiatric nursing; nurses working in MR/DD.
[17] Manpower.
[18] General duty nurse occupational interest group; office nurse occupational interest group; public health occupational interest group.
[19] Nurse practitioners advanced practice.
[20] Nurse practitioners advanced practice.
[21] School nurse teachers specialty group; primary care practitioners specialty group; directors, associates and assistants, nursing practice and services specialty group; continuing education, staff development personnel specialty group.
[22] Specialty group.
[23] Scholarships.
[24] College health.
[25] Inservice education; legistative committee; nursing diagnosis.
[26] Primary care practitioners and/or clinicians.
[27] General duty nurse; nursing education; office nurse.
[28] Emergency health preparedness.
[29] Joint practice group of nurse practitioners and physicians.
[30] Management administrative professional practice group; continuing education providers.

SOURCE: American Nurses' Association, Research and Policy Analysis Department, Statistics Unit. Special tabulation prepared by the American Nurses' Association in cooperation with the state nurses' associations, 1980. Unpublished data.

**Table I-I-4. Constituent Associations of the National Student Nurses'
Association and their Membership, August 1976 and 1977**

State or territory	Number of members		State or territory	Number of members	
	1976	1977		1976	1977
Total	36,299	31,893			
Alabama	1,233	1,083	Montana	181	177
Alaska	...	...	Nebraska	369	401
Arizona	421	291	Nevada	83	97
Arkansas	412	367	New Hampshire	294	294
California	6,536	6,022	New Jersey	1,071	630
Colorado	187	286	New Mexico	333	403
Connecticut	75	16	New York	1,085	767
Delaware	57	68	North Carolina	826	808
District of Columbia	103	68	North Dakota	168	240
Florida	723	797	Ohio	1,285	826
Georgia	704	732	Oklahoma	703	933
Guam	...	...	Oregon	319	210
Hawaii	186	109	Pennsylvania	2,102	1,059
Idaho	233	209	Puerto Rico	...	1
Illinois	934	766	Rhode Island	75	47
Indiana	984	951	South Carolina	534	643
Iowa	396	352	South Dakota	588	604
Kansas	427	379	Tennessee	457	414
Kentucky	451	476	Texas	3,424	2,800
Louisiana	837	738	Utah	263	220
Maine	68	76	Vermont	1	...
Maryland	104	67	Virginia	868	906
Massachusetts	843	524	Virgin Islands	43	30
Michigan	555	625	Washington	456	407
Minnesota	587	560	West Virginia	484	494
Mississippi	1,258	1,224	Wisconsin	897	961
Missouri	1,021	729	Wyoming	55	6

SOURCE: National Student Nurses' Association, 1978. Unpublished data.

Table I-I-5. Members of National Nurses' Associations in
Membership with International Council of Nurses, December 31, 1979

Country	Number of members	Country	Number of members
Argentina	[1]750	Malaysia (West)	950
Australia	30,670	Mauritius	[1]1,187
Austria	4,681	Mexico	[1]500
Bahamas	[1]212	Morocco	[1]200
Barbados	[1]121	Nepal	130
Belgium	1,204	Netherlands	5,158
Bermuda	84	New Zealand	[1]8,384
Bolivia	250	Nicaragua	[1]200
Botswana	210	Nigeria	[1]3,000
Brazil	3,100	Norway	24,416
Burma	[1]420	Pakistan	[1]510
Canada	126,761	Panama	[1]450
Chile	1,900	Paraguay	[1]120
Colombia	[1]500	Peru	[1]815
Costa Rica	987	Philippines	4,500
Cyprus	(2)	Poland	6,000
Denmark	35,395	Portugal	174
Ecuador	[1]240	Puerto Rico	[1]1,516
Egypt	[1]510	Rhodesia (Zimbabwe)	577
Ethiopia	[1]200	Saint Lucia	[1]110
Fiji	[1]1,060	Salvador (El)	450
Finland	22,417	Senegal	[1]300
France	1,935	Sierra Leone	[1]120
Gambia	[1]80	Singapore	[1]1,000
Germany (Federal Rep. of)	6,481	Spain	25,000
Ghana (British)	2,550	Sri Lanka (Ceylon)	200
Greece	[1]1,000	Sudan	[1]255
Guyana	[1]240	Swaziland	210
Haiti	133	Sweden	51,564
Honduras	[1]521	Switzerland	[1]11,725
Hong Kong	[1]1,578	Taiwan (Rep. of China)	[1]2,854
Iceland	1,078	Tanzania	[1]559
India	[1]4,421	Thailand	1,774
Iran	[1]277	Trinidad & Tobago	[1]230
Ireland	[1]6,265	Turkey	[1]514
Israel	[1]9,500	Uganda	[1]100
Italy	1,134	United Kingdom	99,387
Jamaica	[1]1,136	United States	156,712
Japan	157,111	Uruguay	250
Jordan	[1]370	Venezuela	1,980
Kenya	1,000	Western Samoa	[1]300
Korea (South)	[1]6,500	Yugoslavia	[1]4,500
Lebanon	1,000	Zaire	[1]700
Liberia	101	Zambia	[1]339
Luxembourg	25		

[1] Figures do not represent 1979 membership; totals presented are those last registered by member associations.
[2] Information not available.

SOURCE: International Council of Nurses, 1980.

Table I-I-6. Members of National Nurses' Associations in Membership with International Council of Nurses, December 31, 1978

Country	Number of members	Country	Number of members
Argentina	750	Malaysia (West)	1,000
Australia	28,758	Mauritius	1,187
Austria	4,645	Mexico	500
Bahamas	¹212	Morocco	¹200
Barbados	121	Nepal	68
Belgium	1,287	Netherlands	5,529
Bermuda	100	New Zealand	8,384
Bolivia	220	Nicaragua	200
Botswana	200	Nigeria	¹3,000
Brazil	2,500	Norway	19,638
Burma	¹420	Pakistan	¹510
Canada	121,494	Panama	450
Chile	2,309	Paraguay	120
Colombia	500	Peru	¹815
Costa Rica	916	Philippines	2,000
Denmark	34,428	Poland	6,000
Ecuador	¹240	Portugal	62
Egypt	510	Puerto Rico	1,516
Ethiopia	200	Rhodesia (Zimbabwe)	500
Fiji	1,060	Saint Lucia	110
Finland	21,535	Salvador (El)	400
France	1,912	Senegal	300
Gambia	¹80	Sierra Leone	¹120
Germany (Fed. Rep. of)	6,205	Singapore	1,000
Ghana (British)	2,500	Spain	25,000
Greece	1,000	Sri Lanka (Ceylon)	200
Guyana	240	Sudan	¹255
Haiti	139	Swaziland	210
Honduras	¹521	Sweden	69,291
Hong Kong	1,578	Switzerland	11,725
Iceland	1,013	Taiwan (Rep. of China)	2,854
India	4,421	Tanzania	¹559
Iran	277	Thailand	1,724
Ireland	6,265	Trinidad & Tobago	230
Israel	9,500	Turkey	¹514
Italy	1,203	Uganda	¹100
Jamaica	1,136	United Kingdom	81,091
Japan	157,111	United States	155.242
Jordan	370	Uruguay	200
Kenya	1,000	Venezuela	1,940
Korea (South)	6,500	Western Samoa	300
Lebanon	1,000	Yugoslavia	4,500
Liberia	300	Zaire	¹700
Luxembourg	25	Zambia	¹339

¹Figures do not represent 1978 membership; totals presented are those last registered by member associations.
SOURCE: International Council of Nurses, 1980.

Chapter II, Section A
STUDENTS

Annual statistics on students in nursing education are gathered and compiled by the National League for Nursing. NLN statistics include data on student admissions, enrollments, and graduations in basic programs preparing candidates for licensure as registered nurses. Nursing education data are most useful for assessing trends in recruitment into the field of nursing and for analysis and projection of the future supply of registered nurses.

To prepare for licensure as a registered nurse, an individual can attend one of three types of nursing educational programs: diploma, associate degree, and baccalaureate. A nursing diploma is obtained after graduation from a hospital-based program, which is usually 3 years in duration. Basic nursing education provided in a 2-year community or junior college leads to an associate degree in nursing, and that provided through a 4-year collegiate program results in a bachelor's degree in nursing.

In academic year 1977-78, the admissions to all three types of initial nursing educational programs totaled 111,928, a 1.4 percent decrease from the previous year. It should be noted that this figure represents the first decline in total admissions to nursing schools in more than a decade. The last such drop was observed in academic year 1966-67. Decomposition of the 1977-78 admission data according to the type of program showed 20,611 students were admitted to diploma programs, 53,653, to associate degree programs, and 37,664, to baccalaureate and higher degree programs. The relative distributions of these admissions among the programs were 18.4 percent, 47.9 percent, and 33.7 percent, respectively. Over the past 10 years the proportion of admissions to diploma programs has dropped to less than half, while the relative proportions of associate degree and baccalaureate admissions have increased by about two-thirds (62.4 percent) and one-third (35.3 percent), respectively.

The 1977-78 data also revealed a first-time decline (1.4 percent) in admissions to associate degree programs since their introduction in the mid-1950s. A somewhat larger downward trend (7.3 percent) was exhibited in admissions to diploma programs. Only the baccalaureate programs marked growth (1.9 percent) in their admissions over the previous year.

Although total admissions dropped, nursing did not appear to be losing ground as an attractive career choice. Since the preponderance of first-year nursing students were recent high school graduates and female, comparisons over the years between admissions to basic nursing educational programs and the number of female high school graduates has been informative. About 7.1 percent of the 1976-77 female high school graduates were admitted to initial

Total graduates from all initial programs climbed from 78,461 in 1976-77 to 78,697 in 1977-78, continuing a decade-long upward trend; however, the current data portrayed the lowest net gain (0.3 percent) in graduations in comparison to any other year-to-year change since 1966. Of the 1977-78 nursing educational programs in 1977-78. This percentage has remained fairly constant in recent years.

nursing school graduates, almost half (47.1 percent) came from associate degree programs; about one-third (31.1 percent) from baccalaureate programs; and the remaining 21.8 percent earned diplomas. These data reflected the long-term decline in the number of diploma graduates in contrast with the uninterrupted growth in the number of graduates from associate degree and baccalaureate programs. The net year-to-year gains for the latter two programs over the past 5 years, however, might portend sluggish, if any substantial growth in the ensuing years. This picture exacerbates a particular dilemma for nursing when consideration is given to the acute demands in health care for nurses with baccalaureate and higher preparation. More baccalaureate prepared nurses are required for direct patient care roles, for supervisory positions, and to provide an expanded pool from which the master's and doctoral programs in nursing may draw.

The number of enrollments in initial programs preparing individuals for registered nurse licensure is reported annually as of October 15. Enrollments in nursing educational programs continued to dwindle, from 247,739 in 1977 to 242,259 in 1978, a decline of 2.2 percent. This rate marked the third consecutive year that aggregate enrollments were down. Review of enrollments by type of program showed a decrease in both diploma and baccalaureate programs, dropping 9.1 percent and 1.2 percent to 48,059 and 101,239, respectively. For diploma programs these figures portrayed a continuation of a 6-year decelerating pattern, while the negative growth in baccalaureate enrollments was unprecedented—at least over the last two decades. Associate degree programs had a negligible net gain of 574 students, representing a 0.6 percent increase.

The vast majority of nursing students, 197,366, were enrolled in NLN-accredited programs; 44,893 were in nonaccredited programs. It might be noted that NLN accreditation is voluntary, but state accreditation is not. NLN accreditation, aimed at the maintenance of quality nursing education, was granted to 958 programs in 1978. There was some disparity among the various types of nursing programs with respect to NLN accreditation. The 1978 data showed 93.3 percent of the diploma programs, 83.0 percent of the baccalaureate programs, and 50.8 percent of the associate degree programs were accredited by NLN. The relative proportions within each type of program attaining NLN accreditation has been on the upswing in recent years.

NLN periodically compiles data on admissions, graduations, and enrollments of minority groups in nursing. The latest triennial survey was conducted in 1978. Overall, about 87 percent of the initial RN programs responded to the questionnaire. Of the 1,214 responding programs, three-quarters reported having admitted at least one minority student that year. About two-thirds (62 percent) admitted at least one black; and about equal proportions (37 percent and 36 percent) reported admitting at least one Hispanic and one American Indian or Asian. The reporting programs accounted for 101,438 admissions to basic nursing educational programs, of which 11,212, or 11.1 percent were racial/ethnic minorities. While numerically more minority students entered associate degree programs, there was little disparity between the relative proportions of minority admissions to either associate degree or baccalaureate programs (11.8 percent and 12.3 percent, respectively). In contrast, 6.9 percent of the diploma program admissions were racial/ethnic minorities.

In terms of enrollments, about 83 percent of the responding programs reported having at least one minority student. These programs represented 219,582 of the total enrollments in basic programs. Minority enrollments numbered 18,692, or 8.5 percent of the total. Baccalaureate and associate degree programs showed the largest numbers of minority enrollments (8,889 and 7,612 students). The percentages of minority students in these programs were almost twice the rate reported by the diploma programs (9.4 percent and 9.5 percent versus 4.9 percent). Blacks constituted the largest percentages of racial/ethnic minority enrollments in each type of nursing program.

Graduations from the responding programs totaled 70,432 students, of whom 5,724, or 8.1 percent, were minorities. About two-thirds of the basic nursing programs indicated that at least one minority student had graduated in 1978 from their programs. About 10.7 percent of the graduates from associate degree programs were minorities, as were 7.3 percent of the graduates of baccalaureate and 3.9 percent of the graduates of diploma programs.

The NLN survey provided some evidence of slight declines in the relative proportions of male students in initial RN programs from 1975 to 1978. Judgment must be exercised, however, in the interpretation of these trend data because of differential response patterns in each year. In 1975, 7.7 percent of the admissions, 6.0 percent of the enrollments, and 7.3 percent of the graduates from responding programs were men. Comparable figures in 1978 showed men comprised 6.3 percent of the 101,438 admissions, 4.7 percent of the 219,582 enrollments, and 5.5 percent of the 70,432 graduations from the surveyed programs. There was variation in the proportionate representation of men by type of program, with the associate degree programs recording the greatest percentages, followed by the baccalaureate programs.

NLN presented similar data on licensed practical nurses who returned to school to prepare for registered nurse licensure. In 1978, 6,369 LPNs were admitted to the 1,214 programs in the survey. The associate degree programs continued to be the most popular choice for licensed practical nurses. About 11.2 percent of the admissions, 8.3 percent of the enrollees, and 12.4 percent of the graduates of associate degree programs held practical or vocational nurse licenses.

The U.S. Department of Justice, Immigration and Naturalization Service, provided information on the numbers of nurses admitted to the United States as exchange-visitors and trainees. The decade-long trend for reduced numbers of registered nurses, nursing students, and health trainees with exchange-visitor status to enter the country remained almost unabated. From 1977 to 1978, their number declined 43.7 percent to 111 nurses. Admissions to the United States of industrial trainees was more variable. When location of origin was taken into account, declines were observed from almost every continent in the number of exchange-visitors and industrial trainees admitted to this country; however, the largest aggregate decreases were recorded for Asia, North America, and Africa.

Table II-A-1. Admissions of Students to Initial Programs—R.N.[1] in the
United States and Outlying Areas,[2] Academic Years 1968-69 to 1977-78

Academic year[3]	Total number	Diploma		Associate degree		Baccalaureate[4]	
		Number	Percent of total	Number	Percent of total	Number	Percent of total
1977-78 ...	111,928	20,611	18.4	53,653	47.9	37,664	33.7
1976-77 ...	113,479	22,243	19.6	54,289	47.8	36,947	32.6
1975-76 ...	113,311	23,622	20.8	53,033	46.8	36,656	32.3
1974-75 ...	110,068	24,696	22.4	50,180	45.6	35,192	32.0
1973-74 ...	108,210	26,943	24.9	48,595	44.9	32,672	30.2
1972-73 ...	104,713	29,848	28.5	44,387	42.4	30,478	29.1
1971-72 ...	94,154	29,801	31.7	36,996	39.3	27,357	29.1
1970-71 ...	79,282	28,980	36.6	29,889	37.7	20,413	25.7
1969-70 ...	70,428	28,996	41.2	23,797	33.8	17,635	25.0
1968-69 ...	64,157	29,267	45.6	18,907	29.5	15,983	24.9

[1]Includes admissions to programs closed prior to October 15.
[2]Includes Guam, Puerto Rico, and Virgin Islands.
[3]Reporting dates for 1970-71 through 1977-78 are August 1-July 31; reporting dates for 1968-69 and 1969-70
are September 1-August 31.
[4]Includes students admitted to initial programs leading to a master's degree: 1977-78, 122; 1976-77, 109; 1975-
76, 63; 1974-75, 64; 1973-74, 48; 1972-73, 48; 1971-72, 45; 1970-71, 35; 1969-70, 19; 1968-69, 33.
SOURCE: National League for Nursing, *State-Approved Schools of Nursing—R.N., 1979*, and previous
                    years.

Table II-A-2. Percent Change over Previous Year in Admissions of
Students to Initial Programs—R.N.[1] in the United States and Outlying
Areas,[2] Academic Years 1968-69 to 1977-78

Academic year[3]	Total	Diploma	Associate degree	Baccalaureate[4]
1977-78	− 1.4	−7.3	− 1.2	+ 1.9
1976-77	+ 0.1	−5.8	+ 2.4	+ 0.8
1975-76	+ 2.9	−4.3	+ 5.7	+ 4.2
1974-75	+ 1.7	−8.3	+ 3.3	+ 7.7
1973-74	+ 3.3	−9.7	+ 9.5	+ 7.2
1972-73	+11.2	+0.2	+20.0	+11.4
1971-72	+18.8	+2.8	+23.8	+34.0
1970-71	+12.6	−0.1	+25.6	+15.8
1969-70	+ 9.8	−0.9	+25.9	+10.3
1968-69	+ 4.5	−7.5	+27.1	+ 7.3

[1]Includes admissions to programs closed prior to October 15.
[2]Includes Guam, Puerto Rico, and Virgin Islands.
[3]Reporting dates for 1970-71 through 1977-78 are August 1-July 31: reporting dates for 1968-69 and 1969-70
are September 1-August 31.
[4]Includes students admitted to initial programs leading to a master's degree: 1977-78, 122; 1976-77, 109; 1975-
76, 63; 1974-75, 64; 1973-74, 48; 1972-73, 48; 1971-72, 45; 1970-71, 35; 1969-70, 19; 1968-69, 33.
SOURCE: National League for Nursing, *State-Approved Schools of Nursing—R.N., 1979*, and previous
                    years.

**Table II-A-3. Admissions for Academic Years 1971-72 to 1977-78
to Initial Programs—R.N. in the United States and Outlying Areas,[1]
by Accreditation Status on Succeeding January 1**

Type of program and academic year[2]	Total admissions	Accredited			Nonaccredited[3]		
		Programs[4]	Admissions	Percent of total	Programs[4]	Admissions	Percent of total
Total programs							
1977-78 ...	111,928	958	87,955	78.6	416	23,973	21.4
1976-77 ...	113,479	916	85,895	75.7	456	27,584	24.3
1975-76 ...	113,311	950	86,112	76.0	466	27,199	24.0
1974-75 ...	110,068	932	81,844	74.4	480	28,224	25.6
1973-74 ...	108,210	905	77,536	71.7	510	30,674	28.3
1972-73 ...	104,713	898	74,220	70.9	530	30,493	29.1
1971-72 ...	94,154	891	67,788	72.0	535	26,366	28.0
Diploma							
1977-78	20,611	321	19,692	95.5	23	919	4.5
1976-77	22,243	333	21,121	95.0	34	1,122	5.0
1975-76	23,622	384	22,205	94.0	45	1,417	6.0
1974-75	24,696	409	22,980	93.1	52	1,716	6.9
1973-74	26,943	430	24,835	92.2	65	2,108	7.8
1972-73	29,848	466	27,503	92.1	78	2,345	7.9
1971-72	29,801	497	27,000	90.6	91	2,801	9.4
Associate degree							
1977-78 ...	53,653	344	34,238	63.8	333	19,415	36.2
1976-77 ...	54,289	304	32,130	59.2	352	22,159	40.8
1975-76 ...	53,033	294	31,009	58.5	350	22,024	41.5
1974-75 ...	50,180	268	28,236	56.3	353	21,944	43.7
1973-74 ...	48,595	236	25,163	51.8	368	23,432	48.2
1972-73 ...	44,387	207	21,255	47.9	370	23,132	52.1
1971-72 ...	36,996	181	17,759	48.0	361	19,237	52.0
Baccalaureate							
1977-78 ...	37,664	293	[5]34,025	90.3	60	3,639	9.7
1976-77 ...	36,947	279	[5]32,644	88.4	70	4,303	11.6
1975-76 ...	36,656	272	[5]32,898	89.7	71	3,758	10.3
1974-75 ...	35,192	255	30,628	87.0	75	[5]4,564	13.0
1973-74 ...	32,672	239	27,538	84.3	77	[5]5,134	15.7
1972-73 ...	30,478	225	25,462	83.5	82	[5]5,016	16.5
1971-72 ...	27,357	213	[5]23,029	84.2	83	4,328	15.8

[1]Includes Guam, Puerto Rico, and Virgin Islands.
[2]Reporting dates for admissions are August 1-July 31.
[3]Included in this category are programs which applied but were never accredited and those which never applied for accreditation.
[4]Includes programs that closed during the academic year: 1977-78, 26; 1976-77, 27; 1975-76, 43; 1974-75, 37; 1973-74, 43; 1972-73, 55; 1971-72, 49.
[5]Includes students admitted to initial programs leading to a master's degree: 1977-78, 122; 1976-77, 109; 1975-76, 63; 1974-75, 64; 1973-74, 48; 1972-73, 48; 1971-72, 45.

SOURCE: National League for Nursing, unpublished data, 1979; *State-Approved Schools of Nursing—R.N., 1977,* and previous years.

Table II-A-4. Students Admitted to Initial Programs—R.N., Academic Year August 1, 1977-July 31, 1978

State or area	Total	Diploma	Associate degree	Baccalaureate
Total[1]	111,928	20,611	53,653	[2]37,664
United States, total	110,950	20,611	52,991	[2]37,348
Alabama	2,690	172	1,089	1,429
Alaska	77	...	38	39
Arizona	1,059	...	622	437
Arkansas	1,282	107	819	356
California	6,508	378	4,266	1,864
Colorado	883	82	360	441
Connecticut	1,565	357	598	610
Delaware	533	116	171	246
District of Columbia	729	56	63	610
Florida	3,538	212	2,603	723
Georgia	2,285	453	1,474	358
Hawaii	210	...	146	64
Idaho	387	...	289	98
Illinois	5,840	1,768	2,779	1,293
Indiana	2,813	445	1,364	1,004
Iowa	2,099	618	848	633
Kansas	1,239	326	467	446
Kentucky	1,978	120	1,385	473
Louisiana	2,002	321	643	1,038
Maine	609	171	222	216
Maryland	1,990	215	1,206	569
Massachusetts	3,607	1,125	1,322	1,160
Michigan	4,336	824	2,164	1,348
Minnesota	2,234	288	1,183	763
Mississippi	1,448	76	868	504
Missouri	2,515	1,061	896	558
Montana	399	...	105	294
Nebraska	960	437	280	243
Nevada	193	...	131	62
New Hampshire	457	200	93	164
New Jersey	3,441	1,037	1,540	864
New Mexico	464	...	336	128
New York	12,512	1,546	6,441	4,525
North Carolina	2,660	316	1,451	893
North Dakota	433	151	128	154
Ohio	5,530	2,030	2,088	1,412
Oklahoma	1,253	107	655	491
Oregon	967	124	599	244
Pennsylvania	6,640	2,671	1,732	2,237
Rhode Island	861	80	244	537
South Carolina	1,140	34	705	401
South Dakota	646	132	248	266
Tennessee	2,623	559	1,330	734
Texas	5,977	483	2,774	2,720
Utah	518	...	373	145
Vermont	309	...	209	100
Virginia	2,683	590	1,030	1,063
Washington	1,914	87	1,122	705
West Virginia	1,169	135	774	260
Wisconsin	2,609	601	646	1,362
Wyoming	136	...	72	64
Outlying areas, total	978	...	662	316
Guam	51	...	51	...
Puerto Rico	890	...	574	316
Virgin Islands	37	...	37	...

[1] Based on information from 1,379 schools with 1,400 programs.
[2] Includes 122 students admitted to two initial programs leading to a master's degree.

SOURCE: National League for Nursing, *State-Approved Schools of Nursing, R.N., 1979*, pp. 60 and 61.

Table II-A-5. Graduations of Students from Initial Programs—R.N.[1] in the United States and Outlying Areas,[2] Academic Years 1968-69 to 1977-78

Academic year	Total number	Diploma		Associate degree		Baccalaureate[3]	
		Number	Percent of total	Number	Percent of total	Number	Percent of total
1977-78 ...	78,697	17,131	21.8	37,069	47.1	24,497	31.1
1976-77 ...	78,461	18,014	23.0	36,815	46.9	23,632	30.1
1975-76 ...	77,633	19,861	25.6	35,094	45.2	22,678	29.2
1974-75 ...	74,536	21,673	29.1	32,622	43.8	20,241	27.1
1973-74 ...	67,628	21,280	31.5	29,299	43.3	17,049	25.2
1972-73 ...	59,427	21,445	36.1	24,850	41.8	13,132	22.1
1971-72 ...	51,784	21,592	41.7	19,165	37.0	11,027	21.3
1970-71 ...	47,001	22,334	47.5	14,754	31.4	9,913	21.1
1969-70 ...	43,639	22,856	52.4	11,678	26.8	9,105	20.8
1968-69 ...	42,196	25,114	59.5	8,701	20.6	8,381	19.9

[1]Includes graduations from programs closed prior to October 15.
[2]Includes Guam, Puerto Rico, and Virgin Islands.
[3]Includes students graduated from initial programs leading to a master's degree: 1977-78, 49; 1976-77, 54; 1975-76, 46; 1974-75, 41; 1973-74, 41; 1972-73, 42; 1971-72, 25; 1970-71, 15; 1969-70, 21; 1968-69, 23.
SOURCE: National League for Nursing, *State-Approved Schools of Nursing—R.N., 1979*, and previous years.

Table II-A-6. Percent Change over Previous Year in Graduations of Students from Initial Programs—R.N.[1] in the United States and Outlying Areas,[2] Academic Years 1968-69 to 1977-78

Academic year	Total	Diploma	Associate degree	Baccalaureate[3]
1977-78	+ 0.3	− 4.9	+ 0.7	+ 3.7
1976-77	+ 1.1	− 9.3	+ 4.9	+ 4.2
1975-76	+ 4.2	− 8.4	+ 7.6	+12.0
1974-75	+10.2	+ 1.8	+11.3	+18.7
1973-74	+13.8	− 0.8	+17.9	+29.8
1972-73	+14.8	− 0.7	+29.7	+19.1
1971-72	+10.2	− 3.3	+29.9	+11.2
1970-71	+ 7.7	− 2.3	+26.3	+ 8.9
1969-70	+ 3.4	− 9.0	+34.2	+ 8.6
1968-69	+ 1.5	−10.9	+40.0	+17.3

[1]Includes graduations from programs closed prior to October 15.
[2]Includes Guam, Puerto Rico, and Virgin Islands.
[3]Includes students graduated from initial programs leading to a master's degree: 1977-78, 49; 1976-77, 54; 1975-76, 46; 1974-75, 41; 1973-74, 41; 1972-73, 42; 1971-72, 25; 1970-71, 15; 1969-70, 21; 1968-69, 23.
SOURCE: National League for Nursing, *State-Approved Schools of Nursing—R.N., 1979*, and previous years.

CHART 6. STUDENTS GRADUATED FROM INITIAL PROGRAMS OF NURSING EDUCATION—R.N., 1968-69 to 1977-78

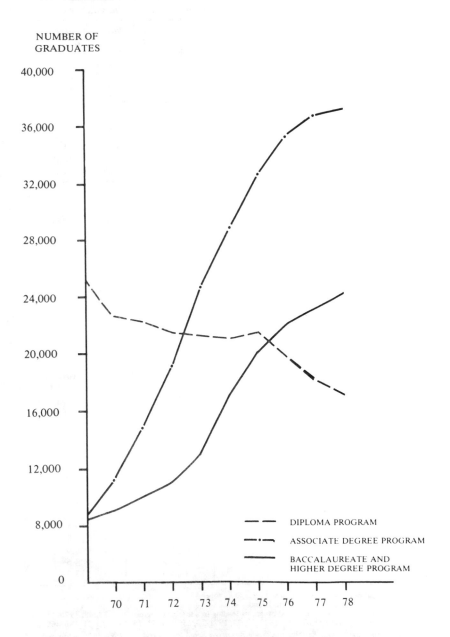

NUMBER OF
GRAPHICS

DIPLOMA PROGRAM

ASSOCIATE DEGREE PROGRAM

BACCALAUREATE AND
HIGHER DEGREE PROGRAM

SOURCE: National League for Nursing, *State-Approved Schools of Nursing—R.N., 1979,* and previous years.

Prepared by American Nurses' Association, Research and Policy Analysis Department, Statistics Unit, 1980.

**Table II-A-7. Graduations for Academic Years 1971-72 to 1977-78 from
Initial Programs—R.N. in the United States and Outlying Areas,[1] by
Accreditation Status on Succeeding January 1**

Type of program and academic year	Total graduations	Accredited			Nonaccredited[2]		
		Programs[3]	Graduations	Percent of total	Programs[3]	Graduations	Percent of total
Total programs							
1977-78	78,697	958	63,582	80.8	416	15,115	19.2
1976-77	78,461	916	61,253	78.1	456	17,208	21.9
1975-76	77,633	950	61,728	79.5	466	15,905	20.5
1974-75	74,536	932	58,478	78.5	480	16,058	21.5
1973-74	67,628	905	52,071	77.0	510	15,557	23.0
1972-73	59,427	898	45,268	76.2	530	14,159	23.8
1971-72	51,784	891	39,659	76.6	535	12,125	23.4
Diploma							
1977-78	17,131	321	16,241	94.8	23	890	5.2
1976-77	18,014	333	16,862	93.6	34	1,152	6.4
1975-76	19,861	384	18,632	93.8	45	1,229	6.2
1974-75	21,673	409	20,217	93.3	52	1,456	6.7
1973-74	21,280	430	19,631	92.3	65	1,649	7.7
1972-73	21,445	466	19,649	91.6	78	1,796	8.4
1971-72	21,592	497	19,575	90.7	91	2,017	9.3
Associate degree							
1977-78	37,069	344	24,082	65.0	333	12,987	35.0
1976-77	36,815	304	22,044	59.9	352	14,771	40.1
1975-76	35,094	294	21,344	60.8	350	13,750	39.2
1974-75	32,622	268	19,090	58.5	353	13,532	41.5
1973-74	29,299	236	16,484	56.3	368	12,815	43.7
1972-73	24,850	207	13,340	53.7	370	11,510	46.3
1971-72	19,165	181	9,619	50.2	361	9,546	49.8
Baccalaureate							
1977-78	24,497	293	[4]23,259	94.9	60	1,238	5.1
1976-77	23,632	279	[4]22,347	94.6	70	1,285	5.4
1975-76	22,678	272	[4]21,752	95.9	71	926	4.1
1974-75	20,241	255	19,171	94.7	75	[4]1,070	5.3
1973-74	17,049	239	15,956	93.6	77	[4]1,093	6.4
1972-73	13,132	225	12,279	93.5	82	[4]853	6.5
1971-72	11,027	213	[4]10,465	94.9	83	562	5.1

[1] Includes Guam, Puerto Rico, and Virgin Islands.
[2] Included in this category are programs which applied but were never accredited and those which never applied for accreditation.
[3] Includes programs that closed during academic year: 1977-78, 26; 1976-77, 27; 1975-76, 43; 1974-75, 37; 1973-74, 43; 1972-73, 55; 1971-72, 49.
[4] Includes students graduated from initial programs leading to a master's degree: 1977-78, 49; 1976-77, 54; 1975-76, 46; 1974-75, 41; 1973-74, 41; 1972-73, 42; 1971-72, 25.
SOURCE: National League for Nursing, unpublished data, 1979; *State-Approved Schools of Nursing—R.N., 1977,* and previous years.

Table II-A-8. Students Graduating from Initial Programs—R.N., Academic Year August 1, 1977-July 31, 1978[1]

State or area	Total	Diploma	Associate degree	Baccalaureate
Total[2]	78,697	17,131	37,069	[3]24,497
United States, total	77,874	17,131	36,556	[3]24,187
Alabama	1,515	158	796	561
Alaska	38	...	25	13
Arizona	730	...	472	258
Arkansas	603	...	455	148
California	5,185	255	3,544	1,386
Colorado	664	93	287	284
Connecticut	952	267	358	327
Delaware	322	83	98	141
District of Columbia	428	42	79	307
Florida	2,352	121	1,806	425
Georgia	1,546	311	904	331
Hawaii	149	...	87	62
Idaho	261	...	209	52
Illinois	4,379	1,387	1,977	1,015
Indiana	2,160	383	1,067	710
Iowa	1,452	478	555	419
Kansas	1,030	354	320	356
Kentucky	1,308	99	881	328
Louisiana	1,161	214	430	517
Maine	390	127	156	107
Maryland	1,475	190	793	492
Massachusetts	3,092	1,181	1,026	885
Michigan	3,111	758	1,530	823
Minnesota	1,804	270	902	632
Mississippi	810	57	497	256
Missouri	1,829	831	647	351
Montana	317	51	71	195
Nebraska	728	337	226	165
Nevada	127	...	75	52
New Hampshire	365	154	79	132
New Jersey	2,370	796	1,058	516
New Mexico	357	...	247	110
New York	8,416	1,599	4,067	2,750
North Carolina	1,903	235	878	790
North Dakota	437	154	75	208
Ohio	4,073	1,602	1,539	932
Oklahoma	780	51	432	297
Oregon	771	102	395	274
Pennsylvania	4,902	2,515	1,056	1,331
Rhode Island	492	66	179	247
South Carolina	826	22	520	284
South Dakota	448	89	189	170
Tennessee	1,620	316	867	437
Texas	3,875	277	1,892	1,706
Utah	422	...	305	117
Vermont	229	...	155	74
Virginia	1,673	459	674	540
Washington	1,393	97	737	559
West Virginia	763	105	502	156
Wisconsin	1,794	445	417	932
Wyoming	47	...	20	27
Outlying areas, total	823	...	513	310
Guam	50	...	50	...
Puerto Rico	759	...	449	310
Virgin Islands	14	...	14	...

[1]Includes 965 graduations from 26 programs closed between October 16, 1977 and October 15, 1978.
[2]Based on information from 1,379 schools with 1,400 programs.
[3]Includes 49 graduations from initial programs who were granted a master's degree.
SOURCE: National League for Nursing, State-Approved Schools of Nursing—R.N., 1979, pp. 60 and 61.

Table II-A-9. Admissions, Graduations, and Enrollments in Initial Programs—R.N. in the United States,[1] and Percent Change over Previous Year, 1968-69 to 1977-78

Academic year[2]	Admissions[3]		Graduations[3]		Enrollments[4]	
	Number	Percent change	Number	Percent change	Number	Percent change
1977-78	110,950	− 1.4	77,874	+ 0.2	239,486	− 2.4
1976-77	112,523	+ 0.3	77,755	+ 0.9	245,390	− 0.7
1975-76	112,174	+ 2.9	77,065	+ 4.3	247,044	− 0.5
1974-75	109,020	+ 1.6	73,915	+10.2	248,171	+ 2.3
1973-74	107,344	+ 3.4	67,061	+13.9	242,551	+ 5.1
1972-73	103,789	+11.2	58,881	+14.8	230,803	+ 9.3
1971-72	93,344	+18.9	51,304	+10.4	211,239	+13.6
1970-71	78,524	+12.7	46,455	+ 7.8	185,869	+14.1
1969-70	69,677	+ 9.9	43,103	+ 3.1	162,924	+ 9.2
1968-69	63,408	+ 4.5	41,801	+ 1.3	149,124	+ 3.5

[1]Excludes Guam, Puerto Rico, and Virgin Islands.
[2]Reporting dates for 1970-71 through 1977-78 are August 1-July 31; reporting dates for 1968-69 and 1969-70 are September 1-August 31.
[3]Includes admissions and graduations from programs closed prior to October 15.
[4]As of October 15, following close of academic year.
SOURCE: National League for Nursing, *State-Approved Schools of Nursing—R.N., 1979,* and previous years.

Table II-A-10. Enrollment in Schools of Nursing—R.N. in the United States and Outlying Areas,[1] by Type of Program and Control of School, October 15, 1978

Type of program[2]	Total	Control of school			
		Hospital	University or senior college	Junior or community college	Independent
Number of schools ...	[3]1,353	338	500	500	15
Number of students, total	242,259	47,077	124,801	67,749	2,632
Diploma	48,059	46,262	...	...	1,797
Associate degree ...	92,961	815	24,397	67,749	...
Baccalaureate	101,239	...	100,404	...	835

[1]Includes Guam, Puerto Rico, and Virgin Islands.
[2]Excludes programs closed prior to October 15.
[3]Includes 21 schools conducting 2 programs each.
SOURCE: National League for Nursing, unpublished data, 1979.

Table II-A-11. Enrollment in Initial Programs—R.N. in the United States and Outlying Areas,[1] 1969-1978

Year, as of October 15	Number of programs[2]	Total number	Enrollment					
			Diploma		Associate degree		Baccalaureate[3]	
			Number	Percent of total	Number	Percent of total	Number	Percent of total
1978	1,374	242,259	48,059	19.8	92,961	38.4	101,239	41.8
1977	1,372	247,739	52,858	21.3	92,387	37.3	102,494	41.4
1976	1,373	249,541	56,091	22.5	92,404	37.0	101,046	40.5
1975	1,375	250,385	60,213	24.1	89,492	35.7	100,680	40.2
1974	1,372	244,486	64,083	26.2	85,452	35.0	94,951	38.8
1973	1,373	232,589	68,760	29.6	78,673	33.8	85,156	36.6
1972	1,377	213,127	71,694	33.6	67,543	31.7	73,890	34.7
1971	1,363	187,551	71,466	38.1	56,300	30.0	59,785	31.9
1970	1,355	164,545	71,055	43.2	44,593	27.1	48,897	29.7
1969	1,339	150,795	72,798	48.3	34,537	22.9	43,460	28.8

[1] Includes Guam, Puerto Rico, and Virgin Islands.
[2] Excludes programs closed prior to October 15.
[3] Includes students enrolled in initial programs leading to a master's degree: 1978, 247; 1977, 174; 1976, 135; 1975, 121; 1974, 107; 1973, 89; 1972, 88; 1971, 71; 1970, 50; 1969, 42.
SOURCE: National League for Nursing, *State-Approved Schools of Nursing—R.N., 1979*, and previous years.

Table II-A-12. Percent Change over Previous Year in Enrollment of Students in Initial Programs—R.N.[1] in the United States and Outlying Areas,[2] 1969-1978

Year, as of October 15	Total	Diploma	Associate degree	Baccalaureate[3]
1978	− 2.2	−9.1	+ 0.6	− 1.2
1977	− 0.7	−5.8	− (4)	+ 1.4
1976	− 0.3	−6.8	+ 3.3	+ 0.4
1975	+ 2.4	−6.0	+ 4.7	+ 6.0
1974	+ 5.1	−6.8	+ 8.6	+11.5
1973	+ 9.1	−4.1	+16.5	+15.2
1972	+13.6	+0.3	+20.0	+23.6
1971	+14.0	+0.6	+26.3	+22.3
1970	+ 9.1	−2.4	+29.1	+12.5
1969	+ 3.6	−6.4	+25.7	+ 7.7

[1] Excludes programs closed prior to October 15.
[2] Includes Guam, Puerto Rico, and Virgin Islands.
[3] Includes students enrolled in initial programs leading to a master's degree: 1978, 247; 1977, 174; 1976, 135; 1975, 121; 1974, 107; 1973, 89; 1972, 88; 1971, 71; 1970, 50; 1969, 42.
[4] Less than 0.1 percent.
SOURCE: National League for Nursing, *State-Approved Schools of Nursing—R.N., 1979*, and previous years.

Table II-A-13. Enrollment as of October 15, 1972 to 1978 in Initial Programs—R.N. in the United States and Outlying Areas,[1] by Accreditation Status on Succeeding January 1

Type of program and year, as of October 15	Total enrollment	Accredited			Nonaccredited[2]		
		Programs[3]	Enrollment	Percent of total	Programs[3]	Enrollment	Percent of total
Total programs							
1978	242,259	958	197,366	81.5	416	44,893	18.5
1977	247,739	916	197,359	79.7	456	50,380	20.3
1976	249,541	918	199,277	79.9	455	50,264	20.1
1975	250,385	904	196,290	78.4	471	54,095	21.6
1974	244,486	874	186,578	76.3	498	57,908	23.7
1973	232,589	861	174,950	75.2	512	57,639	24.8
1972	213,127	855	159,423	74.8	522	53,704	25.2
Diploma							
1978	48,059	321	46,004	95.7	23	2,055	4.3
1977	52,858	333	50,153	94.9	34	2,705	5.1
1976	56,091	352	52,957	94.4	38	3,134	5.6
1975	60,213	382	56,252	93.4	46	3,961	6.6
1974	64,083	401	59,021	92.1	60	5,062	7.9
1973	68,760	431	63,309	92.1	63	5,451	7.9
1972	71,694	462	64,998	90.7	81	6,696	9.3
Associate degree							
1978	92,961	344	59,424	63.9	333	33,537	36.1
1977	92,387	304	55,645	60.2	352	36,742	39.8
1976	92,404	294	55,143	59.7	348	37,261	40.3
1975	89,492	268	51,404	57.4	350	38,088	42.6
1974	85,452	235	44,576	52.2	363	40,876	47.8
1973	78,673	206	38,491	48.9	368	40,182	51.1
1972	67,543	180	31,462	46.6	361	36,081	53.4
Baccalaureate							
1978	101,239	293	[4]91,938	90.8	60	9,301	9.2
1977	102,494	279	[4]91,561	89.3	70	10,933	10.7
1976	101,046	272	[4]91,177	90.2	69	9,869	9.8
1975	100,680	254	88,634	88.0	75	[4]12,046	12.0
1974	94,951	238	82,981	87.4	75	[4]11,970	12.6
1973	85,156	224	73,150	85.9	81	[4]12,006	14.1
1972	73,890	213	[4]62,963	85.2	80	10,927	14.8

[1]Includes Guam, Puerto Rico, and Virgin Islands.
[2]Included in this category are programs which applied but were never accredited and those which never applied for accreditation.
[3]Excludes programs closed prior to October 15.
[4]Includes students enrolled in initial programs leading to a master's degree: 1978, 208; 1977, 174; 1976, 135; 1975, 121; 1974, 95; 1973, 89; 1972, 88.

SOURCE: National League for Nursing, unpublished data, 1979; *State-Approved Schools of Nursing—R.N., 1979*, and previous years.

Table II-A-14. Student Enrollment in Initial Programs—R.N., October 15, 1978

State or area	Total	Diploma	Associate degree	Baccalau-reate
Total[1]	*242,259*	*48,059*	*92,961*	[2]*101,239*
United States, total	*239,486*	*48,059*	*91,527*	[2]*99,900*
Alabama	5,272	416	1,698	3,158
Alaska	298	...	66	232
Arizona	1,980	...	1,021	959
Arkansas	2,182	281	1,068	833
California	12,863	831	7,560	4,472
Colorado	2,125	251	704	1,170
Connecticut	3,704	934	994	1,776
Delaware	1,279	147	312	820
District of Columbia	2,410	153	269	1,988
Florida	6,140	514	4,017	1,609
Georgia	4,097	878	2,270	949
Hawaii	380	...	236	144
Idaho	712	...	490	222
Illinois	13,153	3,974	4,985	4,194
Indiana	6,526	1,112	2,548	2,866
Iowa	4,328	1,501	1,353	1,474
Kansas	2,393	602	806	985
Kentucky	3,571	239	2,390	942
Louisiana	4,287	743	896	2,648
Maine	1,366	367	406	593
Maryland	3,765	570	2,036	1,159
Massachusetts	9,251	2,843	2,578	3,830
Michigan	9,040	1,570	3,894	3,576
Minnesota	4,837	748	2,162	1,927
Mississippi	2,586	138	1,484	964
Missouri	5,660	2,474	1,554	1,632
Montana	945	...	195	750
Nebraska	2,186	1,149	534	503
Nevada	458	...	363	95
New Hampshire	1,094	417	153	524
New Jersey	7,794	2,406	2,608	2,780
New Mexico	936	...	632	304
New York	28,082	3,593	11,943	12,546
North Carolina	5,854	738	2,425	2,691
North Dakota	1,386	340	210	836
Ohio	12,780	4,886	3,817	4,077
Oklahoma	2,281	131	1,150	1,000
Oregon	1,906	341	954	611
Pennsylvania	15,664	6,437	2,911	6,316
Rhode Island	1,952	224	429	1,299
South Carolina	2,583	81	1,157	1,345
South Dakota	1,563	305	424	834
Tennessee	5,539	1,317	2,286	1,936
Texas	11,661	944	4,315	6,402
Utah	1,044	...	662	382
Vermont	685	...	343	342
Virginia	5,617	1,460	1,732	2,425
Washington	3,935	165	1,945	1,825
West Virginia	2,254	320	1,260	674
Wisconsin	6,738	1,519	1,164	4,055
Wyoming	344	...	118	226
Outlying areas	*2,773*	...	*1,434*	*1,339*
Guam	91	...	91	...
Puerto Rico	2,643	...	1,304	1,339
Virgin Islands	39	...	39	...

[1]Based on information from 1,353 schools with 1,374 programs, excluding those closed prior to October 15.
[2]Includes 247 students enrolled in initial programs leading to a master's degree.
SOURCE: National League for Nursing. *State-Approved Schools of Nursing—R.N., 1979*, pp. 60 and 61.

Table II-A-15. Minority Student Admissions in Schools of Nursing
Reporting One or More Such Students, in the United States and
Outlying Areas, 1978

Racial/ethnic background and type of program	Programs receiving questionnaire	Programs returning questionnaire		Admissions in programs returning questionnaire		
		Number	Percent reporting at least one minority student admitted	Total admissions	Minority student admissions	
					Number	Percent
Minority, total	1,401	1,214	75	101,438	11,212	11.1
Diploma	367	311	69	19,241	1,331	6.9
Associate degree	679	580	76	46,755	5,515	11.8
Baccalaureate[1] ...	355	323	80	35,442	4,366	12.3
Blacks	1,401	1,214	62	101,438	7,313	7.2
Diploma	367	311	54	19,241	828	4.3
Associate degree	679	580	62	46,755	3,580	7.7
Baccalaureate[1]	355	323	70	35,442	2,905	8.2
Hispanics	1,401	1,214	37	101,438	2,520	2.5
Diploma	367	311	29	19,241	232	1.2
Associate degree	679	580	38	46,755	1,318	2.8
Baccalaureate[1]	355	323	44	35,442	970	2.7
American Indians/ Orientals	1,401	1,214	36	101,438	1,379	1.4
Diploma	367	311	29	19,241	271	1.4
Associate degree	679	580	36	46,755	617	1.3
Baccalaureate[1]	355	323	42	35,442	491	1.4

[1]Includes basic students and some students who previously graduated from diploma or associate degree programs.

SOURCE: National League for Nursing, "Educational Preparation for Nursing—1978," *Nursing Outlook*, Vol. 27, No. 9, September 1979, pp. 611-613.

Table II-A-16. Minority Student Graduations in Schools of Nursing Reporting One or More Such Students, in the United States and Outlying Areas, 1978

Racial/ethnic background and type of program	Programs receiving questionnaire	Programs returning questionnaire		Graduations from programs returning questionnaire		
		Number	Percent reporting at least one minority student graduated	Total graduations	Minority student graduations	
					Number	Percent
Minority, total	*1,401*	*1,214*	*63*	*70,432*	*5,724*	*8.1*
Diploma	367	311	48	14,802	576	3.9
Associate degree	679	580	69	32,343	3,450	10.7
Baccalaureate[1] ...	355	323	65	23,287	1,698	7.3
Blacks	*1,401*	*1,214*	*50*	*70,432*	*3,279*	*4.7*
Diploma	367	311	36	14,802	320	2.2
Associate degree	679	580	55	32,343	1,967	6.1
Baccalaureate[1]	355	323	57	23,287	992	4.3
Hispanics	*1,401*	*1,214*	*27*	*70,432*	*1,558*	*2.2*
Diploma	367	311	16	14,802	112	0.8
Associate degree	679	580	30	32,343	1,041	3.2
Baccalaureate[1]	355	323	30	23,287	405	1.7
American Indians/ Orientals	*1,401*	*1,214*	*25*	*70,432*	*887*	*1.3*
Diploma	367	311	13	14,802	144	1.0
Associate degree	679	580	28	32,343	442	1.4
Baccalaureate[1]	355	323	31	23,287	301	1.3

[1]Includes basic students and some students who previously graduated from diploma or associate degree programs.

SOURCE: National League for Nursing, "Educational Preparation for Nursing—1978," *Nursing Outlook,* Vol. 27, No. 9, September 1979, pp. 611-613.

Table II-A-17. Minority Student Enrollments[1] in Schools of Nursing Reporting One or More Such Students, in the United States and Outlying Areas, 1978

Racial/ethnic background and type of program	Programs receiving questionnaire	Programs returning questionnaire		Enrollments in programs returning questionnaire		
		Number	Percent reporting at least one minority student enrolled	Total enrollments	Minority student enrollments	
					Number	Percent
Minority, total	1,401	1,214	83	219,582	18,692	8.5
Diploma	367	311	79	44,628	2,191	4.9
Associate degree	679	580	84	80,344	7,612	9.5
Baccalaureate[2]	355	323	87	94,610	8,889	9.4
Blacks	1,401	1,214	72	219,582	12,730	5.8
Diploma	367	311	67	44,628	1,409	3.2
Associate degree	679	580	71	80,344	5,003	6.2
Baccalaureate[2]	355	323	79	94,610	6,318	6.7
Hispanics	1,401	1,214	44	219,582	3,354	1.5
Diploma	367	311	35	44,628	369	0.8
Associate degree	679	580	43	80,344	1,686	2.1
Baccalaureate[2]	355	323	54	94,610	1,299	1.4
American Indians/ Orientals	1,401	1,214	43	219,582	2,608	1.2
Diploma	367	311	36	44,628	413	0.9
Associate degree	679	580	39	80,344	923	1.1
Baccalaureate[2]	355	323	57	94,610	1,272	1.3

[1]Enrollments are as of October 15, 1978.
[2]Includes basic students and some students who previously graduated from diploma and associate degree programs.
SOURCE: National League for Nursing, "Educational Preparation for Nursing—1978," *Nursing Outlook*, Vol. 27, No. 9, September 1979, pp. 611-613.

Table II-A-18. Enrollment[1] in Selected Nursing Programs in Junior and Senior Colleges by Racial/Ethnic Background, Academic Year 1975-76

Type of program	Total enrollment	Racial/ethnic background					
		Minorities					White
		Total	Black	Asian	American Indian	Hispanic	
Nurse anesthetist	272	20	14	5	...	1	252
Nurse-midwife	59	14	14	...	...	...	45
Nurse practitioner	128	17	5	3	1	8	111

[1]May include some post-RN students.
SOURCE: U.S. Department of Health, Education, and Welfare, Public Health Service, Health Resources Administration, *Minorities and Women in the Health Fields*, DHEW Publication No. (HRA) 79-22, October 1978.

Table II-A-19. Male Student Admissions, Enrollments, and Graduations from Schools of Nursing Reporting One or More Male Students, in the United States and Outlying Areas, 1978

Type of program	Programs receiving questionnaire	Programs returning questionnaire		Admissions in programs returning questionnaire		
		Number	Percent reporting at least one male student admitted	Total admissions	Male student admissions	
					Number	Percent
Total	1,401	1,214	79	101,438	6,383	6.3
Diploma	367	311	79	19,241	1,027	5.3
Associate degree	679	580	80	46,755	3,154	6.7
Baccalaureate[1]	355	323	78	35,442	2,202	6.2

Type of program	Programs receiving questionnaire	Programs returning questionnaire		Enrollments in programs returning questionnaire		
		Number	Percent reporting at least one male student enrolled	Total enrollments	Male student enrollments	
					Number	Percent
Total	1,401	1,214	86	219,582	10,428	4.7
Diploma	367	311	88	44,628	1,862	4.2
Associate degree	679	580	85	80,344	4,317	5.4
Baccalaureate[1]	355	323	85	94,610	4,249	4.5

Type of program	Programs receiving questionnaire	Programs returning questionnaire		Graduations from programs returning questionnaire		
		Number	Percent reporting at least one male student graduated	Total graduations	Male student graduations	
					Number	Percent
Total	1,401	1,214	73	70,432	3,902	5.5
Diploma	367	311	68	14,802	655	4.4
Associate degree	679	580	76	32,343	2,076	6.4
Baccalaureate[1]	355	323	74	23,287	1,171	5.0

[1]Includes basic students and some students who were previously graduated from diploma or associate degree programs.

SOURCE: National League for Nursing, "Educational Preparation for Nursing—1978," *Nursing Outlook*, Vol. 27, No. 9, September 1979, pp. 611-613.

**Table II-A-20. Licensed Practical or Vocational Nurse Student
Admissions, Enrollments[1] and Graduations in Initial Programs in the
United States and Outlying Areas, 1978**

| Type of program | Programs receiving questionnaire | Programs returning questionnaire | | Admissions in programs returning questionnaire | | |
| | | Number | Percent reporting at least one LPN/LVN student admitted | Total admissions | LPN/LVN student admissions | |
					Number	Percent
Total	1,401	1,214	80	101,438	6,369	6.3
Diploma	367	311	86	19,241	668	3.5
Associate degree	679	580	84	46,755	5,219	11.2
Baccalaureate ...	355	323	67	35,442	482	1.4

| Type of program | Programs receiving questionnaire | Programs returning questionnaire | | Enrollments in programs returning questionnaire | | |
| | | Number | Percent reporting at least one LPN/LVN student enrolled | Total enrollments | LPN/LVN student enrollments | |
					Number	Percent
Total	1,401	1,214	83	219,582	8,808	4.0
Diploma	367	311	89	44,628	1,398	3.1
Associate degree	679	580	86	80,344	6,674	8.3
Baccalaureate ...	355	323	72	94,610	736	0.8

| Type of program | Programs receiving questionnaire | Programs returning questionnaire | | Graduations from programs returning questionnaire | | |
| | | Number | Percent reporting at least one LPN/LVN student graduated | Total graduations | LPN/LVN student graduations | |
					Number	Percent
Total	1,401	1,214	78	70,432	4,849	6.9
Diploma	367	311	84	14,802	568	3.8
Associate degree	679	580	82	32,343	4,016	12.4
Baccalaureate ...	355	323	66	23,287	265	1.1

[1]Enrollments as of October 15, 1978.
SOURCE: National League for Nursing, 1980. Unpublished data.

Table II-A-21. Earned Degrees Conferred in the United States, 1966-67 to 1986-87

Academic year	Total	Men				Women			
		Total	Baccalaureate[1]	Master's	Doctorate	Total	Baccalaureate[1]	Master's	Doctorate
Projected[2]									
1986-87	1,535,800	817,900	581,200	208,000	28,700	717,900	473,000	231,400	13,500
1985-86	1,545,900	826,300	591,300	206,200	28,800	719,600	482,200	224,400	13,000
1984-85	1,551,400	831,800	599,300	203,700	28,800	719,600	489,500	217,600	12,500
1983-84	1,548,900	833,700	604,300	200,700	28,700	715,200	493,700	209,500	12,000
1982-83	1,537,300	829,900	604,100	197,200	28,600	707,400	494,900	201,100	11,400
1981-82	1,522,300	824,200	602,700	193,100	28,400	698,100	494,000	193,200	10,900
1980-81	1,502,800	817,100	599,500	189,200	28,400	685,700	491,200	184,000	10,500
1979-80	1,476,100	804,700	592,700	184,000	28,000	671,400	485,300	176,100	10,000
1978-79	1,446,500	791,800	584,400	179,800	27,600	654,700	478,200	167,000	9,500
1977-78	1,424,700	785,700	583,500	175,000	27,200	639,000	470,900	159,100	9,000
1976-77	1,399,300	780,000	582,300	170,900	26,800	619,300	459,500	151,300	8,500
Actual									
1975-76	1,334,230	751,332	557,817	167,248	26,267	582,898	430,578	144,523	7,797
1974-75	1,305,382	742,184	553,797	161,570	26,817	563,198	425,052	130,880	7,226
1973-74	1,310,441	761,050	575,843	157,842	27,365	549,391	423,749	119,191	6,451
1972-73	1,270,528	747,719	564,680	154,468	28,571	522,809	407,700	108,903	6,206
1971-72	1,215,680	718,953	541,313	149,550	28,090	496,727	389,371	102,083	5,273
1970-71	1,140,292	676,814	511,138	138,146	27,530	463,478	366,538	92,363	4,577
1969-70	1,069,391	639,688	488,174	121,624	25,890	429,703	343,060	82,667	3,976
1968-69	984,129	588,663	444,380	121,531	22,752	395,466	319,805	72,225	3,436
1967-68	866,548	524,209	390,507	113,519	20,183	342,339	276,190	63,230	2,906
1966-67	768,871	474,604	353,349	103,092	18,163	294,267	237,198	54,615	2,454

[1]Baccalaureate includes first professional degrees such as chiropody, dentistry, law, medicine, optometry, osteopathy, podiatry, theology, and veterinary medicine.

[2]Revised. Intermediate projection used.

SOURCE: U.S. Department of Health, Education, and Welfare, Education Division, National Center for Education Statistics, *Projections of Education Statistics to 1986-87*, Publication No. NCES 78-403, 1978, p. 38.

Table II-A-22. Total and First-time Opening (Fall) Degree-Credit Enrollment,[1] by Sex, United States, 1972-1986

	Total		Men		Women	
Year	Number	Percent change	Number	Percent change	Number	Percent change
Total fall enrollment						
Projected[2]						
1986	12,903,000	+0.2	6,634,000	−0.1	6,269,000	+0.5
1985	12,881,000	+0.2	6,643,000	−0.2	6,238,000	+0.5
1984	12,860,000	+0.3	6,653,000	+0.1	6,207,000	+0.6
1983	12,816,000	+0.7	6,648,000	+0.5	6,168,000	+1.0
1982	12,722,000	+1.1	6,618,000	+0.8	6,104,000	+1.5
1981	12,579,000	+1.6	6,566,000	+1.5	6,013,000	+1.8
1980	12,376,000	+2.5	6,468,000	+1.9	5,908,000	+3.0
1979	12,079,000	+2.5	6,345,000	+2.1	5,734,000	+2.9
1978	11,782,000	+2.5	6,212,000	+1.9	5,570,000	+3.1
1977	11,499,000	+4.4	6,095,000	+4.9	5,404,000	+3.9
Actual						
1976[3]	11,012,000	−1.5	5,811,000	−5.5	5,201,000	+3.3
1975	11,184,859	+9.4	6,148,997	+9.4	5,035,862	+9.4
1974	10,223,729	+6.5	5,622,429	+4.7	4,601,300	+8.8
1973	9,602,123	+4.2	5,371,052	+2.5	4,231,071	+6.4
1972	9,214,860	+3.0	5,238,757	+0.6	3,976,103	+6.3
First-time fall enrollment						
Projected						
1986	(4)	(4)	(4)	(4)	(4)	(4)
1985	1,709,000	−1.3	877,000	−1.6	832,000	−1.1
1984	1,732,000	−3.1	891,000	−3.2	841,000	−3.0
1983	1,787,000	−4.1	920,000	−4.4	867,000	−3.9
1982	1,864,000	−2.5	962,000	−2.4	902,000	−2.5
1981	1,911,000	−1.3	986,000	−1.4	925,000	−1.2
1980	1,936,000	−0.9	1,000,000	−1.0	936,000	−0.8
1979	1,954,000	−0.5	1,010,000	0.0	944,000	−0.1
1978	1,955,000	+1.1	1,010,000	+1.0	945,000	+1.3
1977	1,933,000	+0.6	1,000,000	+0.4	933,000	+0.8
Actual						
1976	(4)	(4)	(4)	(4)	(4)	(4)
1975	1,910,125	+3.0	991,914	+2.0	918,211	+4.1
1974	1,854,442	+5.6	972,707	+4.5	881,735	+6.7
1973	1,756,854	+0.9	930,783	+0.2	826,071	+1.8
1972	1,740,438	−1.4	928,804	−4.0	811,634	+1.7

[1] Includes full and part-time students, resident and extension.
[2] Revised. Intermediate projection used. Data rounded to nearest thousand.
[3] Revised. Data rounded to nearest thousand.
[4] Information not available.

SOURCES: U.S. Department of Health, Education, and Welfare, Education Division, National Center for Education Statistics, *Projections of Education Statistics to 1986-87*, Publication No. NCES 78-403, 1978, p. 20; *Projections of Education Statistics to 1985-86*, Publication No. NCES 77-402, 1977, p. 22.

Table II-A-23. High School Graduates Compared with Population 18 Years of Age, United States, 1966-67 to 1980-81

School year	Population 18 years old[1] (in thousands)	High school graduates (in thousands)			Graduates per 100 persons 18 years of age
		Total[2]	Male	Female	
Projected					
1980-81	4,124	3,043	1,522	1,521	73.8
1979-80	4,188	3,097	1,547	1,550	73.9
1978-79	4,264	3,144	1,570	1,574	73.7
1977-78	4,237	3,160	1,578	1,582	74.6
1976-77	4,232	3,149	1,571	1,578	74.4
Actual					
1975-76	[3]4,244	3,153	1,572	1,581	74.3
1974-75[3]	4,236	3,140	1,545	1,595	74.1
1973-74[3]	4,123	3,081	1,515	1,566	74.7
1972-73[3]	4,049	3,043	1,503	1,540	75.2
1971-72[3]	3,982	3,008	1,490	1,518	75.5
1970-71[3]	3,891	2,944	1,457	1,487	75.7
1969-70	[3]3,796	2,896	1,433	1,463	76.3
1968-69	[3]3,692	2,829	1,402	1,427	76.6
1967-68	[3]3,566	2,702	1,341	1,360	75.8
1966-67	[3]3,535	2,679	1,332	1,348	75.8

[1] Age as of October 1, following graduation. Data from the Bureau of the Census.
[2] Figures may not add to totals due to rounding.
[3] Revised figure.
SOURCE: U.S. Department of Health, Education, and Welfare, Education Division, National Center for Education Statistics, *Projections of Education Statistics to 1986-87*, Publication No. NCES 78-403, 1978, pp. 37 and 158.

Table II-A-24. Registered Nurses and Health Trainees Admitted as Exchange-Visitors, Fiscal Years 1970-1978

Year	Registered nurses	Health trainees[1]
1978	111	(2)
1977	197	(2)
1976	194	(2)
1975	213	13
1974	287	26
1973	419	5
1972	312	70
1971	520	47
1970	755	354

[1] Includes student nurses; prior to fiscal year 1974 the figure is for student nurses only.
[2] Included with registered nurses.
SOURCE: U.S. Department of Justice, Immigration and Naturalization Service, 1980, and previous years.

Table II-A-25. Nurses Admitted as Exchange-Visitors and Industrial Trainees, by Country or Region of Last Permanent Residence, Fiscal Year 1978

Country or region of last permanent residence	Total admitted	Exchange-visitors	Industrial trainees
All countries	121	111	10
Europe	25	21	4
Austria	1	1	...
Belgium	1	1	...
Denmark	2	2	...
Finland	1	1	...
France	1	...	1
Ireland	5	5	...
Netherlands	5	5	...
Poland	1	1	...
Sweden	1	1	...
Switzerland	1	1	...
United Kingdom	6	3	3
Asia	24	24	...
Bangladesh	2	2	...
India	1	1	...
Iran	1	1	...
Japan	1	1	...
Jordan	2	2	...
Korea	1	1	...
Nepal	4	4	...
Philippines	4	4	...
Syria	2	2	...
Taiwan	2	2	...
Thailand	3	3	...
Turkey	1	1	...
Africa	34	34	...
Botswana	4	4	...
Egypt	4	4	...
Ethiopia	1	1	...
Gambia	3	3	...
Ghana	2	2	...
Kenya	4	4	...
Lesotho	3	3	...
Nigeria	6	6	...
South Africa, Republic of ...	1	1	...
Sudan	1	1	...
Togo	2	2	...
Zaire	2	2	...
Zambia	1	1	...
North America	24	19	5
Canada	10	6	4
Mexico	3	3	...
West Indies	10	9	1
Bermuda	1	...	1
Jamaica	7	7	...
St. Christopher	1	1	...
Trinidad & Tobago	1	1	...
Central America	1	1	...
Honduras	1	1	...
South America	14	13	1
Brazil	3	3	...
Colombia	7	6	1
Ecuador	1	1	...
Peru	2	2	...
Surinam	1	1	...

SOURCE: U.S. Department of Justice, Immigration and Naturalization Service, 1980. Unpublished data.

Chapter II, Section B
SCHOOLS OF NURSING

Fundamental to developing quality nursing programs and acquiring the man-power to deliver health services is an adequate nursing educational system. Concomitant with efforts to assist and recruit students into the nursing profession are continuous efforts to improve the quality of nursing education. Among the means to achieve this goal in nursing education are setting of standards, program accreditation, acquisition of funds for construction and rehabilitation of facilities, and development of prepared faculty to teach in the programs.

The nursing educational system has been responding to demands that newly graduated nurses have increasingly advanced skills and preparation to deal with the growing complexities of the health care system. This fact is evidenced by the unabated shift of nursing educational programs out of service institutions into colleges and universities. Data collected annually by the National League for Nursing attest to this trend.

As of October 15, 1978, there was a total of 1,374 programs offered by 1,353 schools, to prepare nurses to take the registered nurse licensure examination. On the average, these programs enrolled 179 students each. The net increase in the number of schools from the previous year was one school, and there was a net gain of two programs. Twenty-one schools in 1978 reported offering two initial programs, both associate degree and baccalaureate.

The diminutive change in the overall number of programs from 1977 to 1978 was not reflective of marginal change in its components but rather was the net effect of substantial counterbalancing shifts among the individual types of programs. The total number of diploma programs decreased by 6.3 percent to 344; the number of associate degree programs increased by 3.2 percent to 677; and the number of baccalaureate programs rose 1.1 percent to 353. These figures represented major changes in the relative mix of programs over the past decade—the number of diploma programs is now about half their number in 1969; the number of associate degree programs grew by 73.6 percent; and the number of baccalaureate programs grew by 39.0 percent.

The type of program continued to be closely related to the type of institution offering the program. The 1978 data showed that out of a total of 344 diploma programs the preponderance (333) were in hospitals, and 11 were operated by independent agencies. Community or junior colleges accounted for 76.2 percent of the associate degree programs, while 0.8 percent were under hospital control. Universities or senior colleges offered either associate degree or baccalaureate programs, with 21 offering both; however, there were more than twice as many baccalaureate programs (328) as there were associate degree programs (151) provided in senior collegiate settings.

There was a close correspondence between the type of institution offering the program and the type of financial support. Most hospital-based programs (86.7 percent) receive private support, while 59.4 percent of the university or senior colleges and 96.4 percent of junior or community colleges receive public support. The trend away from diploma programs is reflected in the shift in the funding of nursing education from private to public sources. The percentage of schools receiving public support continued to increase, reaching 61.0 percent in 1978.

Minimum standards for nursing educational programs are established by each state. All nursing programs must be approved by a state agency, either the state board of nursing or the state education department. State approval signifies that minimum standards have been met and graduates are eligible to take the state licensure examination. In addition to state approval, a program may seek voluntary accreditation by the National League for Nursing. The purpose of national accreditation by NLN is the maintenance of quality nursing education. The proportion of programs with NLN accreditation as of January 1, 1979, was 69.7 percent, up 4 percentage points from the previous year. There were differences among the programs with respect to NLN accreditation. Of the diploma programs, about 43.3 percent were accredited in 1979, while 83.0 percent of the baccalaureate and 50.8 percent of the associate degree programs were NLN-accredited that year.

Table II-B-1. Number of Schools, Initial Programs—RN and Average Enrollment, United States and Outlying Areas,[1] October 15, 1969-1978

Year	Number of schools[2]	Number of programs[3]	Average number of students per school
1978	1,353	1,374	179
1977	1,352	1,372	183
1976	1,349	1,373	185
1975	1,360	1,375	184
1974	1,359	1,372	180
1973	1,359	1,373	171
1972	1,363	1,377	156
1971	1,350	1,363	139
1970	1,343	1,355	122
1969	1,328	1,339	114

[1] Includes Guam, Puerto Rico, and Virgin Islands.
[2] Includes schools which conducted two programs each.
[3] Excludes programs closed prior to October 15.
SOURCE: National League for Nursing, *State-Approved Schools of Nursing—R.N., 1979*, and previous years.

Table II-B-2. Number of Initial Programs—RN in the United States and Outlying Areas,[1] October 15, 1969-1978

Year	Total programs[2]		Diploma		Associate degree		Baccalaureate	
	Number	Percent change	Number	Percent change	Number	Percent change	Number[3]	Percent change
1978	1,374	+0.1	344	-6.3	677	+ 3.2	353	+1.1
1977	1,372	-0.1	367	-5.9	656	+ 2.2	349	+2.3
1976	1,373	-0.1	390	-8.9	642	+ 3.9	341	+3.6
1975	1,375	+0.2	428	-7.2	618	+ 3.3	329	+5.1
1974	1,372	-0.1	461	-6.7	598	+ 4.2	313	+2.6
1973	1,373	-0.3	494	-9.0	574	+ 6.1	305	+4.1
1972	1,377	+1.0	543	-7.5	541	+10.2	293	+2.8
1971	1,363	+0.6	587	-8.4	491	+10.6	285	+5.6
1970	1,355	+1.2	641	-7.8	444	+13.8	270	+6.3
1969	1,339	+3.6	695	-4.5	390	+18.2	254	+8.1

[1] Includes Guam, Puerto Rico, and Virgin Islands.
[2] Excludes programs closed prior to October 15.
[3] Includes one initial program leading to a master's degree from 1969 through 1973, and two initial programs leading to a master's degree from 1974 through 1978.

SOURCE: National League for Nursing, State-Approved Schools of Nursing—R.N., 1979, and previous years.

Table II-B-3. Number of Schools Offering Initial Programs—RN in the United States and Outlying Areas,[1] October 1973-1978

	Number of schools					
Type of program	1973	1974	1975	1976	1977	1978
Total	1,359	1,363	1,360	1,349	1,352	1,353
One program	1,345	1,350	1,345	1,325	1,332	1,332
Diploma	493	461	426	388	367	344
Associate degree	561	588	603	618	636	656
Baccalaureate[2]...	291	301	316	319	329	332
Two programs	14	13	15	24	20	21
Diploma and baccalaureate	1	...	...	...	...	...
Diploma and associate degree	...	...	2	2	...	...
Associate degree and baccalaureate	13	13	13	22	20	21

[1] Includes Guam, Puerto Rico, and Virgin Islands.
[2] Includes one initial program leading to a master's degree in 1973, and two initial programs leading to a master's degree from 1974 through 1978.
SOURCE: National League for Nursing, 1979. Unpublished data.

Table II-B-4. Type of Control of Schools Offering Initial Programs—RN in the United States and Outlying Areas,[1] October 15, 1978

		Type of control			
Type of program	Number of schools	Hospital	University or senior college	Junior or community college	Independent
Total	1,353	338	500	500	15
One program	1,332	338	479	500	15
Diploma	344	333	...	...	11
Associate degree	656	5	151	500	...
Baccalaureate	[2]332	...	328	...	4
Two programs	21	...	21	...	...
Associate degree and baccalaureate ...	21	...	21	...	...

[1] Includes Guam, Puerto Rico, and Virgin Islands.
[2] Includes two initial programs leading to a master's degree.
SOURCE: National League for Nursing, 1979. Unpublished data.

Table II-B-5. Type of Support and Control of Schools Offering Initial Programs—RN in the United States and Outlying Areas,[1] October 15, 1978

Control	Total schools	Public support		Private support	
		Number	Percent	Number	Percent
Total	[2]1,353	826	61.0	527	39.0
Hospital	338	45	13.3	293	86.7
University or senior college	500	297	59.4	203	40.6
Junior or community college	500	482	96.4	18	3.6
Independent	15	2	13.3	13	86.7

[1] Includes Guam, Puerto Rico, and Virgin Islands.
[2] Includes 21 schools conducting two programs each.
SOURCE: National League for Nursing, 1979. Unpublished data.

Table II-B-6. Enrollments in Schools Offering Initial Programs—RN in the United States and Outlying Areas,[1] October 15, 1978

Type of program	Number of schools	Number of students			
		Total	Diploma	Associate degree	Baccalaureate
Total	1,353	242,259	48,059	92,961	101,239
One program	1,332	231,474	48,059	87,990	95,425
Diploma	344	48,059	48,059	...	...
Associate degree	656	87,990	...	87,990	...
Baccalaureate[2] ..	332	95,425	...	...	95,425
Two programs ...	21	10,785	...	4,971	5,814
Associate degree and baccalaureate	21	10,785	...	4,971	5,814

[1] Includes Guam, Puerto Rico, and Virgin Islands.
[2] Includes students in two initial programs leading to a master's degree.
SOURCE: National League for Nursing, 1979. Unpublished data.

CHART 7. SCHOOLS OF NURSING OFFERING INITIAL
PROFESSIONAL PROGRAMS, BY TYPE OF CONTROL,
OCTOBER 15, 1978

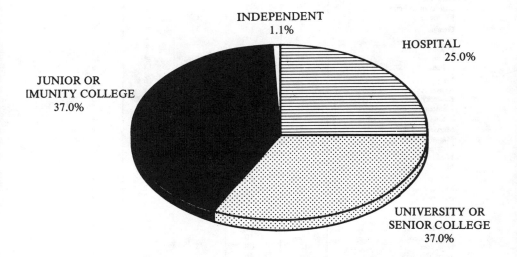

INDEPENDENT
1.1%

HOSPITAL
25.0%

JUNIOR OR
[MUNITY COLLEGE
37.0%

UNIVERSITY OR
SENIOR COLLEGE
37.0%

Type of control

SOURCE: National League for Nursing, 1979. Unpublished data.

Prepared by American Nurses' Association, Research and Policy Analysis Department, Statistics Unit, 1980.

Table II-B-7. Number of Schools and Number of Initial Programs—RN, October 15, 1978

State or area	Number of schools	Number of programs			
		Total	Diploma	Associate degree	Baccalaureate
Total	[1]1,353	[2]1,374	344	677	[3]353
United States, total	1,340	1,358	344	666	[3]348
Alabama	29	31	4	17	10
Alaska	2	2	...	1	1
Arizona	14	14	...	12	2
Arkansas	18	19	1	11	7
California	84	84	4	61	19
Colorado	12	12	2	7	3
Connecticut	19	19	5	7	7
Delaware	7	7	2	3	2
District of Columbia	7	7	1	1	5
Florida	31	31	1	22	8
Georgia	32	33	5	21	7
Hawaii	4	5	...	4	1
Idaho	6	6	...	5	1
Illinois	80	80	31	34	15
Indiana	27	30	7	14	9
Iowa	33	33	9	16	8
Kansas	24	24	6	11	7
Kentucky	27	28	2	20	6
Louisiana	16	16	3	6	7
Maine	9	9	4	3	2
Maryland	23	23	4	13	6
Massachusetts	51	52	22	19	11
Michigan	46	46	10	24	12
Minnesota	23	23	4	10	9
Mississippi	21	22	2	14	6
Missouri	34	35	12	16	7
Montana	4	4	...	2	2
Nebraska	12	12	6	2	4
Nevada	4	4	...	3	1
New Hampshire	8	8	5	1	2
New Jersey	41	41	21	13	7
New Mexico	10	10	...	9	1
New York	107	108	28	48	32
North Carolina	46	46	7	28	11
North Dakota	9	9	3	2	4
Ohio	68	68	31	25	12
Oklahoma	18	18	1	10	7
Oregon	16	16	1	13	2
Pennsylvania	97	97	55	19	23
Rhode Island	7	7	2	2	3
South Carolina	12	14	1	10	3
South Dakota	8	8	2	3	3
Tennessee	27	28	7	15	6
Texas	54	54	6	31	17
Utah	4	5	...	2	3
Vermont	3	4	...	3	1
Virginia	37	37	15	15	7
Washington	23	23	2	15	6
West Virginia	17	17	2	11	4
Wisconsin	26	26	8	10	8
Wyoming	3	3	...	2	1
Outlying areas, total	13	16	...	11	5
Guam	1	1	...	1	...
Puerto Rico	11	14	...	9	5
Virgin Islands	1	1	...	1	...

[1]Includes 21 schools conducting 2 programs each.
[2]Excludes programs closed prior to October 15.
[3]Includes two initial programs leading to a master's degree.
SOURCE: National League for Nursing, *State-Approved Schools of Nursing—R.N., 1979*, p. 60.

Table II-B-8. Initial Programs—RN in the United States and Outlying Areas,[1] 1969-1978, by Accreditation Status on Succeeding January 1

Year, as of October 15	Total programs, as of October 15[2]	Accredited							No accreditation status[3]						
		Total	Diploma		Associate degree		Baccalaureate		Total	Diploma		Associate degree		Baccalaureate	
			Number	Percent accredited	Number	Percent accredited	Number	Percent accredited		Number	Percent non-accredited	Number	Percent non-accredited	Number	Percent non-accredited
1978	1,374	958	321	93.3	344	50.8	[4]293	83.0	416	23	6.7	333	49.2	60	17.0
1977	1,372	902	333	90.7	293	44.7	[4]276	79.1	470	34	9.3	363	55.3	73	20.9
1976	1,373	918	352	90.3	294	45.8	[4]272	79.8	455	38	9.7	348	54.2	69	20.2
1975	1,375	904	382	89.3	268	43.4	254	77.2	471	46	10.7	350	56.6	[4]75	22.8
1974	1,372	874	401	87.0	235	39.3	238	76.0	498	60	13.0	363	60.7	[4]75	24.0
1973	1,373	861	431	87.2	206	35.9	224	73.4	512	63	12.8	368	64.1	[5]81	26.6
1972	1,377	855	462	85.1	180	33.3	[5]213	72.7	522	81	14.9	361	66.7	80	27.3
1971	1,363	840	489	83.3	153	31.2	[5]198	69.5	523	98	16.7	338	68.8	87	30.5
1970	1,355	836	521	81.3	128	28.8	[5]187	69.3	519	120	18.7	316	71.2	83	30.7
1969	1,339	819	556	80.0	90	23.1	[5]173	68.1	520	139	20.0	300	76.9	81	31.9

[1]Includes Guam, Puerto Rico, and Virgin Islands.
[2]Excludes programs closed prior to October 15.
[3]Included in this category are programs which applied but were never accredited and those which never applied for accreditation.
[4]Includes two initial programs leading to a master's degree.
[5]Includes one initial program leading to a master's degree.

SOURCE: National League for Nursing, *State-Approved Schools of Nursing—R.N. 1979*, and previous years.

Table II-B-9. Accreditation Status of Initial Programs—RN, January 1, 1979[1]

		Accredited			No accreditation status[2]		
State or area	Total number of programs	Diploma programs	Associate degree programs	Baccalaureate programs	Diploma programs	Associate degree programs	Baccalaureate programs
Total	[3]1,374	321	344	[3]293	23	333	60
United States, total ...	[3]1,358	321	338	[3]291	23	328	57
Alabama	31	4	8	8	...	9	2
Alaska	2	...	1	1	...	...	...
Arizona	14	...	8	2	...	4	...
Arkansas	19	...	5	2	1	6	5
California	84	4	23	19	...	38	...
Colorado	12	2	2	3	...	5	...
Connecticut	19	5	5	6	...	2	1
Delaware	7	1	2	1	1	1	1
District of Columbia	7	1	1	4	...	...	1
Florida	31	1	4	6	...	18	2
Georgia	33	5	16	4	...	5	3
Hawaii	5	...	1	1	...	3	...
Idaho	6	...	5	1	...	...	...
Illinois	80	30	12	12	1	22	3
Indiana	30	7	12	8	...	2	1
Iowa	33	9	...	6	...	16	2
Kansas	24	6	4	6	...	7	1
Kentucky	28	1	11	4	1	9	2
Louisiana	16	3	4	6	...	2	1
Maine	9	4	2	1	...	1	1
Maryland	23	4	7	3	...	6	3
Massachusetts	52	22	13	9	...	6	2
Michigan	46	10	5	9	...	19	3
Minnesota	23	4	9	8	...	1	1
Mississippi	22	1	2	4	1	12	2
Missouri	35	12	6	6	...	10	1
Montana	4	...	...	2	...	2	...
Nebraska	12	6	2	2	...	...	2
Nevada	4	...	1	1	...	2	...
New Hampshire	8	3	1	2	2	...	...
New Jersey	41	18	11	7	3	2	...
New Mexico	10	...	4	1	...	5	...
New York	108	24	33	28	4	15	4
North Carolina	46	5	4	11	2	24	...
North Dakota	9	3	1	3	...	1	1
Ohio	68	31	14	9	...	11	3
Oklahoma	18	1	9	6	...	1	1
Oregon	16	1	6	2	...	7	...
Pennsylvania	97	51	9	18	4	10	5
Rhode Island	7	2	2	3	...	...	...
South Carolina	14	...	6	3	1	4	...
South Dakota	8	2	2	3	...	1	...
Tennessee	28	7	13	6	...	2	...
....	54	6	22	16	...	9	1
....	5	...	2	2	...	...	1
Vermont	4	...	3	1	...	...	...
Virginia	37	13	7	7	2	8	...
Washington	23	2	9	6	...	6	...
West Virginia	17	2	6	3	...	5	1
Wisconsin	26	8	3	8	...	7	...
Wyoming	3	...	...	1	...	2	...
Outlying areas, total ...	16	...	6	2	...	5	3
Guam	1	...	...	...	...	1	...
Puerto Rico	14	...	5	2	...	4	3
Virgin Islands	1	...	1	...	...	...	...

[1]Accreditation status is as of January 1, 1979, but the number of programs in existence is as of October 15, 1978, excluding those closed prior to October 15.

[2]Included in this category are programs which applied but were never accredited and those which never applied for accreditation.

[3]Includes two initial programs leading to a master's degree.

SOURCE: National League for Nursing, *State-Approved Schools of Nursing—R.N., 1979*, p. 60.

Chapter II, Section C
REGISTERED NURSE EDUCATION

Major changes taking place in the health care system are having tremendous implications for nursing. The growing complexity of health care dictates a commitment toward continuing education for all health professionals, including nurses. In the nursing profession, certain positions often require post-basic educational preparation. Teaching, administration, and research in nursing have historically required advanced academic credentials. Nursing's expanded knowledge base, new opportunities for clinical specialties, and supervisory positions necessitate formal education beyond initial training as a nurse. While continuing education may take many forms, this chapter provides information on registered nurses enrolled in programs leading to academic degrees.

According to the 1978 statistics compiled by the National League for Nursing, there were 39,457 registered nurse students enrolled in baccalaureate and higher degree programs in nursing. This figure represents a 9 percent rise over the previous year, when enrollments totaled 36,192 nurses; however, this increase was about half the annual percentage gains observed in the previous 6 years. The majority of nurses (64.8 percent) enrolled in colleges and universities were in baccalaureate nursing programs; 33.2 percent were in master's degree programs, and 2.0 percent were studying for a doctorate. Changes in enrollments among the component programs from 1977 to 1978 exhibited lower rates of increase (9.9 percent and 7.9 percent) for the baccalaureate and master's degree programs than those in the previous years. The doctoral enrollments showed negative growth, down from large growth spurts of around 25 percent in prior years. In 1978, there were 18,134 nurses enrolled on a full-time basis ånd 21,323 nurses continuing their formal education part-time. More nurses in academic nursing programs were part-timers. The trend for part-time enrollments has risen steadily from 38 percent in 1970 to 54 percent of the overall matriculation figures in 1978. With the marginal exception of the master's degree students, each program showed a proclivity toward part-time enrollment: 56.1 percent of the baccalaureate, 54.6 percent of the doctoral, and 49.9 percent of the master's candidates were enrolled less than full-time.

For master's degree students, NLN also compiled information on the nursing focus and functional purpose of the curriculum in which the registered nurses were enrolled for full-time study. The 1978 data revealed medical-surgical nursing as the primary focus area for about a quarter of the registered nurses, followed by maternal-child health nursing (17.6 percent) and psychiatric-mental health nursing practice (16.1 percent). While medical-surgical nursing has traditionally dominated as the focus of advanced nursing preparation, 1978 marked the first time maternal-child health nursing held second place status. In previous years, psychiatric-mental health nursing ranked second. In terms of the functional purpose of the degree, almost three-quarters of the master's students indicated advanced clinical practice, regardless of the focus area of the degree. In descending order, teaching was chosen by 13.4 percent of the master's candidates; 5 percent chose administration; 2.6 percent, supervision;

2.6 percent, supervision and teaching; 0.8 percent, other; and 1.2 percent did not report a functional area.

Graduations in 1978 from baccalaureate and master's degree programs recorded gains of 12.9 percent and 11.5 percent over the previous year, while the number of earned doctorates declined by 10.2 percent. In 1978, there were 6,146 bachelor's, 4,271 master's, and 53 doctoral degrees awarded to registered nurses. In 1978 the graduates from master's programs in nursing continued to be concentrated in medical-surgical nursing, which encompassed about one-third of those earning degrees. The second largest group of graduates (17.1 percent) focused on psychiatric-mental health, followed by maternal-child health (16.3 percent) and public health nursing (6.6 percent).

The Association of Schools of Public Health provided data on the admissions and enrollments in public health nursing programs offered by schools of public health. In 1978, about 3.0 percent of the total admissions to schools of public health were nurses entering public health nursing programs. The 112 nurses admitted to such programs in 1978 marked a 26 percent gain from the previous year. Nurse enrollments in public health nursing programs totaled 168 in 1978.

Data from the 1977 national sample survey of registered nurses conducted by the American Nurses' Association under contract with the Division of Nursing, Public Health Service, U.S. Department of Health and Human Services, estimated there were 165,979 registered nurses enrolled in formal educational programs in 1977. These data indicate a vast majority of nurses were continuing their formal training outside schools of nursing. It is estimated that 67.8 percent were enrolled in baccalaureate programs and 25.6 percent in master's and higher degree programs. A small proportion (6.0 percent) reported seeking an associate degree. Based on the median age of this group, it was speculated that some older diploma nurses may have elected the associate degree route as re-entry into formal education to update their nursing skills or to obtain a more general educational background.

Table II-C-1. Registered Nurse Students Enrolled in Colleges and Universities, by Type of Nursing Program, Fall 1969-1978

Year	Total number enrolled	Baccalaureate		Master's		Doctoral	
		Number	Percent	Number	Percent	Number	Percent
1978	39,457	25,563	64.8	13,105	33.2	789	2.0
1977	36,192	23,259	64.3	12,143	33.6	790	2.2
1976	30,672	19,231	62.7	10,809	35.2	632	2.1
1975	26,022	15,854	60.9	9,662	37.1	506	1.9
1974	21,924	13,518	61.7	7,924	36.1	482	2.2
1973	18,872	11,711	62.1	6,786	36.0	375	2.0
1972	15,967	9,223	57.8	6,342	39.7	402	2.5
1971	13,398	7,700	57.5	5,405	40.3	293	2.2
1970	12,769	7,692	60.2	4,765	37.3	312	2.4
1969	13,058	8,329	63.8	4,443	34.0	286	2.2

SOURCES: National League for Nursing, *Some Statistics on Baccalaureate and Higher Degree Programs in Nursing, 1976-77, NLN Nursing Data Book*, 1978, and unpublished data, 1980.

Table II-C-2. Percent Change Each Year in Registered Nurse Students Enrolled in Colleges and Universities, by Type of Program, Fall 1969-1978

Year	Total enrollment	Baccalaureate	Master's	Doctoral
1978	+ 9.0	+ 9.9	+ 7.9	− 0.1
1977	+18.0	+20.9	+12.3	+25.0
1976	+17.9	+21.3	+11.9	+24.9
1975	+18.7	+17.3	+21.9	+ 5.0
1974	+16.2	+15.4	+16.8	+28.5
1973	+18.2	+27.0	+ 7.0	− 6.7
1972	+19.2	+19.8	+17.3	+37.2
1971	+ 4.9	+ 0.1	+13.4	− 6.1
1970	− 2.2	− 7.6	+ 7.2	+ 9.1
1969	+ 7.7	+ 6.1	+10.6	+10.9

SOURCES: National League for Nursing, *Some Statistics on Baccalaureate and Higher Degree Programs in Nursing, 1976-77, NLN Nursing Data Book*, 1978, and unpublished data, 1980.

Table II-C-3. Registered Nurse Students Enrolled in Colleges and Universities for Full-time and Part-time Study, Fall 1969-1978

Year	Number of colleges and universities	Enrollment				
		Total	Full-time		Part-time	
			Number	Percent	Number	Percent
1978	537	39,457	18,134	46	21,323	54
1977	516	36,192	16,853	47	19,339	53
1976	473	30,672	15,774	51	14,898	49
1975	329	26,022	13,262	51	12,760	49
1974	315	21,924	11,479	52	10,445	48
1973	280	18,872	10,660	56	8,212	44
1972	267	15,967	10,084	63	5,883	37
1971	240	13,398	8,772	65	4,626	35
1970	216	12,769	7,878	62	4,891	38
1969	201	13,058	7,672	59	5,386	41

SOURCES: National League for Nursing, *Some Statistics on Baccalaureate and Higher Degree Programs in Nursing, 1976-77*, and previous years; *NLN Nursing Data Book*, 1978, and unpublished data, 1980.

Table II-C-4. Registered Nurse Students Granted Academic Degrees in Nursing from Colleges and Universities, 1968-69 to 1977-78

Academic year[1]	Total number of graduates	Baccalaureate		Master's		Doctoral	
		Number	Percent	Number	Percent	Number	Percent
1977-78	10,470	6,146	58.7	4,271	40.8	53	0.5
1976-77	9,334	5,445	58.3	3,830	41.0	59	0.6
1975-76	8,258	4,759	57.6	3,437	41.6	62	0.8
1974-75	6,559	3,791	57.8	2,694	41.1	74	1.1
1973-74	5,692	3,003	52.8	2,643	46.4	46	0.8
1972-73	5,176	2,681	51.8	2,446	47.3	49	0.9
1971-72	4,499	2,337	51.9	2,135	47.5	27	0.6
1970-71	4,338	2,214	51.0	2,083	48.0	41	1.0
1969-70	4,428	2,413	54.5	1,988	44.9	27	0.6
1968-69	3,981	2,176	54.6	1,766	44.4	39	1.0

[1] Reporting dates for baccalaureate programs prior to 1970-71 and for graduate programs prior to 1971-72 were September 1 through August 31. The current reporting dates are August 1 to July 31.

SOURCES: National League for Nursing, *NLN Nursing Data Book*, 1978, and unpublished data, 1980.

CHART 8. REGISTERED NURSE STUDENTS GRANTED
ACADEMIC DEGREES, 1974-75 to 1977-78

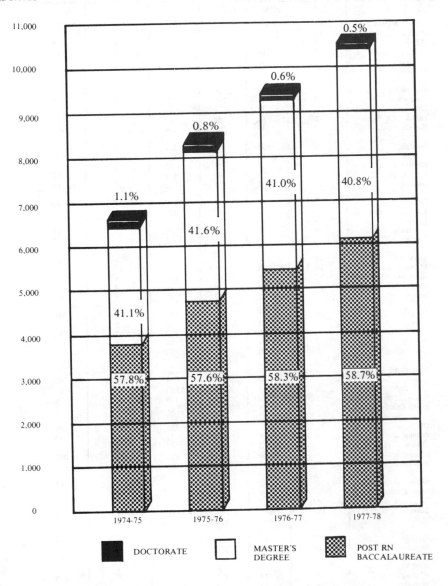

NUMBER OF
GRADUATES

SOURCE: National League for Nursing. *NLN Nursing Data Book*. 1978 and unpublished data. 1980.

Prepared by American Nurses' Association. Research and Policy Analysis Department. Statistics Unit. 1980.

**Table II-C-5. Number of Registered Nurse Students Enrolled[1]
in and Graduated[2] from Baccalaureate Programs in Colleges
and Universities, 1978**

| State or area | Enrollment, fall 1978 | | | | Graduations 1977-78 | |
	Number of institutions	Total	Full-time	Part-time	Number of institutions	Number of graduates
Total	399	25,563	11,215	14,348	323	6,146
United States, total ...	395	25,437	11,171	14,266	320	6,122
Alabama	13	863	456	407	10	141
Alaska	1	57	15	42	1	5
Arizona	2	104	104	...	2	18
Arkansas	6	45	34	11	2	8
California	24	1,647	650	997	21	745
Colorado	6	839	220	619	4	142
Connecticut	7	394	118	276	4	71
Delaware	1	35	9	26	1	1
District of Columbia	5	82	49	33	4	36
Florida	7	510	302	208	6	202
Georgia	9	508	186	322	6	250
Hawaii	1	12	12	...	1	6
Idaho	2	37	21	16	2	17
Illinois	16	797	383	414	14	252
Indiana	11	762	311	451	10	219
Iowa	9	276	119	157	7	99
Kansas	8	166	52	114	6	45
Kentucky	7	441	238	203	7	67
Louisiana	8	129	58	71	5	17
Maine	1	20	17	3	1	5
Maryland	5	276	193	83	3	128
Massachusetts	14	735	495	240	13	280
Michigan	12	848	247	601	9	165
Minnesota	10	262	228	34	9	122
Mississippi	4	85	42	43	5	67
Missouri	12	1,212	221	991	8	288
Montana	2	53	48	5	2	34
Nebraska	3	250	128	122	3	93
Nevada	2	69	16	53	1	16
New Hampshire ...	2	370	16	354	1	14
New Jersey	8	781	495	286	7	177
New Mexico	2	70	44	26	1	7
New York	39	6,790	2,948	3,842	30	929
North Carolina	11	218	109	109	11	70
North Dakota	3	33	22	11	3	11
Ohio	16	970	337	633	12	144
Oklahoma	6	78	45	33	5	15
Oregon	3	123	40	83	3	40
Pennsylvania	29	1,434	539	895	22	297
Rhode Island	3	267	69	198	3	67
South Carolina	4	192	121	71	3	62
South Dakota	3	19	14	5	2	7
Tennessee	9	402	177	225	7	40
Texas	19	687	365	322	14	268
Utah	3	132	113	19	3	56
Vermont	1	14	9	5	1	2
Virginia	8	327	234	93	7	125
Washington	6	230	187	43	6	62
West Virginia	4	262	106	156	4	68
Wisconsin	7	513	202	311	7	119
Wyoming	1	11	7	4	1	3
Puerto Rico	4	126	44	82	3	24

[1]Enrollments as of October 15, 1978.
[2]Graduations between August 1, 1977 and July 31, 1978.
SOURCE: National League for Nursing, 1979. Unpublished data.

Table II-C-6. Full-time Enrollments in Master's Programs, by Nursing Focus and Functional Purpose of Curriculum, Fall 1978

| Nursing focus | Total | Administration | | Supervision | Teaching | Supervision and teaching | Advanced clinical practice | Other | Not specified |
		Service	Education						
Total	6,561	327	2	172	882	170	4,878	53	77
Medical-surgical	1,768	...	...	20	318	...	1,430	...	...
Maternal-child	1,158	...	...	11	163	...	984	...	...
Maternal-child	467	...	...	1	71	...	395	...	...
Maternity	156	...	...	4	25	...	127	...	...
Pediatrics	535	...	...	6	67	...	462	...	...
Psychiatric-mental health	1,059	...	...	5	108	...	946	...	...
Public health nursing	472	32	...	16	42	...	382	...	...
Other[1]	2,027	295	2	120	251	170	1,136	53	...
None	77	...	...	...	...	...	...	...	77

[1] Includes sciences, fundamentals, inservice, combined majors, and rehabilitation.
SOURCE: National League for Nursing, 1980. Unpublished data.

Table II-C-7. Number of Registered Nurse Students Enrolled[1] in Master's and Doctoral Programs in Colleges and Universities, Fall 1978

	Enrollment							
	Master's program				Doctoral program			
State or area	Number of institutions	Total	Full-time	Part-time	Number of institutions	Total	Full-time	Part-time
Total	118	13,105	6,561	6,544	20	789	358	431
United States, total	116	13,087	6,543	6,544	20	789	358	431
Alabama	1	271	136	135	1	45	31	14
Alaska	...	...	...	...	...	...	...	...
Arizona	2	224	101	123	1	10	9	1
Arkansas	2	78	19	59	...	...	...	...
California	8	1,080	663	417	1	42	42	...
Colorado	1	201	191	10	1	2	2	...
Connecticut	2	226	191	35	...	...	...	...
Delaware	1	51	26	25	...	...	...	...
District of Columbia ...	1	370	219	151	1	81	34	47
Florida	2	98	65	33	...	...	...	...
Georgia	3	266	150	116	...	...	...	...
Hawaii	1	66	66	...	...	...	...	...
Idaho	...	...	...	...	...	...	...	...
Illinois	7	809	307	502	2	51	41	10
Indiana	3	365	129	236	1	10	6	4
Iowa	1	72	44	28	...	...	...	...
Kansas	2	288	31	257	...	...	...	...
Kentucky	1	75	64	11	...	...	...	...
Louisiana	3	79	49	30	...	...	...	...
Maine	...	...	...	...	...	...	...	...
Maryland	1	354	201	153	...	...	...	...
Massachusetts	5	486	352	134	1	38	7	31
Michigan	3	281	158	123	2	48	44	4
Minnesota	2	210	147	63	...	...	...	...
Mississippi	3	90	57	33	...	...	...	...
Missouri	3	208	110	98	...	...	...	...
Montana	1	18	17	1	...	...	...	...
Nebraska	1	107	46	61	...	...	...	...
Nevada	...	...	...	...	...	...	...	...
New Hampshire	...	...	...	...	...	...	...	...
New Jersey	2	264	97	167	...	...	...	...
New Mexico	...	...	...	...	...	...	...	...
New York	13	2,261	913	1,348	2	285	41	244
North Carolina	5	264	131	133	...	...	...	...
North Dakota	...	...	...	...	...	...	...	...
Ohio	5	462	279	183	1	18	16	2
Oklahoma	1	94	19	75	...	...	...	...
Oregon	2	113	44	69	...	...	...	...
Pennsylvania	4	643	307	336	2	37	15	22
Rhode Island	1	43	21	22	...	...	...	...
South Carolina	2	159	56	103	...	...	...	...
South Dakota	...	...	...	...	...	...	...	...
Tennessee	3	193	153	40	...	...	...	...
Texas	8	1,184	332	852	2	100	53	47
Utah	2	166	131	35	1	14	9	5
Vermont	...	...	...	...	...	...	...	...
Virginia	2	192	124	68	...	...	...	...
Washington	1	310	221	89	1	8	8	...
West Virginia	1	39	16	23	...	...	...	...
Wisconsin	4	327	160	167	...	...	...	...
Wyoming	...	...	...	...	...	...	...	...
Puerto Rico	2	18	18	...	...	...	...	...

[1] Enrollments as of October 15, 1978.

SOURCE: National League for Nursing, 1979. Unpublished data.

Table II-C-8. Graduations From Master's Programs, by Nursing Focus and Functional Purpose of Curriculum, Academic Years 1972-73 to 1977-78

Academic year[1]	Total	Nursing focus					
		Medical-surgical	Maternal-child	Psychiatric-mental health	Public health nursing	Other[2]	None
1977-78	4,271	1,271	695	732	284	1,275	14
1976-77	3,830	1,007	579	678	364	1,155	47
1975-76	3,437	969	524	620	329	82'	174
1974-75	2,694	811	487	551	359	46	19
1973-74	2,643	776	470	568	282	2'	318
1972-73	2,446	781	389	601	309	...	304

Academic year[1]	Total	Functional purpose of curriculum							
		Administration		Supervision	Teaching	Supervision and teaching	Advanced clinical practice	Other	Not specified
		Service	Education						
1977-78	4,271	268	2	146	974	157	2,675	35	14
1976-77	3,830	219	7	43	944	6	2,468	96	47
1975-76	3,437	174	15	120	895	18	2,016	25	174
1974-75	2,694	172	7	38	769	27	1,632	30	19
1973-74	2,643	166	5	89	864	6	1,504	...	9
1972-73	2,446	149	6	109	760	16	1,351	...	55

[1] Reporting dates are August 1 through July 31.
[2] Includes sciences, fundamentals, inservice, combined majors, and rehabilitation.
SOURCE: National League for Nursing. *Some Statistics on Baccalaureate and Higher Degree Programs in Nursing, 1976-77,* and previous years, *NLN Nursing Data Book, 1978,* and unpublished data, 1980.

Table II-C-9. Graduations from Master's Programs, by Nursing Focus and Functional Purpose of Curriculum, Academic Year 1977-78

| Nursing focus | Total | Administration | | Supervision | Teaching | Supervision and teaching | Advanced clinical practice | Other | Not specified |
		Service	Education						
Total	4,271	268	2	146	974	157	2,675	35	14
Medical-surgical	1,271	...	...	4	389	...	878	...	...
Maternal-child	695	...	...	1	185	...	509	...	...
Maternal-child	348	...	...	...	114	...	234	...	...
Maternity	84	...	...	1	25	...	58	...	...
Pediatrics	263	...	...	...	46	...	217	...	...
Psychiatric-mental health	732	...	...	4	121	...	607	...	...
Public health nursing	284	20	...	18	67	3	176	...	...
Other[1]	1,275	248	2	119	212	154	505	35	...
None	14	...	...	...	...	...	...	...	14

[1]Includes sciences, fundamentals, inservice, combined majors, and rehabilitation.
SOURCE: National League for Nursing, 1980. Unpublished data.

Table II-C-10. Registered Nurse Students Granted Master's and Doctoral Degrees in Nursing from Colleges and Universities, August 1, 1977-July 31, 1978

State or area	Master's		Doctoral	
	Number of institutions	Number of graduates	Number of institutions	Number of graduates
Total	109	4,271	11	53
United States, total...	107	4,255	11	53
Alabama	1	64	...	...
Alaska	...	...	...	...
Arizona	2	54	...	...
Arkansas	2	18	...	...
California	8	327	1	5
Colorado	1	99	...	...
Connecticut	2	75	...	...
Delaware	1	4	...	...
District of Columbia	1	99	1	5
Florida	2	39	...	...
Georgia	3	223	...	...
Hawaii	1	16	...	...
Idaho	...	...	...	...
Illinois	7	273	1	1
Indiana	3	76	...	...
Iowa	1	31	...	...
Kansas	2	19	...	...
Kentucky	1	31	...	...
Louisiana	3	33	...	...
Maine	...	...	...	...
Maryland	1	106	...	...
Massachusetts	4	363	1	1
Michigan	3	117	2	3
Minnesota	2	93	...	...
Mississippi	3	45	...	...
Missouri	3	75	...	...
Montana	1	4	...	...
Nebraska	1	23	...	...
Nevada	...	...	...	...
New Hampshire ...	...	...	...	...
New Jersey	2	34	...	...
New Mexico	...	...	...	...
New York	11	771	1	27
North Carolina	5	86	...	...
North Dakota	...	...	...	...
Ohio	3	128	1	1
Oklahoma	1	33	...	...
Oregon	1	16	...	...
Pennsylvania	4	203	1	3
Rhode Island	1	24	...	...
South Carolina	2	32	...	...
South Dakota	...	...	...	...
Tennessee	2	76	...	...
Texas	6	310	2	7
Utah	2	23	...	...
Vermont	...	...	...	...
Virginia	2	43	...	...
Washington	1	83	...	...
West Virginia	1	6	...	...
Wisconsin	4	80	...	...
Wyoming	...	...	...	...
Puerto Rico	2	16	...	...

SOURCE: National League for Nursing, 1980. Unpublished data.

**Table II-C-11. Admissions to Schools of Public Health and Public Health
Nursing Programs, 1974-75 to 1978-79**

		Schools of public health	
		Public health nursing programs	
	Total	Admissions	
Year	admissions	Number	Percent
1978-79	3,735	112	3.0
1977-78	3,427	89	2.6
1976-77	3,317	79	2.4
1975-76	2,708	81	3.0
1974-75	2,980	143	4.8

SOURCE: Association of Schools of Public Health. Unpublished data, 1980.

**Table II-C-12. Enrollments in Schools of Public Health and Public
Health Nursing Programs, 1974-75 to 1978-79**

		Schools of public health	
		Public health nursing programs	
	Total	Enrollments	
Year	enrollments	Number	Percent
1978-79	7,106	168	2.4
1977-78	6,463	143	2.2
1976-77	6,217	115	1.8
1975-76	6,020	240	4.0
1974-75	5,072	146	2.9

SOURCE: Association of Schools of Public Health. Unpublished data, 1980.

Table II-C-13. Estimated Number and Median Age of Registered Nurses[1] Enrolled in an Educational Program by Type of Degree Sought, September 1977

Type of degree sought	(n)	N	Median age
Total	1,845	165,979	34.3
Associate degree	101	9,899	40.5
Baccalaureate	1,253	112,504	34.1
Master's degree and above ...	472	42,536	33.8
Not reported	19	1,041	

[1] Includes only registered nurses actively licensed in September 1977 who worked in the United States if employed in nursing, or lived in the United States if not employed in nursing and who responded to the question on age.

NOTE: "N" corresponds to the weighted population estimate derived from the sample and "n" refers to the actual number of surveys upon which the sample was based. Because of rounding, sum of estimated numbers (N) may not add to total.

SOURCE: Roth, Aleda V., et al. *1977 National Sample Survey of Registered Nurses: A Report on the Nurse Population and Factors Affecting Their Supply*, final report on Contract No. (HRA 231-76-0085) between the American Nurses' Association and the Division of Nursing, U.S. Department of Health and Human Services, NTIS Publication No. HRP-0900603, 1979.

Table II-C.14. Estimated Number and Percent of Registered Nurses[1] Enrolled in an Educational Program by Type of Enrollment and Type of Degree Sought, September 1977

Type of degree sought	Total			Type of enrollment								
				Full-time			Part-time			Full/part-time not reported		
	(n)	N	Percent	(n)	N	Percent	(n)	N	Percent	(n)	N	Percent
Total	1,845	165,979	100.0	387	35,989	21.7	1,449	129,446	78.0	9	544	0.3
Associate degree	101	9,899	100.0	13	1,121	11.3	88	8,777	88.7	...	...	...
Baccalaureate	1,253	112,504	100.0	230	21,022	18.7	1,022	91,427	81.3	1	56	(2)
Master's degree	393	35,214	100.0	112	10,911	31.0	281	24,303	69.0	...	...	...
Doctorate	79	7,322	100.0	31	2,900	39.6	48	4,421	60.4	...	...	...
Not reported	19	1,041	100.0	1	35		10	518		8	488	...

[1] Includes only registered nurses actively licensed in September 1977 who worked in the United States if employed in nursing, or lived in the United States if not employed in nursing.
[2] Less than 0.1 percent

NOTE: "N" corresponds to the weighted population estimate derived from the sample and "n" refers to the actual number of surveys upon which the sample was based. Because of rounding, sums of estimated numbers (N) and estimated percents may not add to totals.

SOURCE: Roth, Aleda V., et al. 1977 National Sample Survey of Registered Nurses: A Report on the Nurse Population and Factors Affecting Their Supply, final report on Contract No. (HRA 231-76-0085) between the American Nurses' Association and the Division of Nursing, U.S. Department of Health and Human Services, NTIS Publication No. HRP-0900603, 1979.

Chapter II, Section D
FINANCIAL ASSISTANCE

Financial assistance to nursing students in the form of scholarships and loans is made available through several sources, including the federal government, some state governments, and private sources. These funds have been specifically set aside for students in the field of nursing. Students desiring detailed information about financial assistance should write directly to individual schools of nursing.

Federal support for psychiatric nursing has been provided from the National Institute of Mental Health, an agency of the U.S. Department of Health, Education, and Welfare (now the Department of Health and Human Services). The number of NIMH trainee stipends in psychiatric nursing awarded in 1979-80 totaled 890, a decrease of 13.5 percent from the previous year. The components of change, however, varied by type of program, revealing the overall decline could be attributed to substantially reduced aid for continuing education training, since assistance in the form of stipends from NIMH showed increases for formal education. In 1979-80, 44 stipends were given to baccalaureate students, 779 to master's candidates, 37 to predoctoral students, and 30 for other stipends. These figures reflected the following changes over the previous year among the programs: 12.8 percent, 9.1 percent, 76.2 percent, and −88.2 percent, respectively.

The Rehabilitation Services Administration of the Division of Manpower Development awarded five Rehabilitation Nursing Traineeships in 1979-80, equalling the number awarded in each of the two prior years. In fiscal year 1977-78, 77 nurses were supported through Public Health Traineeships. The Public Health Traineeships were reduced by 17 from fiscal year 1977. Maternal and Child Health Service funds for advanced study in maternal and pediatric nursing rose almost 32 percent in academic year 1977-78 over the previous year to 381 fellowships. There was only a slight increase (1.3 percent) in 1978-79 to 386 fellowships. Academic year 1978-79 marked the largest number of maternal and pediatric nursing fellowships awarded in a single year over the past decade.

Table II-D-1. National Institute of Mental Health Trainee Stipends in Psychiatric Nursing, by Academic Year of Training, 1970-71 to 1979-80

Academic year	Total	Baccalaureate	Master's	Predoctoral	Other
1979-80	890	44	779	37	[1]30
1978-79	1,029	39	714	[2]21	255
1977-78	1,092	134	740	[2]69	149
1976-77	1,252	165	882	[2]59	[1]146
1975-76	1,210	189	931	[2]50	[3]40
1974-75	1,272	281	940	[2]51	...
1973-74	1,224	201	982	[2]41	...
1972-73	1,368	310	1,019	[2]39	...
1971-72	1,407	333	1,014	[2]60	...
1970-71	1,432	257	1,065	[2,4]110	...

[1] Training in continuing education.
[2] Includes postmaster's trainee stipends for training in research and special areas.
[3] Clinical specialist on a conference grant.
[4] Includes 15 stipends for short term training.

SOURCE: U.S. Department of Health and Human Services, Public Health Service, National Institute of Mental Health, Division of Manpower and Training Programs, 1980, and previous years. Unpublished data.

Table II-D-2. Public Health Traineeships, 1968-69 to 1977-78

Fiscal year[1]	Number of trainees	Fiscal year[1]	Number of trainees
1977-78	77	1972-73	266
1976-77	94	1971-72	[3]208
1975-76	147	1970-71	364
1974-75	233	1969-70	291
1973-74	[2]26	1968-69	320

[1] Data reflects number of nurses supported during a given year, July 1 through June 30.
[2] Public Health Traineeship Awards for training in fiscal year 1974 were made only to enrolled trainees to permit them to complete their training.
[3] First year that Public Health Traineeship Awards were made under the Public Health Special Purpose Traineeship Program. Prior to this time awards were made under a separate program.

SOURCE: U.S. Department of Health, Education, and Welfare, Public Health Service, Health Resources Administration, Bureau of Health Manpower, Division of Associated Health Professions, 1978, and previous years. Unpublished data.

Table II-D-3. Maternal and Child Health Service[1] Funds for Advanced Study in Maternal and Pediatric Nursing, 1969-70 to 1978-79

Academic year	Fellowships awarded	Academic year	Fellowships awarded
1978-79	386	1973-74	302
1977-78	381	1972-73	253
1976-77	289	1971-72	120
1975-76	311	1970-71	109
1974-75	347	1969-70	93

[1] Formerly Children's Bureau.
SOURCE: U.S. Department of Health and Human Services, Public Health Service, Health Services Administration, Bureau of Community Health Services, 1980, and previous years. Unpublished data.

Table II-D-4. Rehabilitation Nursing Traineeships, 1970-71 to 1979-80

Fiscal year	Traineeships awarded	Fiscal year	Traineeships awarded
1979-80	5	1974-75	8
1978-79	5	1973-74	13
1977-78	5	1972-73	17
1976-77	6	1971-72	23
1975-76	9	1970-71	55

SOURCE: U.S. Department of Health and Human Services, Division of Manpower Development, Rehabilitation Services Administration, 1980, and previous years. Unpublished data.

Chapter III, Section A
EMPLOYMENT CONDITIONS IN HOSPITALS AND RELATED FACILITIES

Included within this section are data from the Bureau of Labor Statistics, U.S. Department of Labor's latest comprehensive survey of employment conditions in hospitals and nursing and personal care homes, as well as information from the 1979 National Survey of Hospitals and Medical School Salaries, and the 1977 national sample survey of registered nurses.

The 1978 BLS hospital survey covered all private (nongovernment) and state and local government hospitals employing 100 workers or more within 23 standard metropolitan statistical areas (SMSAs). Excluded from the scope of the survey were hospitals operated by the federal government. Average hourly salaries paid to registered nurses in seven nursing positions within these hospitals were computed for each SMSA in the study. Summary earnings statistics are presented in the narrative for full-time registered nurses in nonfederal hospitals. The tables provide more detailed breakdowns for the government and nongovernment components. For directors of nursing, those in the New York City area, earning on the average of $14.03 per hour, had the highest wages, while their counterparts in the Seattle-Everett, Washington area had the lowest hourly earnings ($9.49). Salaries of nursing supervisors ranged from $7.61 per hour for those in the Atlanta, Georgia area to $10.25 in San Francisco-Oakland, California. These two geographic areas also had the low and high average hourly earnings for general duty nurses, although the spread was not as great, from $5.84 to $8.32.

Among the metropolitan areas covered in the survey, almost all nurses employed in nonfederal hospitals had insurance protection for hospitalization and surgical and medical benefits paid for wholly or partially by the hospital. There was more diversity among the areas in the coverage provided by the hospitals for other types of insurance protection, such as life, accidental death and dismemberment, sickness and accident, major medical, and dental. After one year of service, nurses generally received at least 2 weeks paid vacation. Five years of service marked the point at which the majority of nurses earned at least 3 weeks of paid vacation. The Northeastern area appeared to have more liberal provisions for paid vacations. Most nonfederal hospitals offered at least eight paid holidays per year. As was true with paid vacations, the Northeastern geographic area appeared to have the most generous holiday provisions; the majoriy of hospitals in this region offered at least 10 paid holidays.

The University of Texas Medical Branch at Galveston conducted a 1979 National Survey of Hospitals and Medical School Salaries. The July 1979 survey consisted of 37 hospitals, 12 medical schools, and 29 medical centers. Calculation of monthly salaries was based upon a standard 40-hour week, exclusive of the cash value of fringe benefits. The average monthly starting salary for staff nurses in all institutions combined was $1,041, representing a 5.9 percent increase since July 1978. This figure reflected the average monthly salary that would normally be paid to fill vacant staff nurse positions in the various institutions.

The average monthly recruiting salary for head nurses was $1,242; for clinical nurse specialists, $1,333 per month; and for nurse anesthetists, $1,523. The percent increase since 1978 in the average starting salaries for head nurses equalled that of the staff nurses, but was slightly exceeded by the gains of clinical nurse specialists (6.0 percent). Average maximum monthly salaries recorded in 1979 were $1,363 for staff nurses, $1,603 for head nurses, $1,675 for clinical nurse specialists, and $1,965 for nurse anesthetists.

Data from the 1977 national sample survey of registered nurses reported the average earnings of all registered nurses in hospitals and nursing homes for selected types of positions. Nationally, in 1977 nurses holding administrative positions averaged $1,461 monthly; nurse supervisors, $1,183; head nurses, $1,121; and general duty nurses, $1,021. Staff nurses in nursing home settings averaged $881 per month.

The BLS collected data on earnings and supplementary benefits of nurses in nongovernment nursing and personal care facilities in 21 SMSAs in September 1978. For full-time general duty nurses, the average hourly earnings ranged from $5.25 in Buffalo, New York, to $8.16 in the New York City area. Average earnings for head nurses working full-time ranged from $4.99 per hour in the Kansas City area to $9.25 per hour in the New York City area. For the most part, at least 50 percent of the nursing and personal care homes offered hospitalization, surgical, and medical insurance coverage. Those in the Northeastern area were the most likely to provide such coverage. With respect to the number of paid holidays, most facilities gave at least 7 days, although there was much variation in the number of paid holidays among the SMSAs.

Table III-A-1. Average Hourly Earnings¹ and Number of Full-time Registered Nurses in Nonfederal Hospitals, by Metropolitan Area,² September 1978

Metropolitan area	Director of nursing		Supervisor of nurses		Nursing instructor		Head nurse		General duty nurse		Clinical nursing specialist		Nurse anesthetist	
	Number	Average hourly earnings	Number	Average hourly earnings	Number	Average hourly earnings	Number	Average hourly earnings	Number	Average hourly earnings	Number	Average hourly earnings	Number	Average hourly earnings
Atlanta, GA	30	$10.59	159	$7.61	88	$6.42	354	$7.15	2,811	$5.84	36	$7.62	51	$10.62
Baltimore, MD	24	12.65	392	8.89	133	8.37	752	7.77	3,832	6.65	146	7.89	75	10.37
Boston, MA	62	12.58	647	8.73	361	8.39	1,024	7.87	8,725	6.61	177	9.00	120	10.27
Buffalo, NY	16	11.26	166	8.29	98	7.41	493	7.37	2,576	6.08	12	7.84	15	8.76
Chicago, IL	93	13.24	846	9.43	343	8.77	1,875	8.56	15,187	7.12	306	8.56	211	10.29
Cleveland, OH	35	11.06	224	8.87	87	7.65	502	8.16	3,648	7.06	...	...	...	...
Dallas-Fort Worth, TX	37	10.26	185	7.80	65	7.21	517	7.08	4,165	6.04	12	7.35	120	9.31
Denver-Boulder, CO	27	11.34	175	9.06	55	7.99	433	7.82	3,463	6.54	65	8.15	28	9.41
Detroit, MI	75	12.78	495	9.29	200	8.58	936	8.37	6,160	7.41	47	9.14	260	10.99
Houston, TX	48	10.40	317	8.25	74	8.30	838	7.59	3,720	6.74	...	...	74	10.87
Kansas City, MO-KS	12	11.99	155	8.49	114	8.06	305	7.65	2,629	6.34	75	6.96	...	...
Los Angeles-Long Beach, CA	132	12.79	823	10.02	267	9.08	1,624	9.13	14,717	7.69	191	9.52	77	11.64
Memphis, TN-AR-MS	...	...	...	...	...	...	...	...	...	...	...	...	...	...
Miami, FL	27	12.16	216	8.97	93	8.86	709	7.95	2,629	6.52	139	6.61	41	9.56
Milwaukee, WI	27	12.14	171	8.93	152	8.01	346	7.83	2,540	6.60	23	8.69	27	9.44
Minneapolis-St. Paul, MN-WI	21	12.41	137	8.67	14	7.98	415	7.95	4,101	6.74	...	...	266	9.39
New York, NY-NJ	130	14.03	1,730	9.76	412	9.51	3,966	8.57	21,967	7.59	...	...	...	...
Philadelphia, PA-NJ	77	12.16	668	8.39	313	7.96	1,209	7.60	9,248	6.54	77	8.46	154	9.06
Portland, OR-WA	23	11.52	142	8.71	107	8.43	327	7.98	2,453	6.96	19	8.02	92	10.41
St. Louis, MO-IL	48	11.44	261	8.42	264	7.73	540	7.81	5,895	6.44	68	7.80	150	10.59
San Francisco-Oakland, CA	61	13.09	313	10.25	105	9.77	572	9.54	5,648	8.32	29	10.01	47	9.93
Seattle-Everett, WA	29	9.49	101	9.23	12	8.11	333	8.23	3,413	7.13	22	8.90	...	...
Washington, DC-MD-VA	29	13.65	238	9.28	99	8.47	493	8.37	4,588	6.71	105	9.05	77	10.64

¹Excludes premium pay for overtime, work on weekends, holidays and late shifts.
²Standard Metropolitan Statistical Areas as defined by the U.S. Office of Management and Budget through February 1974. All metropolitan areas consist of one or more counties.

SOURCE: U.S. Department of Labor, Bureau of Labor Statistics, *Industry Wage Survey: Hospitals, September 1978.* Individual releases, 1979.

Table III-A-2. Average Hourly Earnings[1] and Number of Full-time Registered Nurses in Nongovernment Hospitals, by Metropolitan Area,[2] September 1978

Metropolitan area	Director of nursing		Supervisor of nurses		Nursing instructor		Head nurse		General duty nurse		Clinical nursing specialist		Nurse anesthetist	
	Number	Average hourly earnings	Number	Average hourly earnings	Number	Average hourly earnings	Number	Average hourly earnings	Number	Average hourly earnings	Number	Average hourly earnings	Number	Average hourly earnings
Atlanta, GA	19	$10.44	98	$7.52	52	$6.14	184	$7.23	1,571	$5.80	24	$7.77	75	$10.37
Baltimore, MD	17	12.12	208	9.06	100	8.27	494	7.72	3,209	6.60	132	7.79	112	10.44
Boston, MA	41	13.93	453	9.18	304	8.54	770	8.14	7,585	6.60	167	9.08		
Buffalo, NY	10	11.48	102	8.34	87	7.38	232	7.51	2,027	6.15	7	7.78	198	10.20
Chicago, IL	84	13.27	689	9.28	297	8.59	1,530	8.54	13,689	7.07	213	8.48		
Cleveland, OH	28	10.94	172	8.84	70	7.71	410	8.16	3,140	7.07			102	9.12
Dallas-Fort Worth, TX	27	10.15	142	7.88	46	7.19	392	7.06	3,094	6.03	7	7.45	24	9.21
Denver-Boulder, CO	21	11.06	133	8.93	55	7.99	352	7.67	2,674	6.49	25	8.19	216	11.06
Detroit, MI	61	12.84	372	9.52	161	8.66	759	8.46	5,613	7.42	44	9.25	56	9.94
Houston, TX	44	10.38	280	8.19	52	7.94	719	7.55	3,100	6.69				
Kansas City, MO-KS	9	11.65	114	8.54	104	8.13	211	7.79	987	6.35			38	12.31
Los Angeles-Long Beach, CA	119	12.63	641	9.82	187	9.22	1,325	9.13	11,229	7.74	84	9.93		
Memphis, TN-AR-MS														
Miami, FL	19	12.04	173	8.84	51	8.23	558	7.85	2,060	6.64	124	6.64	24	9.43
Milwaukee, WI	25	12.05	137	8.82	117	7.93	237	7.96	2,184	6.56	22	8.66	23	9.59
Minneapolis-St. Paul, MN-WI	17	12.30	86	8.35			310	7.92	2,857	6.74			221	9.28
New York, NY-NJ	100	14.55	966	10.04	375	9.53	2,259	8.95	17,427	7.68				
Philadelphia, PA-NJ	66	12.11	593	8.38	292	7.85	1,106	7.58	9,021	6.53	70	8.43	152	9.06
Portland, OR-WA	21	11.42	129	8.68			287	7.91	1,984	6.94	9	7.55	91	10.42
St. Louis, MO-IL	38	11.57	197	8.42	219	7.75	396	7.93	5,167	6.48	34	8.20	118	10.47
San Francisco-Oakland, CA	35	13.13	209	10.20	84	9.74	333	9.60	3,535	8.41	20	9.92	31	10.32
Seattle-Everett, WA	23	8.45	74	9.18	8	8.35	223	8.27	2,429	7.13	11	8.87		
Washington, DC-MD-VA	25	13.30	220	9.08	89	8.32	444	8.33	4,152	6.67	91	8.99		

[1]Excludes premium pay for overtime, work on weekends, holidays and late shifts.

[2]Standard Metropolitan Statistical Areas as defined by the U.S. Office of Management and Budget through February 1974. All metropolitan areas consist of one or more counties.

SOURCE: U.S. Department of Labor, Bureau of Labor Statistics, Industry Wage Survey: Hospitals, September 1978. Individual releases, 1979.

Table III-A-3. Average Hourly Earnings¹ and Number of Full-time Registered Nurses in State and Local Government Hospitals, by Metropolitan Area,² September 1978

Metropolitan area	Director of nursing		Supervisor of nurses		Nursing instructor		Head nurse		General duty nurse		Clinical nursing specialist		Nurse anesthetist	
	Number	Average hourly earnings	Number	Average hourly earnings	Number	Average hourly earnings	Number	Average hourly earnings	Number	Average hourly earnings	Number	Average hourly earnings	Number	Average hourly earnings
Atlanta, GA	11	$10.85	61	$7.75	36	$6.82	170	$7.06	1,240	$5.89	…	…	…	…
Baltimore, MD	7	13.94	184	8.71	33	8.68	258	7.84	623	6.89	…	…	…	…
Boston, MA	21	9.94	194	7.69	57	7.61	254	7.05	1,140	6.63	10	$7.68	8	$7.91
Buffalo, NY	6	10.89	64	8.22	…	…	261	7.24	549	5.82	…	…	13	8.58
Chicago, IL	…	…	157	10.05	…	…	345	8.63	1,498	7.54	…	…	…	…
Cleveland, OH	7	11.54	52	8.98	…	…	92	8.19	508	6.98	22	7.31	7	9.43
Dallas-Fort Worth, TX	10	10.56	43	7.54	…	…	125	7.14	1,071	6.08	…	…	18	10.35
Denver-Boulder, CO	6	12.30	42	9.49	…	…	81	8.47	789	6.71	…	…	…	…
Detroit, MI	14	12.51	123	8.59	39	8.26	177	7.98	547	7.29	…	…	44	10.66
Houston, TX	…	…	…	…	…	…	119	7.79	620	6.98	…	…	…	…
Kansas City, MO-KS	…	…	41	8.36	…	…	94	7.35	642	6.31	…	…	…	…
Los Angeles-Long Beach, CA	13	14.32	182	10.74	…	…	299	9.15	3,488	7.50	107	9.19	39	10.98
Memphis, TN-AR-MS	…	…	25	7.52	…	…	45	6.98	…	…	…	…	…	…
Miami, FL	…	…	…	…	…	…	…	…	…	…	…	…	…	…
Milwaukee, WI	…	…	…	…	…	…	…	…	1,244	6.73	…	…	…	…
Minneapolis-St. Paul, MN-WI	30	12.30	51	9.21	37	9.26	105	8.03	…	…	…	…	45	9.95
New York, NY-NJ	11	12.49	…	…	21	9.46	1,707	8.08	…	…	…	…	…	…
Philadelphia, PA-NJ	…	…	75	8.47	…	…	103	7.89	227	6.92	…	…	…	…
Portland, OR-WA	…	…	…	…	…	…	…	…	…	…	…	…	…	…
St. Louis, MO-IL	10	10.93	64	8.42	45	7.66	144	7.49	728	6.17	…	…	32	11.03
San Francisco-Oakland, CA	26	13.05	124	10.33	21	9.92	296	9.42	2,444	8.14	9	10.21	16	9.19
Seattle-Everett, WA	…	…	…	…	…	…	49	8.75	436	7.04	…	…	…	…
Washington, DC-MD-VA	…	…	18	11.69	10	9.84	…	…	…	…	14	9.47	…	…

¹Excludes premium pay for overtime, work on weekends, holidays and late shifts.

²Standard Metropolitan Statistical Areas as defined by the U.S. Office of Management and Budget through February 1974. All metropolitan areas consist of one or more counties.

SOURCE: U.S. Department of Labor, Bureau of Labor Statistics, *Industry Wage Survey: Hospitals, September 1978.* Individual releases, 1979.

NURSES IN NONFEDERAL HOSPITALS, BY TYPE OF POSITION
FOR SELECTED METROPOLITAN AREAS, 1978

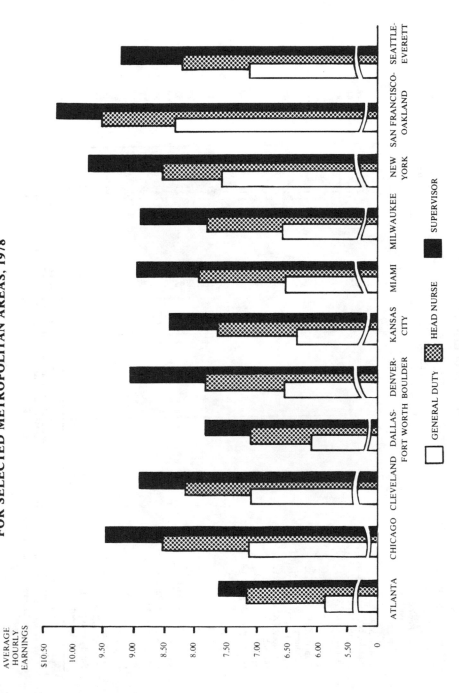

SOURCE: U.S. Department of Labor, Bureau of Labor Statistics, *Industry Wage Survey: Hospitals,*
          September 1978. Individual releases, 1979.

Table III-A-4. Retirement Plans[1] for Professional and Technical Employees[2] in Nonfederal Hospitals, by Metropolitan Area,[3] September 1978
(Percent of Employees)

Region and metropolitan area	Retirement pension, social security, or both	Pension (other than social security)		Combination of pension and social security	
		Contributory	Noncontributory	Contributory	Noncontributory
Northeast					
Boston, MA	100	21	12	4	61
Buffalo, NY	100	...	...	27	72
New York, NY-NJ	100	...	7	11	81
Philadelphia, PA-NJ	100	...	...	14	85
South					
Atlanta, GA	100	...	14	18	41
Baltimore, MD	100	...	...	28	72
Dallas-Fort Worth, TX	100	7	6	18	49
Houston, TX	100	9	14	62	...
Memphis, TN-AR-MS	100	83	...	17	...
Miami, FL	100	...	20	13	54
Washington, DC-MD-VA	100	8	...	16	70
North Central					
Chicago, IL	100	10	19	21	45
Cleveland, OH	100	15	10	26	49
Detroit, MI	100	...	13	7	73
Kansas City, MO-KS	100	...	...	27	63
Milwaukee, WI	100	...	...	31	69
Minneapolis-St. Paul, MN-WI	100	1	...	44	55
St. Louis, MO-IL	100	...	...	...	98
West					
Denver-Boulder, CO	100	15	3	7	69
Los Angeles-Long Beach, CA	100	4	14	32	37
Portland, OR-WA	100	...	...	20	75
San Francisco-Oakland, CA	100	8	11	12	69
Seattle-Everett, WA	100	...	...	51	45

[1]Includes only those plans for which at least part of the cost is borne by the employer. "Noncontributory plans" include only those plans financed entirely by the employer.
[2]Includes physicians, registered nurses, licensed practical nurses, and various other medical professional and technical occupations.
[3]Standard Metropolitan Statistical Areas as defined by the U.S. Office of Management and Budget through February 1974. All metropolitan areas consist of one or more counties.
SOURCE: U.S. Department of Labor. Bureau of Labor Statistics. *Industry Wage Survey: Hospitals, September 1978.* Individual releases, 1979.

Table III-A-5. Insurance Provisions for Professional and Technical Employees[1] in Nonfederal Hospitals, by Metropolitan Area,[2] September 1978 (Percent of Employees)

Region and metropolitan area	Life	Accidental death and dismemberment	Sickness and accident	Type of insurance plan				
				Hospitalization[3]	Surgical[3]	Medical[3]	Major medical[3]	Dental
Northeast								
Boston, MA	98	79	7	100	100	100	100	17
Buffalo, NY	100	68	7	100	100	100	84	35
New York, NY-NJ	100	91	44	100	100	98	98	91
Philadelphia, PA-NJ	100	95	39	100	100	100	100	50
South								
Atlanta, GA	100	66	15	100	100	100	100	7
Baltimore, MD	81	66	30	100	100	100	100	30
Dallas-Fort Worth, TX	100	87	9	100	100	100	99	...
Houston, TX	100	65	[4]100	100	100	100	100	...
Memphis, TN-AR-MS	94	25	14	100	100	100	100	...
Miami, FL	100	98	11	100	100	100	100	20
Washington, DC-MD-VA	94	93	30	100	100	100	100	22
North Central								
Chicago, IL	97	71	52	100	100	100	100	8
Cleveland, OH	100	97	31	100	100	100	75	22
Detroit, MI	100	89	80	100	100	95	76	79
Kansas City, MO-KS	88	67	2	99	99	99	99	10
Milwaukee, WI	100	79	25	100	100	100	100	23
Minneapolis-St. Paul, MN-WI	79	50	57	100	100	100	100	22
St. Louis, MO-IL	91	63	38	96	96	96	96	12
West								
Denver-Boulder, CO	86	62	5	100	100	100	100	19
Los Angeles-Long Beach, CA	97	60	20	99	99	99	100	60
Portland, OR-WA	83	78	33	100	100	100	100	97
San Francisco-Oakland, CA	90	77	[4]100	100	100	100	100	73
Seattle-Everett, WA	87	87	[4]100	100	100	100	100	95

[1] Includes physicians, registered nurses, licensed practical nurses, and various other medical professional and technical occupations.
[2] Standard Metropolitan Statistical Areas as defined by the U.S. Office of Management and Budget through February 1974. All metropolitan areas consist of one or more counties.
[3] May include some care provided outside of insurance.
[4] Includes sickness and accident insurance or sick leave or both.

SOURCE: U.S. Department of Labor, Bureau of Labor Statistics, *Industry Wage Survey: Hospitals, September 1978.* Individual releases, 1979.

Table III-A-6. Paid Vacation Provisions[1] for Professional and Technical Employees[2] in Nonfederal Hospitals, by Metropolitan Area,[3] September 1978
(Percent of Employees)

Region and metropolitan area	Weeks after one year of service				Weeks after five years of service			Weeks after ten years of service			Weeks after twenty-five years of service[4]		
	At least one but less than 2	At least 2 but less than 3	At least 3 but less than 4	4 or more	At least 2 but less than 3	At least 3 but less than 4	4 or more	At least 2 but less than 3	At least 3 but less than 4	4 or more	At least 3 but less than 4	At least 4 but less than 5	5 or more
Northeast													
Boston, MA	...	18	82	...	...	57	43	...	2	98	2	59	39
Buffalo, NY	10	91	...	...	...	48	52	...	11	89	...	69	31
New York, NY-NJ	6	7	88	...	(5)	8	92	...	3	98	1	35	64
Philadelphia, PA-NJ	(5)	64	31	4	17	65	18	2	52	45	10	63	26
South													
Atlanta, GA	...	97	3	...	9	92	...	5	84	12	35	61	...
Baltimore, MD	...	62	32	6	16	53	18	...	16	84	...	45	54
Dallas-Fort Worth, TX	...	100	...	...	15	86	...	3	87	10	69	31	...
Houston, TX	...	66	34	...	25	75	...	1	50	49	30	54	16
Memphis, TN-AR-MS	...	100	...	...	10	89	...	6	68	25	...	25	68
Miami, FL	...	82	18	1	39	53	8	35	37	28	29	57	10
Washington, DC-MD-VA	...	84	10	6	...	75	24	...	31	69	12	53	35
North Central													
Chicago, IL	...	45	48	7	8	66	27	...	13	87	...	51	49
Cleveland, OH	...	38	62	...	21	49	30	...	34	66	4	53	43
Detroit, MI	1	88	1	10	3	85	11	...	49	51	5	83	12
Kansas City, MO-KS	1	96	3	...	37	63	...	...	99	1	27	73	...
Milwaukee, WI	...	89	11	...	...	89	11	...	59	41	...	70	30
Minneapolis-St. Paul, MN-WI	...	88	13	...	...	32	68	...	15	86	...	86	14
St. Louis, MO-IL	...	90	10	...	26	73	...	...	88	12	5	83	12
West													
Denver-Boulder, CO	8	75	17	...	5	87	...	...	63	29	18	74	...
Los Angeles-Long Beach, CA	...	94	5	1	3	89	8	3	23	74	4	86	9
Portland, OR-WA	...	100	...	...	...	100	...	...	17	83	...	100	...
San Francisco-Oakland, CA	...	95	5	...	11	19	81	...	11	88	...	18	82
Seattle-Everett, WA	...	100	...	...	...	89	...	...	30	70	...	100	...

[1]Vacation payments such as percent of annual earnings were converted to an equivalent basis. Periods of service were chosen arbitrarily and do not necessarily reflect individual establishment provisions for progression. For example, the changes in provisions indicated at 10 years may include changes which occurred between 5 and 10 years.

[2]Includes physicians, registered nurses, licensed practical nurses, and various other medical professional and technical occupations.

[3]Standard Metropolitan Statistical Areas as defined by the U.S. Office of Management and Budget through February 1974. All metropolitan areas consist of one or more counties.

[4]Vacation provisions were virtually the same after longer periods of service.

[5]Less than 0.5 percent.

SOURCE: U.S. Department of Labor, Bureau of Labor Statistics. *Industry Wage Survey: Hospitals, September 1978.* Individual releases. 1979.

Table III-A-7. Paid Holiday Provisions[1] for Professional and Technical Employees[2] in Nonfederal Hospitals, by Metropolitan Area,[3] September 1978 (Percent[4] of Employees)

Region and metropolitan area	Employees with paid holidays	Number of holidays						
		5 days or less	6 days	7 days	8 days	9 days	10 days	11 days or more
Northeast								
Boston, MA	100	...	...	...	...	...	12	86
Buffalo, NY	100	...	...	...	...	...	29	71
New York, NY-NJ	100	...	...	...	(5)	2	6	91
Philadelphia, PA-NJ	100	...	...	6	12	15	29	35
South								
Atlanta, GA	100	2	30	41	25	...	...	3
Baltimore, MD	100	...	...	...	1	65	11	23
Dallas-Fort Worth, TX	100	5	44	48	...	...	...	3
Houston, TX	100	...	17	52	12	11	7	1
Memphis, TN-AR-MS	100	...	...	6	...	...	68	25
Miami, FL	99	4	6	30	14	12	...	33
Washington, DC-MD-VA	100	...	...	3	15	69	9	4
North Central								
Chicago, IL	98	...	5	11	28	32	3	15
Cleveland, OH	100	...	13	4	...	44	24	9
Detroit, MI	100	...	...	16	18	34	20	...
Kansas City, MO-KS	100	...	1	41	48	7	...	3
Milwaukee, WI	100	...	22	31	32	15	...	...
Minneapolis-St. Paul, MN-WI	100	...	...	1	72	14	7	6
St. Louis, MO-IL	100	...	...	2	59	21	7	12
West								
Denver-Boulder, CO	100	...	...	38	44	3	...	15
Los Angeles-Long Beach, CA	100	...	2	6	47	13	3	28
Portland, OR-WA	100	...	...	40	30	14	1	15
San Francisco-Oakland, CA	100	...	...	...	...	7	65	29
Seattle-Everett, WA	100	...	...	...	80	...	...	20

[1] Paid holidays were limited to full-day paid holidays.
[2] Includes physicians, registered nurses, licensed practical nurses, and various other medical professional and technical occupations.
[3] Standard Metropolitan Statistical Areas as defined by the U.S. Office of Management and Budget through February 1974. All metropolitan areas consist of one or more counties.
[4] Percentages may not add to totals due to rounding.
[5] Less than 0.5 percent

SOURCE: U.S. Department of Labor, Bureau of Labor Statistics, *Industry Wage Survey: Hospitals, September 1978.* Individual releases, 1979.

Table III-A-8. Mean Monthly Salary of Registered Nurses[1] Employed Full-time in Hospitals and Nursing Homes for Selected Types of Positions, by Region[2] of Employment, September 1977

Region of employment

Description	Total United States			Pacific			Mountain			West North Central			East North Central		
	(n)	Mean monthly salary	Sampling error	(n)	Mean monthly salary	Sampling error	(n)	Mean monthly salary	Sampling error	(n)	Mean monthly salary	Sampling error	(n)	Mean monthly salary	Sampling error
Hospital															
Administrator	186	$1,461	30.70	16	(3)	(3)	14	(3)	(3)	30	$1,306	57.22	25	$1,437	79.88
Supervisor	414	1,183	18.76	33	$1,223	53.84	28	$1,157	46.75	51	1,112	40.08	61	1,215	53.69
Head nurse	688	1,121	9.33	62	1,248	40.31	59	1,131	22.83	69	1,076	24.72	97	1,168	23.34
General duty	2,935	1,021	5.30	358	1,170	12.34	285	998	15.97	359	960	9.96	392	1,031	10.83
Nurse clinician	36	1,200	33.64	3	(3)	(3)	2	(3)	(3)	3	(3)	(3)	8	(3)	(3)
Nurse specialist	45	1,206	54.13	4	(3)	(3)	5	(3)	(3)	4	(3)	(3)	6	(3)	(3)
Nurse anesthetist	117	1,647	55.79	10	(3)	(3)	7	(3)	(3)	11	(3)	(3)	21	1,890	87.99
Nursing home															
General duty	171	881	31.47	17	(3)	(3)	20	(3)	(3)	20	(3)	(3)	24	(3)	(3)

Region of employment

Description	West South Central			East South Central			South Atlantic			Middle Atlantic			New England		
	(n)	Mean monthly salary	Sampling error	(n)	Mean monthly salary	Sampling error	(n)	Mean monthly salary	Sampling error	(n)	Mean monthly salary	Sampling error	(n)	Mean monthly salary	Sampling error
Hospital															
Administrator	24	(3)	(3)	17	(3)	(3)	29	$1,345	73.81	16	(3)	(3)	15	(3)	(3)
Supervisor	50	$1,088	24.44	34	$1,112	34.80	88	1,175	35.50	33	$1,217	46.65	36	$1,303	47.32
Head nurse	62	1,070	21.53	52	1,007	32.29	154	1,066	20.27	78	1,136	25.21	55	1,018	27.35
General duty	234	1,022	21.31	221	955	11.98	505	958	8.87	331	1,009	10.83	250	986	17.40
Nurse clinician	2	(3)	(3)	1	(3)	(3)	8	(3)	(3)	6	(3)	(3)	3	(3)	(3)
Nurse specialist	6	(3)	(3)	4	(3)	(3)	7	(3)	(3)	6	(3)	(3)	3	(3)	(3)
Nurse anesthetist	9	(3)	(3)	11	(3)	(3)	32	1,510	34.13	9	(3)	(3)	7	(3)	(3)
Nursing home															
General duty	7	(3)	(3)	5	(3)	(3)	28	690	59.12	22	(3)	(3)	28	866	54.64

[1]Includes only registered nurses actively licensed and working in the United States in September 1977.

[2]States included in each region are: Pacific—Alaska, California, Hawaii, Oregon, Washington; Mountain—Arizona, Colorado, Idaho, Montana, Nevada, New Mexico, Utah, Wyoming; West North Central—Iowa, Kansas, Minnesota, Missouri, Nebraska, North Dakota, South Dakota; East North Central—Illinois, Indiana, Michigan, Ohio, Wisconsin; West South Central—Arkansas, Louisiana, Oklahoma, Texas; East South Central—Alabama, Kentucky, Mississippi, Tennessee; South Atlantic—Delaware, District of Columbia, Florida, Georgia, Maryland, North Carolina, South Carolina, Virginia, West Virginia; Middle Atlantic—New Jersey, New York, Pennsylvania; New England—Connecticut, Maine, Massachusetts, New Hampshire, Rhode Island, Vermont.

[3]Insufficient number of cases to compute mean.

SOURCE: Roth, Aleda V., et al. 1977 National Sample Survey of Registered Nurses: A Report on the Nurse Population and Factors Affecting Their Supply, final report on Contract No. (HRA 231-76-0085) between the American Nurses' Association and the Division of Nursing. U.S. Department of Health and Human Services, NTIS Publication No. HRP-0900603, 1979.

Table III-A-9. Salaries of Registered Nurse Employees in the United States, by Type of Institution and Position, July 1979

Type of institution and position	Starting monthly salary[1]				Maximum monthly salary[2]			
	Lowest	Highest	Midpoint	Average	Lowest	Highest	Midpoint	Average
Institutions combined								
Clinical nurse specialist	$ 950	$2,141[1]	$1,300	$1,333	$ 926	$2,383	$1,679	$1,675
Nurse anesthetist	985	2,083	1,513	1,523	1,386	2,675	1,926	1,965
Head nurse	985	1,925	1,220	1,242	1,139	2,016	1,584	1,603
Staff nurse	825	1,450	1,039	1,041	1,111	1,967	1,348	1,363
Hospitals								
Clinical nurse specialist	990	2,141	1,296	1,366	1,038	2,141	1,588	1,637
Nurse anesthetist	1,214	1,915	1,539	1,549	1,638	2,675	1,937	1,967
Head nurse	1,002	1,925	1,260	1,282	1,140	2,016	1,584	1,620
Staff nurse	927	1,450	1,052	1,068	1,118	1,967	1,347	1,368
Medical schools								
Clinical nurse specialist	950	1,465	(3)	1,234	1,320	1,791	(3)	1,512
Nurse anesthetist	1,732	1,852	(3)	1,792	2,420	2,420	(3)	2,420
Head nurse	1,121	1,332	1,167	1,201	1,139	1,729	1,465	1,467
Staff nurse	825	1,173	981	1,009	1,159	1,587	1,325	1,332
Medical centers								
Clinical nurse specialist	1,004	1,594	1,302	1,322	926	2,383	1,810	1,773
Nurse anesthetist	985	2,083	1,429	1,455	1,386	2,509	1,920	1,909
Head nurse	985	1,456	1,219	1,200	1,290	1,993	1,680	1,628
Staff nurse	896	1,152	1,004	1,019	1,111	1,711	1,384	1,366

[1]Salaries normally paid in order to fill vacancies in a particular job class.
[2]Highest reported salaries actually paid to employees in a particular job class.
[3]Insufficient number of cases to compute salary.

SOURCE: University of Texas Medical Branch at Galveston, *1979 National Survey of Hospital and Medical School Salaries.*

Table III-A-10. Average Hourly Earnings and Number of Registered Nurses in Nongovernment Nursing and Personal Care Facilities,[1] by Metropolitan Area,[1] September 1978

Metropolitan area	General duty nurse						Head nurse					
	Total		Full-time		Part-time[2]		Total		Full-time		Part-time[2]	
	Number	Average hourly earnings	Number	Average hourly earnings	Number	Average hourly earnings	Number	Average hourly earnings	Number	Average hourly earnings	Number	Average hourly earnings
Atlanta, GA	193	$5.31	111	$5.33	82	$5.29	[3]15	$5.69	14	$5.71	...	...
Baltimore, MD	342	5.75	85	5.87	257	5.71	[3]75	6.55	62	6.70	...	...
Boston, MA	1,702	5.59	470	5.59	1,232	5.59	399	6.07	259	6.13	140	$5.95
Buffalo, NY	402	5.31	167	5.25	235	5.35	62	6.14	38	5.98	24	6.40
Chicago, IL	1,391	6.11	879	6.12	512	6.09	170	6.77	143	6.82	27	6.49
Cleveland, OH	544	5.83	230	5.84	314	5.82	[3]130	6.78	93	6.98	...	...
Dallas-Fort Worth, TX	253	5.57	151	5.61	102	5.52	...	...	...	...	...	...
Denver-Boulder, CO	642	5.43	333	5.46	309	5.39	[3]19	5.63	16	5.62	...	...
Detroit, MI	856	5.85	318	5.85	538	5.85	115	6.86	104	6.84	11	7.03
Houston, TX	110	6.25	70	6.10	40	6.51	...	...	...	...	...	...
Kansas City, MO-KS	171	5.51	89	5.73	82	5.28	26	4.99	26	4.99	...	...
Los Angeles-Long Beach, CA	1,785	7.22	893	7.24	892	7.20	371	8.96	371	8.96	...	...
Miami, FL	220	5.27	161	5.29	59	5.19	[3]33	6.20	31	6.20	...	...
Minneapolis-St. Paul, MN-WI	1,295	6.31	443	6.34	852	6.30	92	6.87	76	6.86	16	6.91
Milwaukee, WI	602	6.61	131	6.73	471	6.57	143	7.45	106	7.48	37	7.36
New York, NY-NJ	3,734	8.07	2,164	8.16	1,570	7.96	[3]580	9.25	578	9.25	...	...
Philadelphia, PA-NJ	1,658	5.83	641	5.99	1,017	5.73	242	6.30	212	6.34	30	6.03
St. Louis, MO-IL	583	5.71	225	5.82	358	5.64	74	6.31	74	6.31	...	...
San Francisco-Oakland, CA	1,114	6.81	563	6.95	551	6.65	110	7.49	98	7.55	12	6.93
Seattle-Everett, WA	919	5.95	467	6.02	452	5.89	[3]64	6.47	62	6.47	...	...
Washington, DC-MD-VA	584	5.78	302	5.88	282	5.67	69	6.34	62	6.34	7	6.38

[1] Standard Metropolitan Statistical Areas as defined by the U.S. Office of Management and Budget through February 1974. All metropolitan areas consist of one or more counties.

[2] Part-time employees are those working a schedule regularly calling for fewer hours than the establishment's full-time employees in the same general type of work.

[3] Includes employees not reported separately.

SOURCE: U.S. Department of Labor, Bureau of Labor Statistics, *Industry Wage Survey: Nursing and Personal Care Facilities, September 1978.* Individual releases, 1979.

Table III-A-11. Retirement Plans[1] for Professional and Technical Employees[2] in Nongovernment Nursing and Personal Care Facilities, by Metropolitan Area,[3] May 1976 and September 1978 (Percent of Employees)

Region and metropolitan area	Retirement plans	
	May 1976	September 1978
Northeast		
Boston, MA	23	27
Buffalo, NY	47	51
New York, NY-NJ	76	73
Philadelphia, PA-NJ	34	29
South		
Atlanta, GA	15	17
Baltimore, MD	25	24
Dallas-Fort Worth, TX	22	12
Houston, TX	...	23
Miami, FL	18	16
Washington, DC-MD-VA	35	48
North Central		
Chicago, IL	21	29
Cincinnati, OH-KY-IN	23	...
Cleveland, OH	22	41
Detroit, MI	12	24
Kansas City, MO-KS	15	19
Minneapolis-St. Paul, MN-WI	12	19
Milwaukee, WI	22	25
St. Louis, MO-IL	16	20
West		
Denver-Boulder, CO	2	...
Los Angeles-Long Beach, CA	8	9
San Francisco-Oakland, CA	13	5
Seattle-Everett, WA	19	21

[1] Includes only those plans for which the employer pays at least part of the cost and excludes legally required plans such as workers' compensation and social security. However, plans required by state temporary disability insurance laws are included if the employer contributes more than is required or if the employees receive benefits in excess of the legal requirements.
[2] Includes registered nurses, licensed practical nurses, dietitians, physical therapists, and occupational therapists for both years, and activities directors for 1978 only. The 1978 data reflect full-time employees only.
[3] Standard Metropolitan Statistical Areas as defined by the U.S. Office of Management and Budget through February 1974. All metropolitan areas consist of one or more counties.

SOURCES: U.S. Department of Labor, Bureau of Labor Statistics, *Industry Wage Survey: Nursing Homes and Related Facilities, May 1976,* Bulletin 1964; *Industry Wage Survey: Nursing and Personal Care Facilities, September 1978.* Individual releases, 1979.

Table III-A-12. Insurance Provisions for Full-time Professional and Technical Employees[1] in Nongovernment Nursing and Personal Care Facilities, by Metropolitan Area,[2] September 1978
(Percent of Employees)

Region and metropolitan area	Life	Accidental death and dismemberment	Sickness and accident	Type of insurance plan				
				Hospitalization	Surgical	Medical	Major medical	Dental
Northeast								
Boston, MA	54	48	21	91	91	91	88	...
Buffalo, NY	52	44	6	92	92	92	66	11
New York, NY-NJ	93	93	80	96	96	96	91	87
Philadelphia, PA-NJ	58	38	19	80	77	77	45	...
South								
Atlanta, GA	69	42	3	74	74	74	71	3
Baltimore, MD	77	74	39	92	92	92	85	8
Dallas-Fort Worth, TX	38	28	³53	55	55	55	50	...
Houston, TX	74	34	2	79	79	79	79	...
Miami, FL	84	59	10	80	80	74	74	...
Washington, DC-MD-VA	62	33	14	86	86	86	61	...
North Central								
Chicago, IL	90	56	23	93	93	93	81	24
Cleveland, OH	68	65	40	69	69	69	66	...
Detroit, MI	74	64	31	68	68	68	19	2
Kansas City, MO-KS	42	34	16	68	68	68	68	13
Milwaukee, WI	52	45	16	100	100	100	100	...
Minneapolis-St. Paul, MN-WI	71	36	8	73	73	73	73	1
St. Louis, MO-IL	58	55	14	61	61	61	61	5
West								
Denver-Boulder, CO	7	7	³25	21	21	21	21	3
Los Angeles-Long Beach, CA	62	35	³100	90	90	90	90	18
San Francisco-Oakland, CA	31	26	³100	100	100	100	96	53
Seattle-Everett, WA	42	35	³100	85	91	91	88	...

[1] Includes registered nurses, licensed practical nurses, dietitians, physical therapists, occupational therapists, and activities directors.

[2] Standard Metropolitan Statistical Areas as defined by the U.S. Office of Management and Budget through February 1974. All metropolitan areas consist of one or more counties.

[3] Includes sickness or accident insurance or sick leave or both.

SOURCE: U.S. Department of Labor, Bureau of Labor Statistics, *Industry Wage Survey: Nursing and Personal Care Facilities, September 1978.* Individual releases, 1979.

Table III-A-13. Paid Holiday Provisions[1] for Full-time Professional and Technical Employees[2] in Nongovernment Nursing and Personal Care Facilities, by Metropolitan Area,[3] September 1978 (Percent[4] of Employees)

Region and metropolitan area	Employees with paid holidays	Number of holidays						
		5 days or less	6 days	7 days	8 days	9 days	10 days	11 days or more
Northeast								
Boston, MA	99	...	5	12	12	30	37	3
Buffalo, NY	100	...	1	23	20	22	22	12
New York, NY-NJ	100	(5)	...	1	3	3	3	90
Philadelphia, PA-NJ	100	2	14	13	25	16	8	18
South								
Atlanta, GA	99	44	35	9	6	5	...	...
Baltimore, MD	100	3	12	11	18	44	8	3
Dallas-Fort Worth, TX	81	55	16	10	...	...	...	...
Houston, TX	88	35	22	8	17	6	...	...
Miami, FL	100	2	7	46	22	19	4	...
Washington, DC-MD-VA	99	...	31	26	4	36	3	...
North Central								
Chicago, IL	100	3	20	59	8	...	...	...
Cleveland, OH	90	10	8	15	27	21	2	...
Detroit, MI	100	2	29	30	20	10	4	4
Kansas City, MO-KS	91	6	59	21	4	2	...	...
Milwaukee, WI	97	...	32	43	7	12	...	...
Minneapolis-St. Paul, MN-WI	100	...	7	74	14	5	...	...
St. Louis, MO-IL	97	13	27	32	14	7	3	...
West								
Denver-Boulder, CO	100	72	23	4	1	...	...	...
Los Angeles-Long Beach, CA	96	28	36	24	4	1	2	...
San Francisco-Oakland, CA	100	...	11	11	25	25	35	3
Seattle-Everett, WA	74	13	...	36	6	8	...	...

[1] Paid holidays were limited to full-day paid holidays.
[2] Includes registered nurses, licensed practical nurses, dietitians, physical therapists, occupational therapists, and activities directors.
[3] Standard Metropolitan Statistical Areas as defined by the U.S. Office of Management and Budget through February 1974. All metropolitan areas consist of one or more counties.
[4] Percentages may not add to totals due to rounding.
[5] Less than 0.5 percent.

SOURCE: U.S. Department of Labor, Bureau of Labor Statistics, *Industry Wage Survey: Nursing and Personal Care Facilities, September 1978* Individual releases, 1979.

Table III-A-14. Paid Vacation Provisions[1] for Full-time Professional and Technical Employees[2] in Nongovernment Nursing and Personal Care Facilities, by Metropolitan Area,[3] September 1978 (Percent of Employees)

Region and metropolitan area	Amount of vacation													
	Weeks after one year of service				Weeks after five years of service			Weeks after ten years of service			Weeks after twenty years of service[4]		
	At least one but less than 2	At least 2 but less than 3	At least 3 but less than 4	4 or more	At least 2 but less than 3	At least 3 but less than 4	4 or more	At least 2 but less than 3	At least 3 but less than 4	4 or more	At least 2 but less than 3	At least 3 but less than 4	4 or more
Northeast													
Boston, MA	31	59	7	3	18	70	10	13	38	48	13	34	52
Buffalo, NY	52	48	...	...	11	89	...	9	18	73	1	24	75
New York, NY-NJ	...	13	41	45	1	4	95	1	4	96	1	4	96
Philadelphia, PA-NJ	30	63	3	3	27	59	14	15	52	33	11	43	46
South													
Atlanta, GA	60	39	...	...	58	42	...	27	59	14	27	37	36
Baltimore, MD	24	72	2	2	25	68	7	14	50	37	14	47	40
Dallas-Fort Worth, TX	61	39	...	...	53	31	...	38	45	(5)	38	42	3
Houston, TX	45	55	...	...	58	41	...	47	43	9	43	31	25
Miami, FL	42	56	...	2	5	91	2	4	53	42	4	51	45
Washington, DC-MD-VA	24	76	...	...	39	52	8	14	64	23	5	66	29
North Central													
Chicago, IL	59	38	1	3	9	82	10	6	28	66	6	26	68
Cleveland, OH	41	50	...	...	51	49	...	22	52	27	18	41	40
Detroit, MI	66	29	5	...	14	85	1	4	62	34	4	55	41
Kansas City, MO-KS	51	49	...	...	36	53	...	34	51	6	32	44	16
Milwaukee, WI	14	86	...	...	25	63	12	6	55	38	3	43	53
Minneapolis-St. Paul, MN-WI	40	60	...	...	46	45	9	7	73	20	7	62	31
St. Louis, MO-IL	78	22	...	...	44	49	...	8	69	16	8	61	24
West													
Denver-Boulder, CO	72	23	4	...	23	72	3	24	58	18	22	60	18
Los Angeles-Long Beach, CA	72	26	...	...	32	61	...	23	55	16	23	51	21
San Francisco-Oakland, CA	59	38	3	...	7	80	13	7	16	76	2	16	81
Seattle-Everett, WA	24	74	...	...	48	51	...	33	42	24	33	40	26

[1] Vacation payments such as percent of annual earnings were converted to an equivalent time basis. Periods of service were chosen arbitrarily and do not necessarily reflect individual establishment provisions for progression. For example, the changes in provisions indicated at 10 years may include changes which occurred between 5 and 10 years.

[2] Includes registered nurses, licensed practical nurses, dietitians, physical therapists, occupational therapists, and activities directors.

[3] Standard Metropolitan Statistical Areas as defined by the U.S. Office of Management and Budget through February 1974. All metropolitan areas consist of one or more counties.

[4] Vacation periods are virtually the same after longer periods of service.

[5] Less than 0.5 percent.

SOURCE: U.S. Department of Labor, Bureau of Labor Statistics. *Industry Wage Survey: Nursing and Personal Care Facilities, September 1978.* Individual releases, 1979.

Table III-A-15. Average Hourly Earnings[1] of Registered Nurses Employed Full-time and Part-time in Nursing Homes, by Selected Nursing Home Characteristics, 1977

	Registered nurse	
	Full-time	Part-time
Nursing home characteristics	Average hourly earnings	Average hourly earnings
Total	$5.59	$5.32
Ownership		
Proprietary	5.49	5.31
Voluntary nonprofit	5.54	5.33
Government	6.07	5.42
Certification		
Skilled nursing facility	5.90	5.52
Skilled nursing facility and		
intermediate care facility	5.59	5.22
Intermediate care facility	5.04	5.28
Not certified	5.51	5.21
Bed size		
Less than 50 beds	5.14	5.64
50-99	5.39	5.07
100-199	5.48	5.23
200 beds or more	6.22	5.83
Location		
Region		
Northeast	5.80	5.33
North Central	5.45	5.17
South	5.34	5.22
West	5.72	5.69
Standard federal administrative region		
Region I	5.49	5.30
Region II	6.22	5.67
Region III	5.37	5.00
Region IV	5.14	5.02
Region V	5.61	5.25
Region VI	5.68	(2)
Region VII	4.83	(2)
Region VIII	(2)	(2)
Region IX	6.01	6.15
Region X	(2)	(2)
Type of facility		
Nursing care	5.57	5.30
Other	5.91	5.52

[1] Includes only nurses who reported salary.
[2] Insufficient number of cases to compute average hourly earnings.

SOURCE: U.S. Department of Health, Education, and Welfare, Public Health Service, Office of Health Research, Statistics, and Technology, National Center for Health Statistics, *The National Nursing Home Survey: 1977 Summary for the United States*, Vital and Health Statistics, Series 13, No. 43. DHEW Publication No. (PHS) 79-1794, 1979, p. 19.

Table III-A-16. Average Hourly Earnings[1] of Registered Nurses Employed Full-time and Part-time in Nursing Homes, by Selected Employee Characteristics, 1977

Employee characteristics	Registered nurse	
	Full-time	Part-time
	Average hourly earnings	Average hourly earnings
Total	$5.59	$5.32
Racial/ethnic background		
White (not Hispanic)	5.53	5.26
Black (not Hispanic)	6.49	(2)
Hispanic	(2)	(2)
Other	(2)	(2)
Sex		
Male.................................	(2)	(2)
Female...............................	5.58	5.31
Age group		
Under 35 years	5.34	5.18
35-44	5.71	5.31
45-54	5.84	5.54
55 years and over	5.51	5.29
Years of education		
Less than 12 years.....................	(2)	(2)
12	(2)	(2)
13-14	5.47	5.24
15-16	5.57	5.31
17 years or more	5.87	5.47
Years of current employment		
Less than 2 years......................	5.37	5.23
2-4	5.59	5.33
5-9	5.88	5.58
10 years or more	6.13	5.27
Years of total experience		
Less than 5 years......................	5.14	5.23
5-9	5.75	5.32
10-14	5.84	5.31
15 years or more	5.87	5.45
Benefits		
Paid vacation, sick leave	5.64	5.37
Other leave[3]	5.72	5.39
Pension	6.16	5.92
Health, life insurance	5.84	5.76
Direct medical benefits	6.05	6.18
Meals	5.72	5.32
Employment arrangement		
Contract.............................	(2)	(2)
On staff	5.61	5.25

[1]Includes only nurses who reported salary.
[2]Insufficient number of cases to compute average hourly earnings.
[3]Includes civil and personal leave (jury duty, military reserves, voting, funerals) and release time for attending training institutes.

SOURCE: U.S. Department of Health, Education, and Welfare, Public Health Service, Office of Health Research, Statistics, and Technology, National Center for Health Statistics, *The National Nursing Home Survey: 1977 Summary for the United States*, Vital and Health Statistics, Series 13, No. 43, DHEW Publication No. (PHS) 79-1794, 1979, p. 22.

Chapter III, Section B
SALARIES IN COMMUNITY HEALTH AGENCIES

The National League for Nursing's Division of Home Health Agencies and Community Health Services annually conducts surveys of nurse salaries in selected community health agencies. The 1979 survey compiled data on the salary rates of full-time nursing personnel from 643 of 1,096 agencies. The total responding agencies (213 city and county health units, 250 nonofficial agencies, 28 combination services, 117 boards of education, and 35 state health departments) employed 19,300 full-time registered nurses.

Nurse executive directors in local official health agencies earned $2,542 more in 1979 than their counterparts in nonofficial agencies. The median annual salary for the former group in 1979 was $23,200 and for the latter, $20,658, representing 8.2 percent and 9.0 percent increases, respectively, over those salaries paid in 1978. There were also differences among the agencies in the median salaries of nursing supervisors. Supervisor salaries in boards of education in 1979 ranked first, at $20,150 annually, which was 11.4 percent above the median for supervisors in local official health agencies and 24.2 percent above the median for those in nonofficial agencies. Corresponding percentage increases in the median salaries from 1978 to 1979 were 9.8 percent for those in boards of education, 5.4 percent in local official agencies, and 8.7 percent in nonofficial agencies.

While similar patterns with respect to aggregate median salaries among the various agencies emerged for staff nurses, the proportionate gains between 1978 and 1979 differed. The 1979 median annual salary of staff nurses employed by boards of education was $15,436, amounting to a 4.4 percent increase since 1978. For those working in local official and nonofficial agencies, the median annual salaries were $14,342 and $13,287. The relative gains since 1978 for these two groups of staff nurses were 5.6 percent and 10.1 percent.

The NLN survey defined a "fully qualified" public health nurse as "one who has completed an NLN-accredited collegiate or university nursing program which includes preparation in public health nursing." The median annual salary of such a nurse in 1979 was $14,705 for those in local official agencies, 8.7 percent higher than that of other registered nurses in the same setting. For fully qualified nurses in nonofficial agencies, comparisons showed their median salary was $13,635, 7.0 percent greater than that of those without the appropriate credentials.

An apparent departure from past trends, showing a direct correspondence between the population of the area being served and the median annual salaries of the registered nurses, was observed in the 1978 and 1979 salary data for supervisors and staff nurses. For example, nurse supervisors in local official agencies with a population base of 50,000 to 249,999 persons had lower median salaries than those in local official agencies serving a population of less than 50,000 persons. Similarly, staff nurses in those agencies serving a population of 250,000-499,999 persons had a median annual salary of $12,590, which was $622 less than their counterparts in local agencies serving a population of 50,000 to 249,999 persons. On the other hand, the proportional relationship between size of the population served and median salaries held for nurse executive directors in both local official and nonofficial health agencies.

Salaries of public health nurses showed regional differences. Western states paid the highest salaries to staff nurses in public health, and the Southern states paid the lowest wages within each agency classification. Without exception, however, within each region the highest median annual salaries of staff nurses were those in boards of education.

Salary data for school nurses in academic year 1979-80 was reported by the Educational Research Service (ERS), based upon a national stratified panel sample of public school systems. According to ERS, the mean highest annual salary of school nurses in fall 1979 was $15,865. It should be noted that this figure is reasonably close to the NLN survey result of $15,436, as the median annual salary of staff nurses employed by boards of education as of April 1979; the salary ranges are more diverse, however. Differences between the studies were due to the dates of the survey, the statistical measures, the response rates, and methods used to gather the data; hence, they are not strictly comparable.

State government salary ranges for public health nurses and state directors of health are supplied by the U.S. Office of Personnel Management. The 1979 U.S. minimum annual salary for public health nurses employed by state governments was $12,272, compared to $11,605 in 1978. Starting annual salaries in 1979 ranged from $9,720 in Mississippi to $19,548 in Alaska. The 1979 starting salaries for state directors of public health nursing were lowest in Louisiana ($16,284) and highest in Alaska ($36,120). The U.S. minimum average salary for state directors in 1979 was $20,883. Between 1978 and 1979 the minimum average salary of state directors increased 5.8 percent and the top of the range increased 9.4 percent.

Table III-B-1. Median Annual Salaries of Registered Nurses in Selected Community Health Agencies,[1] by Type of Agency and Position, as of April 1, 1975-1979

Type of agency and position	Median annual salary				
	1975	1976	1977	1978	1979
Local official health agency					
Nurse director	$17,500	$18,100	$19,675	$21,450	$23,200
Supervising nurse	14,413	15,260	16,531	17,156	18,091
Staff nurse	11,495	12,160	13,104	13,584	14,342
Nonofficial agency					
Nurse director	16,400	18,007	18,060	18,950	20,658
Supervising nurse	12,714	13,463	14,588	14,918	16,222
Staff nurse	10,148	10,932	11,645	12,071	13,287
Board of education[2]					
Supervising nurse	15,700	17,600	18,375	18,350	20,150
Staff nurse	11,605	12,901	13,998	14,789	15,436

[1]The number of community health agencies reporting in each year is: 1975-770; 1976-703; 1977-675; 1978-679; 1979-643.
[2]Nurse director classification rarely used in boards of education.
SOURCE: National League for Nursing, "Salaries in Community Health Agencies—1979," *Nursing Outlook*, Vol. 27, No. 12, December 1979, p. 797, and previous years.

Table III-B-2. Median Annual Salaries of Staff Nurses in Selected Community Health Nursing Services, by Type of Agency and Classification, 1975-1979

Type of agency and position	Median annual salary				
	1975	1976	1977	1978	1979
Local official health agency					
All staff nurses	*$11,495*	*$12,160*	*$13,104*	*$13,584*	*$14,342*
Public health nurse, fully qualified[1]	12,033	12,830	13,808	13,692	14,705
Other registered nurse ...	10,626	11,470	12,460	13,067	13,526
Nonofficial agency					
All staff nurses	*10,148*	*10,932*	*11,645*	*12,071*	*13,287*
Public health nurse, fully qualified[1]	10,715	11,400	12,130	12,613	13,635
Other registered nurse ...	9,815	10,543	11,099	11,819	12,738

[1]Public health nurse, fully qualified is defined as a nurse who has completed a collegiate or university program in nursing approved by NLN, including preparation in public health nursing.
SOURCE: National League for Nursing, "Salaries in Community Health Agencies—1979," *Nursing Outlook*, Vol. 27, No. 12, December 1979, p. 797, and previous years.

Table III-B-3. Median Annual Salaries and Middle Range of Salaries of Registered Nurses in Selected Community Health Agencies, by Position, Type of Agency, and Population of Area Served, April 1, 1979

Type of agency and population group	Nurse director		Supervising nurse		Staff nurse	
	Median	Middle range	Median	Middle range	Median	Middle range
Local official health agency						
All population groups	$23,200	$20,500-27,200	$18,091	$16,342-20,581	$14,342	$12,520-16,004
Under 50,000	19,100	16,900-20,200	16,725	13,175-17,173	12,933	11,573-13,650
50,000-249,999	22,550	20,513-25,975	16,675	15,085-18,275	13,212	11,711-15,759
250,000-499,999	23,950	21,375-26,175	17,525	15,315-19,625	12,590	11,453-15,110
500,000 and over	26,700	24,000-31,850	19,700	17,600-21,187	15,252	13,856-16,526
Nonofficial agency						
All population groups	20,658	17,863-25,082	16,222	14,550-18,436	13,287	11,822-14,891
Under 50,000	17,025	15,063-19,075	12,250	10,825-14,275	11,100	9,322-12,330
50,000-249,999	19,650	17,425-22,095	15,783	14,067-18,333	12,542	11,428-14,386
250,000-499,999	25,300	20,050-28,250	15,583	14,517-16,938	12,184	11,274-13,367
500,000 and over	28,150	23,775-32,025	17,413	15,261-19,054	14,522	13,025-15,775
Board of education						
All population groups	(1)	(1)	20,150	15,038-25,003	15,436	11,524-18,075
Under 50,000	…	…	16,850	10,675-20,825	14,050	10,775-19,025
50,000-249,999	…	…	19,500	14,600-21,900	13,023	10,642-16,237
250,000-499,999	…	…	20,500	(2)	15,036	11,225-18,079
500,000 and over	…	…	25,050	24,413-27,938	17,256	13,625-18,375

[1] Nurse director classification rarely used in boards of education.
[2] Too few cases to compute middle range.

SOURCE: National League for Nursing, "Salaries in Community Health Agencies—1979," *Nursing Outlook*, Vol. 27, No. 12, December 1979, p. 798.

CHART 10. MEDIAN ANNUAL SALARIES OF NURSES IN SELECTED COMMUNITY HEALTH AGENCIES, 1977, 1978, 1979

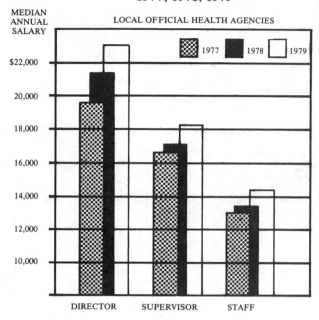

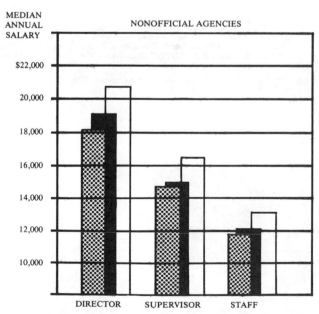

SOURCE: National League for Nursing, *Nursing Outlook*, Vol. 27, No. 12, December 1979, and previous years.

Table III-B-4. Median Annual Salaries of Staff Nurses in Selected
Community Health Agencies, by Type of Agency and HEW Region,[1]
April 1, 1977-1979

Year and type of agency	All regions	HEW region			
		I	II	III	IV
1977					
Local official health agency	$13,104	$13,526	$10,876	$13,370	$15,070
Nonofficial health agency ...	11,645	11,423	11,081	12,281	12,407
Board of education	13,998	14,540	12,430	13,944	15,483
1978					
Local official health agency	13,584	13,515	11,799	14,452	15,442
Nonofficial health agency ...	12,071	11,872	11,574	12,795	14,217
Board of education	14,789	15,899	13,118	14,493	16,647
1979					
Local official health agency	14,342	14,034	12,385	15,333	15,453
Nonofficial health agency ...	13,287	12,818	12,458	14,008	15,928
Board of education	15,436	15,400	13,587	16,075	18,093

[1]The states included in each region are: *Region I*—Connecticut, Delaware, District of Columbia, Maine, Maryland, Massachusetts, New Hampshire, New Jersey, New York, Pennsylvania, Rhode Island, Vermont, Virginia and West Virginia; *Region II*—Alabama, Arkansas, Florida, Georgia, Kentucky, Louisiana, Mississippi, New Mexico, North Carolina, Oklahoma, South Carolina, Tennessee and Texas; *Region III*—Illinois, Indiana, Iowa, Kansas, Michigan, Minnesota, Missouri, Nebraska, Ohio and Wisconsin; *Region IV*—Alaska, Arizona, California, Colorado, Hawaii, Idaho, Montana, Nevada, North Dakota, Oregon, South Dakota, Utah, Washington and Wyoming.

SOURCE: National League for Nursing, "Salaries in Community Health Agencies—1979," *Nursing Outlook*, Vol. 27, No. 12, December 1979, p. 798, and previous years.

Table III-B-5. Employment and Median Annual Salaries of Full-time Registered Nurses in Selected Community Health Agencies,[1] April 1976-1979

Item	Director of professional services[2]	Assistant director	Educational director	Other administrator	Consultant	Assistant supervisor	Nurse practitioner
April 1976							
Number of agencies with position	(3)	160	58	118	84	120	(3)
Number of full-time employees	(3)	254	67	234	761	457	(3)
Median annual salary	(3)	$18,900	$16,150	$13,825	$15,660	$15,236	(3)
April 1977							
Number of agencies with position	42	143	58	100	69	100	64
Number of full-time employees	42	210	67	234	585	397	268
Median annual salary	$17,900	$19,900	$15,650	$15,825	$16,712	$15,347	$14,700
April 1978							
Number of agencies with position	22	186	65	143	75	110	70
Number of full-time employees	22	277	87	375	605	404	390
Median annual salary	$20,300	$19,875	$15,925	$15,546	$16,693	$15,743	$14,917
April 1979							
Number of agencies with position	27	197	65	160	82	134	64
Number of full-time employees	27	326	78	391	574	494	411
Median annual salary	$19,300	$20,433	$17,167	$16,939	$18,160	$16,741	$15,715

[1] Includes nonofficial agencies, official state and local health agencies, and combination services.
[2] In agencies where executive director is a nonnurse.
[3] No such classification listed in 1976.

SOURCE: National League for Nursing, "Salaries in Community Health Agencies—1979," *Nursing Outlook*, Vol. 27, No. 12, December 1979, p. 799, and previous years.

Table III-B-6. Mean of Highest, Mean, and Lowest Salaries Paid by School Systems to Public School Professional Personnel, by Type of Position and Enrollment Grouping, 1979-80 School Year

Enrollment grouping and type of salary	Type of position			
	School nurse	Librarian	Teacher	Counselor
Total, all reporting systems				
Mean of highest	$15,865	$19,455	$20,861	$21,269
Mean of mean	13,788	16,764	15,913	18,847
Mean of lowest	11,754	13,624	10,657	15,321
25,000 or more				
Mean of highest	18,338	20,769	21,595	22,218
Mean of mean	14,430	17,106	16,119	19,070
Mean of lowest	10,947	11,987	10,715	13,768
10,000 to 24,999				
Mean of highest	17,168	21,088	21,954	22,663
Mean of mean	14,234	17,549	16,624	19,591
Mean of lowest	11,261	13,353	10,776	15,065
2,500 to 9,999				
Mean of highest	15,667	19,994	21,390	21,843
Mean of mean	13,948	17,095	16,281	19,241
Mean of lowest	12,149	13,941	10,699	15,519
300 to 2,499				
Mean of highest	12,975	16,347	18,800	18,279
Mean of mean	12,505	15,356	14,683	17,333
Mean of lowest	12,092	14,341	10,466	16,292

SOURCE: *Salaries Paid Professional Personnel in Public Schools, 1979-80.* Part II of National Survey of Salaries and Wages in Public Schools, (Educational Research Service, Inc., 1980), pp. 22-27. The three volume set is available from ERS (1800 North Kent Street, Arlington, Virginia, 22209) for $20 per volume or $55 for the entire set.

Table III-B-7. Mean of Mean Salaries[1] Paid by School Systems to Public School Professional Personnel, by Type of Position and Geographic Region,[2] 1979-80 School Year

Geographic region	Type of position			
	School nurse	Librarian	Teacher	Counselor
Total, all regions	$13,788	$16,764	$15,913	$18,847
New England	11,511	16,237	15,441	17,822
Mideast	16,040	17,249	17,009	20,181
Southeast	10,460	14,116	13,394	15,768
Great Lakes	13,052	17,349	16,459	19,539
Plains	11,433	15,426	14,578	17,893
Southwest	12,678	15,537	14,264	17,725
Rocky Mountains	13,125	16,776	15,345	18,255
Far West	17,885	20,343	18,826	21,722

[1] Data subject to wide sampling and response variation and should be used only as a general indicator.
[2] States included in each region are: *New England*—Connecticut, Maine, Massachusetts, New Hampshire, Rhode Island, Vermont; *Mideast*—Delaware, District of Columbia, Maryland, New Jersey, New York, Pennsylvania; *Southeast*—Alabama, Arkansas, Florida, Georgia, Kentucky, Louisiana, Mississippi, North Carolina, South Carolina, Tennessee, Virginia, West Virginia; *Great Lakes*—Illinois, Indiana, Michigan, Ohio, Wisconsin; *Plains*—Iowa, Kansas, Minnesota, Missouri, Nebraska, North Dakota, South Dakota; *Southwest*—Arizona, New Mexico, Oklahoma, Texas; *Rocky Mountains*—Colorado, Idaho, Montana, Utah, Wyoming; *Far West*—Alaska, California, Hawaii, Nevada, Oregon, Washington.
SOURCE: *Salaries Paid Professional Personnel in Public Schools, 1979-80.* Part II of National Survey of Salaries and Wages in Public Schools, (Educational Research Service, Inc., 1980), p. 17. The three volume set is available from ERS (1800 North Kent Street, Arlington, Virginia, 22209) for $20 per volume or $55 for the entire set.

Table III-B-8. State Government Salary Ranges for Public Health Nurses,[1] August 1, 1979

State	Salary range Minimum	Salary range Maximum	State	Salary range Minimum	Salary range Maximum
United States, average ...	$12,272	$16,395			
Alabama	11,973	14,482	Missouri[9]	$13,236	$17,244
Alaska[2,3]	19,548	23,508	Montana[2]	12,941	17,079
Arizona	12,244	15,663	Nebraska	11,882	16,252
Arkansas	11,986	17,420	Nevada[2]	12,606	17,274
California	17,339	20,849	New Hampshire[2]	11,492	13,935
Colorado	14,220	18,144	New Jersey[10]	10,875	14,677
Connecticut[2]	10,835	13,223	New Mexico[9]	11,712	19,068
Delaware[2]	11,628	15,836	New York[8]	...	...
District of Columbia[4] ...	...	...	North Carolina[2]	11,316	15,468
Florida[5]	11,022	14,446	North Dakota	10,992	15,456
Georgia[2,6]	11,100	14,898	Ohio[2]	11,980	15,579
Hawaii[2]	11,964	14,940	Oklahoma[2]	10,020	13,080
Idaho[2,7]	11,592	15,540	Oregon	12,852	16,380
Illinois	12,564	16,272	Pennsylvania	12,284	15,963
Indiana	14,976	22,438	Rhode Island[2]	12,345	14,318
Iowa	13,998	17,950	South Carolina	11,612	16,458
Kansas[2]	10,884	14,232	South Dakota	10,005	14,768
Kentucky[8]	...	...	Tennessee	11,100	14,676
Louisiana[9]	11,244	16,812	Texas[11]	12,000	15,108
Maine	12,480	16,141	Utah	12,012	17,532
Maryland	11,697	15,322	Vermont	10,920	17,290
Massachusetts[8]	...	...	Virginia	10,992	14,328
Michigan[8]	...	...	Washington[12]	12,492	15,936
Minnesota	13,718	17,017	West Virginia	11,568	18,864
Mississippi	9,720	14,940	Wisconsin	15,723	20,189
			Wyoming[2]	12,816	17,172

[1] This class usually requires graduation from an accredited school of nursing, state registration, and a program of study in public health or appropriate public health nursing experience.
[2] Longevity payments are authorized but not included in the range reported.
[3] Additional salary for cost-of-living is paid in remote areas.
[4] Not reported.
[5] Salary rate effective September 1, 1979.
[6] Hiring at advanced steps may be done if nurse has a B.S. in nursing.
[7] Special conditions may affect salary range.
[8] No comparable class within scope of definition.
[9] Appointments are frequently made above the minimum of the range.
[10] Salaries currently under negotiation.
[11] Salaries will be increased by 5.1 percent, effective September 1, 1979.
[12] Employees will receive a second salary increase, effective October 1, 1979.
SOURCE: U.S. Office of Personnel Management, Intergovernmental Personnel Programs Division, *State Salary Survey, August 1, 1979,* p. 59.

Table III-B-9. State Government Salary Ranges for State Directors of Public Health Nursing,[1] August 1, 1979

State	Salary range		State	Salary range	
	Minimum	Maximum		Minimum	Maximum
United States, average ...	$20,883	$28,335			
Alabama	21,073	27,274	Missouri	$20,676	$27,156
Alaska[2,3]	36,120	43,404	Montana[2]	20,074	26,391
Arizona	21,034	28,618	Nebraska	16,949	23,485
Arkansas	18,642	27,144	Nevada[2]	20,764	28,808
California	25,132	30,326	New Hampshire[2]	16,856	20,647
Colorado	23,148	31,008	New Jersey	18,602	25,115
Connecticut[2,4]	22,261	27,326	New Mexico[9]	17,304	28,164
Delaware[2]	18,004	24,668	New York	27,800	33,800
District of Columbia[5]	...	...	North Carolina[2]	20,388	28,428
Florida[6]	21,987	30,130	North Dakota	19,716	27,732
Georgia[2]	22,176	30,246	Ohio[2]	20,717	28,995
Hawaii[2]	18,756	23,652	Oklahoma[2]	17,340	23,100
Idaho[7]	...	...	Oregon	23,064	29,448
Illinois	20,856	31,128	Pennsylvania	21,614	27,853
Indiana	20,748	31,668	Rhode Island[7]	...	...
Iowa	20,405	27,123	South Carolina	24,466	34,677
Kansas[2]	19,572	25,644	South Dakota	19,532	30,582
Kentucky[2]	16,860	27,420	Tennessee	18,768	27,144
Louisiana	16,284	23,760	Texas	27,400	...
Maine	18,034	23,982	Utah	22,800	33,276
Maryland	21,189	27,832	Vermont[7]	...	...
Massachusetts	20,286	25,244	Virginia	20,500	28,000
Michigan[2,8]	21,422	26,851	Washington[7]	...	...
Minnesota	20,504	27,729	West Virginia[8]	18,864	30,744
Mississippi	19,440	31,080	Wisconsin	21,980	30,785
			Wyoming[2]	20,508	27,480

[1] This class usually requires a bachelor's degree including public health nursing, graduate training in public health nursing, registration to practice nursing in the state, and extensive public health nursing experience, including some administrative and supervisory responsibilities.
[2] Longevity payments are authorized but not included in the range reported.
[3] Additional salary for cost-of-living is paid in remote areas.
[4] Special conditions may affect salary range.
[5] Not reported.
[6] Salary rate effective September 1, 1979.
[7] No comparable class within scope of definition.
[8] Salaries will be increased by seven percent, effective October 1, 1979.
[9] Appointments are frequently made above the minimum of the range.

SOURCE: U.S. Office of Personnel Management, Intergovernmental Personnel Programs Division, *State Salary Survey, August 1, 1979*, p. 60.

Chapter III, Section C
SALARIES OF NURSE FACULTY MEMBERS

Salaries of nurse faculty are periodically gathered from schools belonging to the American Association of Colleges of Nursing and reported by AACN. The 1979-80 AACN data was collected from 206 schools, 85 percent of those receiving the questionnaire; the response rate for the 1978-79 survey was 83 percent. The 1979-80 study showed nurse faculty with the academic rank of professor and with doctoral preparation earned an average of $28,196 during the academic year, a substantial increase (11.2 percent) over the previous year, when the salaries averaged $25,363. Doctorally prepared professors earned 12.2 percent more than their counterparts with lesser preparation, according to the 1979-80 data.

Nurses at the associate professor level with doctoral preparation earned an average of $22,894 in 1979-80, an increase of 7.6 percent over 1978-79. In an academic year, these nurses earned 11.1 percent more than nurse faculty with comparable rank but not holding a doctorate.

Academic year earnings for assistant professors averaged $19,575 for those with doctoral preparation and $17,148 for those without doctorates. Corresponding gains between 1978 and 1979 were 7.7 percent and 6.9 percent, respectively. Nurse instructors with doctorates had a mean salary of $16,513, while those without such preparation had a mean salary of $14,545 in the academic year 1979-80.

The AACN also collected salary data on deans of member nursing programs. Returns from 187 schools, representing a response rate of 81 percent for the 1978-79 study, were received. The median salary of deans of AACN member programs was $35,700 in 1978-79. There was wide regional variation, with those in the Western states having the highest median salaries and those in the Midwest reporting the lowest ($40,900 versus $33,800). Deans in public institutions had the highest median annual salary ($39,000). Those in secular private institutions earned $36,000, while the median salary for the deans in religious private institutions was $27,000. Salaries of deans in schools varied by the type of program offered. Schools having baccalaureate, master's, and doctoral programs showed the median salary of the dean to be 19.9 percent higher than that for schools having baccalaureate and master's programs, and 63 percent higher than schools with only a baccalaureate program.

**Table III-C-1. Mean Annual Salary of Nursing Faculty in AACN[1]
Member Schools, by Academic Rank, and Educational Preparation,
1978-79 and 1979-80**

Academic rank and educational preparation	Academic year		Calendar year	
	1978-79	1979-80	1978-79	1979-80
Professor				
Doctoral preparation	$25,363	$28,196	$30,999	$34,461
Nondoctoral preparation	22,298	25,130	27,253	30,713
Associate professor				
Doctoral preparation	21,271	22,894	25,998	27,981
Nondoctoral preparation	18,933	20,602	23,140	25,180
Assistant professor				
Doctoral preparation	18,172	19,575	22,210	23,925
Nondoctoral preparation	16,047	17,148	19,613	20,958
Instructor				
Doctoral preparation	18,300	16,513	20,155	20,183
Nondoctoral preparation	13,429	14,545	16,413	17,777

[1] American Association of Colleges of Nursing.

SOURCE: American Association of Colleges of Nursing, *Report on Nursing Faculty Salaries in Colleges and Universities, 1979-1980, Revised Edition,* p. 4.

CHART 11. MEAN ANNUAL SALARY EARNED DURING
ACADEMIC YEAR, BY NURSE FACULTY ACCORDING
TO ACADEMIC RANK AND EDUCATIONAL PREPARATION,
1978-79 and 1979-80

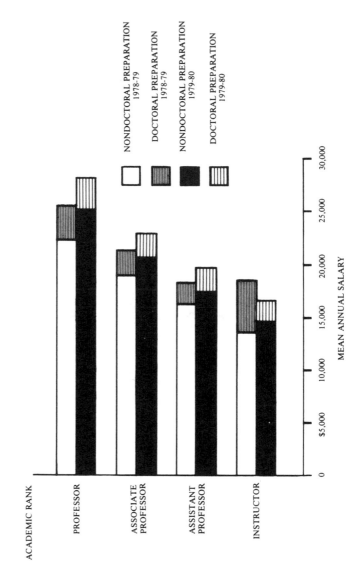

SOURCE: American Association of Colleges of Nursing, *Report on Nursing Faculty Salaries in Colleges
and Universities, 1979-1980, Revised Edition.*

Table III-C-2. Mean Annual Salary of Nursing Faculty With Doctoral Preparation in AACN[1] Member Schools, by Academic Rank, Institutional Control, and Region, Academic Year 1979-80

Academic rank and institutional classification	United States	Region[2]			
		North Atlantic	Midwestern	Southern	Western
Professor					
Public and private school ...	$28,196	$29,658	$28,169	$26,679	$29,144
Public school	28,225	30,926	28,132	26,498	29,487
Secular private school	29,671	29,298	30,121	30,297	...
Religious private school ...	24,980	25,819	26,524	21,890	24,674
Associate professor					
Public and private school ..	22,894	23,427	23,021	22,420	22,706
Public school	22,996	24,912	22,793	22,701	22,807
Secular private school	23,583	23,434	25,750	22,039	...
Religious private school ...	20,886	19,775	21,942	20,160	21,365
Assistant professor					
Public and private school ...	19,575	19,531	20,596	19,039	18,857
Public school	19,786	20,745	20,419	19,237	18,862
Secular private school	19,324	19,161	22,548	18,004	...
Religious private school ...	18,491	17,817	20,384	...	(3)
Instructor					
Public and private school ...	16,513	17,219	18,090	15,864	15,200
Public school	16,242	...	18,090	15,864	15,200
Secular private school	16,410	16,410	...	...	...
Religious private school ...	(3)	(3)	...	...	...

[1] American Association of Colleges of Nursing.
[2] The states included in each region are: *North Atlantic*—Connecticut, Maine, Massachusetts, New Hampshire, New Jersey, New York, Pennsylvania, Rhode Island, Vermont; *Midwestern*— Illinois, Indiana, Iowa, Kansas, Michigan, Minnesota, Missouri, Nebraska, North Dakota, Ohio, South Dakota, Wisconsin; *Southern*— Alabama, Arkansas, Delaware, District of Columbia, Florida, Georgia, Kentucky, Louisiana, Maryland, Mississippi, North Carolina, Oklahoma, South Carolina, Tennessee, Texas, Virginia, West Virginia; *Western*—Alaska, Arizona, California, Colorado, Hawaii, Idaho, Montana, Nevada, New Mexico, Oregon, Utah, Washington, Wyoming.
[3] Insufficient number of cases to compute mean.

SOURCE: American Association of Colleges of Nursing, *Report on Nursing Faculty Salaries in Colleges and Universities, 1979-80, Revised Edition*, pp. 16-20.

Table III-C-3. Mean Annual Salary of Nursing Faculty Without Doctoral Preparation in AACN[1] Member Schools, by Academic Rank, Institutional Control, and Region, Academic Year 1979-80

Academic rank and institutional classification	United States	Region[2]			
		North Atlantic	Midwestern	Southern	Western
Professor					
Public and private school ...	$25,130	$27,426	$23,648	$23,381	$27,571
Public school	25,798	(3)	24,861	23,473	28,442
Secular private school ...	27,188	28,400	....	(3)	....
Religious private school ...	19,990	(3)	20,412	(3)	18,562
Associate professor					
Public and private school ...	20,602	22,191	19,975	20,166	20,843
Public school	21,247	23,182	21,168	20,462	21,839
Secular private school	20,358	21,603	19,959	18,473	16,965
Religious private school ...	18,265	20,421	17,696	19,019	16,944
Assistant professor					
Public and private school ...	17,148	17,562	17,125	16,926	17,187
Public school	17,433	19,016	17,488	17,026	17,481
Secular private school	17,097	17,121	17,992	16,220	13,587
Religious private school ...	16,017	15,931	15,876	16,404	16,163
Instructor					
Public and private school ...	14,545	14,539	14,607	14,434	14,688
Public school	14,684	15,372	14,564	14,401	15,073
Secular private school	14,726	14,303	15,934	14,418	11,031
Religious private school	13,818	13,581	13,729	14,776	13,495

[1] American Association of Colleges of Nursing.
[2] For states in each region, see Table III-C-2.
[3] Insufficient number of cases to compute mean.

SOURCE: American Association of Colleges of Nursing, *Report on Nursing Faculty Salaries in Colleges and Universities, 1979-1980, Revised Edition*, pp. 16-20.

Table III-C-4. Mean Annual Salary of Nursing Faculty with Doctoral Preparation in AACN[1] Member Schools, by Academic Rank, Institutional Control, and Region, Academic Year 1978-79

Academic rank and institutional classification	United States	Region[2]			
		North Atlantic	Midwestern	Southern	Western
Professor					
Public and private school ...	$25,363	$24,667	$25,515	$25,161	$26,014
Public school	25,493	24,450	25,600	24,932	26,392
Secular private school	25,752	25,026	27,511	26,879	....
Religious private school ...	22,623	22,667	23,539	...	19,830
Associate professor					
Public and private school ...	21,271	20,917	21,841	21,183	20,713
Public school	21,428	21,213	21,983	21,302	20,642
Secular private school	21,150	21,063	21,457	21,219	[3]
Religious private school ...	20,220	19,375	21,094	17,734	21,265
Assistant professor					
Public and private school ...	18,172	17,838	19,065	18,569	17,067
Public school	18,322	17,897	19,192	18,769	17,140
Secular private school	18,157	18,248	[3]	17,114	....
Religious private school ...	16,616	15,644	17,903	[3]	16,152
Instructor					
Public and private school ...	16,491	17,930	14,439	...	17,103
Public school	16,467	[3]	[3]	...	17,103
Secular private school	[3]	[3]	...	...	...
Religious private school ...	[3]	[3]	[3]	...	...

[1] American Association of Colleges of Nursing.
[2] For states in each region, see Table III-C-2.
[3] Insufficient number of cases to compute mean.

SOURCE: American Association of Colleges of Nursing, *Report on Nursing Faculty Salaries in Colleges and Universities, 1978-1979*, pp. 14-18.

Table III-C-5. Mean Annual Salary of Nursing Faculty in AACN[1] Member Schools with Baccalaureate Programs Only, by Academic Rank, Institutional Control, and Educational Preparation, Academic Years 1978-79 and 1979-80

Academic rank and institutional classification	Mean annual salary			
	1978-79		1979-80	
	Doctoral preparation	Nondoctoral preparation	Doctoral preparation	Nondoctoral preparation
Professor				
Public and private school	$23,364	$22,455	$26,734	$25,653
Public school	23,289	23,236	26,293	26,679
Secular private school	(2)	...	35,100	...
Religious private school	21,866	18,747	24,682	20,780
Associate professor				
Public and private school	20,111	17,966	20,924	20,052
Public school	20,462	18,499	22,176	21,454
Secular private school	21,268	18,191	21,637	18,946
Religious private school	18,747	16,898	18,798	18,086
Assistant professor				
Public and private school	17,525	15,566	18,908	16,608
Public school	17,556	15,764	19,679	17,406
Secular private school	19,929	16,753	17,139	15,771
Religious private school	15,848	14,775	16,639	15,792
Instructor				
Public and private school	(2)	12,918	(2)	14,127
Public school	(2)	13,223	...	14,840
Secular private school	...	13,099	(2)	13,324
Religious private school	(2)	12,507	...	13,427

[1] American Association of Colleges of Nursing.
[2] Insufficient number of cases to compute mean.

SOURCES: American Association of Colleges of Nursing, *Report on Nursing Faculty Salaries in Colleges and Universities, 1978-1979*, p. 24; *Report on Nursing Faculty Salaries in Colleges and Universities, 1979-1980, Revised Edition*, p. 26.

**Table III-C-6. Mean Annual Salary of Nursing Faculty in AACN[1]
Member Schools with 250 or More Full-Time Baccalaureate Students,
by Academic Rank, Institutional Control, and Educational Preparation,
Academic Years 1978-79 and 1979-80**

| | Mean annual salary | | | |
| | 1978-79 | | 1979-80 | |
Academic rank and institutional classification	Doctoral preparation	Nondoctoral preparation	Doctoral preparation	Nondoctoral preparation
Professor				
Public and private school	*$25,384*	*$22,334*	*$28,450*	*$25,945*
Public school	25,765	23,429	28,674	27,170
Secular private school	24,568	21,641	28,660	27,188
Religious private school	22,631	17,962	25,669	19,808
Associate professor				
Public and private school	*21,268*	*18,979*	*22,946*	*20,784*
Public school	21,560	19,669	23,071	21,474
Secular private school	20,320	18,508	23,444	20,363
Religious private school	20,378	16,669	21,161	18,308
Assistant professor				
Public and private school	*18,093*	*16,058*	*19,569*	*17,147*
Public school	18,373	16,271	19,895	17,407
Secular private school ....·	17,067	16,251	18,892	17,221
Religious private school	16,527	14,916	18,491	15,978
Instructor				
Public and private school	*16,854*	*13,452*	*16,490*	*14,539*
Public school	17,183	13,651	16,359	14,685
Secular private school	...	13,470	(2)	14,773
Religious private school	(2)	12,605	(2)	13,711

[1] American Association of Colleges of Nursing.
[2] Insufficient number of cases to compute mean.

SOURCES: American Association of Colleges of Nursing, *Report on Nursing Faculty Salaries in Colleges and Universities, 1978-1979*, p. 26; *Report on Nursing Faculty Salaries in Colleges and Universities, 1979-1980, Revised Edition*, p. 28.

Table III-C-7. Mean Annual Salary of Nursing Faculty in AACN[1] Member Schools with Less Than 250 Full-Time Baccalaureate Students, by Academic Rank, Institutional Control, and Educational Preparation, Academic Years 1978-79 and 1979-80

Academic rank and institutional classification	Mean annual salary			
	1978-79		1979-80	
	Doctoral preparation	Nondoctoral preparation	Doctoral preparation	Nondoctoral preparation
Professor				
Public and private school	$25,335	$22,231	$27,322	$23,749
Public school	24,255	22,612	26,501	24,007
Secular private school	28,035	(2)	32,418	...
Religious private school	...	(2)	23,431	20,660
Associate professor				
Public and private school	21,186	18,785	22,608	20,134
Public school	20,829	19,279	22,679	20,728
Secular private school	22,343	18,598	23,745	19,783
Religious private school	19,520	16,479	20,182	18,174
Assistant professor				
Public and private school	18,608	15,991	19,606	17,128
Public school	18,014	16,102	19,158	17,503
Secular private school	20,932	16,925	20,605	16,577
Religious private school	(2)	14,754	...	16,113
Instructor				
Public and private school	(2)	13,339	16,575	14,557
Public school	(2)	13,529	15,851	14,681
Secular private school	(2)	13,777	(2)	14,649
Religious private school	...	12,354	...	14,075

[1] American Association of Colleges of Nursing.
[2] Insufficient number of cases to compute mean.

SOURCES: American Association of Colleges of Nursing, *Report on Nursing Faculty Salaries in Colleges and Universities, 1978-1979*, p. 25; *Report on Nursing Faculty Salaries in Colleges and Universities, 1979-1980, Revised Edition*, p. 27.

Table III-C-8. Mean Annual Salary of Nursing Faculty in AACN[1] Member Schools with 100 or More Full-Time Master's Students, by Academic Rank, Institutional Control, and Educational Preparation, Academic Years 1978-79 and 1979-80

| Academic rank and institutional classification | Mean annual salary | | | |
| | 1978-79 | | 1979-80 | |
	Doctoral preparation	Nondoctoral preparation	Doctoral preparation	Nondoctoral preparation
Professor				
Public and private school	$25,441	$23,636	$28,704	$27,421
Public school	26,014	24,400	28,680	27,741
Secular private school	19,586	19,627	29,537	25,717
Religious private school	22,667	...	24,644	...
Associate professor				
Public and private school	20,935	19,423	22,924	21,237
Public school	21,263	19,631	22,816	21,288
Secular private school	19,556	17,222	24,141	21,982
Religious private school	19,670	18,655	20,098	20,054
Assistant professor				
Public and private school	17,828	16,047	19,366	17,436
Public school	18,012	16,108	19,358	17,502
Secular private school	16,993	15,733	19,916	17,742
Religious private school	14,750	15,566	17,783	16,295
Instructor				
Public and private school	17,178	13,629	17,160	14,710
Public school	17,178	13,804	17,312	14,777
Secular private school	...	13,313	(2)	14,667
Religious private school	...	12,350	...	14,385

[1] American Association of Colleges of Nursing.
[2] Insufficient number of cases to compute mean.

SOURCES: American Association of Colleges of Nursing, *Report on Nursing Faculty Salaries in Colleges and Universities, 1978-1979*, p. 27; *Report on Nursing Faculty Salaries in Colleges and Universities, 1979-1980, Revised Edition*, p. 29.

**Table III-C-9. Mean Annual Salary of Nursing Faculty in AACN[1]
Member Schools with Students in Doctoral Programs in Nursing, by
Academic Rank, Institutional Control, and Educational Preparation,
Academic Year 1979-80**

Academic rank and institutional classification	Mean annual salary	
	Doctoral preparation	Nondoctoral preparation
Professor		
Public and private school	*$28,800*	*$27,375*
Public school	28,661	27,668
Secular private school	29,396	25,717
Religious private school	(2)	...
Associate professor		
Public and private school	*23,260*	*21,151*
Public school	22,752	21,251
Secular private school	24,581	20,675
Religious private school	18,600	(2)
Assistant professor		
Public and private school	*19,344*	*17,491*
Public school	19,280	17,502
Secular private school	19,620	17,769
Religious private school	18,425	16,296
Instructor		
Public and private school	*16,793*	*14,870*
Public school	16,505	14,785
Secular private school	(2)	14,973
Religious private school	...	15,068

[1] American Association of Colleges of Nursing.
[2] Insufficient number of cases to compute mean.

SOURCE: American Association of Colleges of Nursing, *Report on Nursing Faculty Salaries in Colleges
and Universities, 1979-1980, Revised Edition*, p. 30.

Table III-C-10. AAUP Weighted Average Salary[1] for Men, and Weighted Average Salary for Women as a Percentage of Men's, by Rank, Category of Institutions,[2] and Affiliation, 1978-79

Academic rank	Average salary—men				Average salary—women as a percentage of men's			
	All combined	Public	Private independent	Church-related	All combined	Public	Private independent	Church-related
Total								
Professor	$26,660	$26,890	$28,340	$21,500	91.2	92.6	86.8	90.7
Associate	20,190	20,630	20,070	17,580	95.1	96.4	92.6	92.0
Assistant	16,630	17,020	16,340	14,840	95.1	95.8	94.1	93.4
Instructor	13,820	14,310	12,960	12,000	94.2	94.1	95.0	95.6
Lecturer	15,620	15,710	15,200	14,820	88.8	89.1	90.4	81.8
AAUP Category I[3]								
Professor	28,770	28,190	31,270	26,860	91.1	92.4	88.4	86.8
Associate	21,270	21,200	21,840	20,700	95.4	96.0	93.5	91.3
Assistant	17,380	17,360	17,510	17,210	94.7	94.7	96.3	91.4
Instructor	13,960	13,910	14,200	14,000	95.3	95.1	97.6	95.7
Lecturer	16,150	16,310	15,330	14,450	88.7	88.2	92.8	87.0
AAUP Category IIA[4]								
Professor	24,650	25,100	24,880	21,110	97.0	97.6	90.9	92.4
Associate	19,870	20,160	19,680	18,000	96.1	97.4	92.5	90.6
Assistant	16,500	16,750	16,200	15,290	96.0	97.0	93.2	91.8
Instructor	13,440	13,730	12,760	12,280	96.4	96.6	97.1	94.0
Lecturer	13,980	13,870	13,360	16,100	92.7	92.2	(5)	82.5
AAUP Category IIB[6]								
Professor	21,650	23,300	23,180	19,780	96.3	95.4	98.8	93.6
Associate	17,460	19,260	17,760	16,330	94.8	95.2	96.5	94.1
Assistant	14,750	16,090	14,830	14,000	95.0	96.2	95.6	95.2
Instructor	12,330	13,400	12,310	11,690	94.5	94.0	95.5	95.5
Lecturer	14,990	14,990	16,380	13,610	84.7	92.7	76.4	71.9
AAUP Category III[7]								
Professor	23,000	23,380	18,040	14,120	100.1	99.3	87.1	(5)
Associate	19,690	19,900	16,330	14,230	98.8	99.1	92.8	(5)
Assistant	16,710	16,900	13,570	12,170	97.1	97.1	98.3	(5)
Instructor	15,130	15,380	11,300	9,320	91.1	92.2	95.2	105.2
Lecturer	13,960	13,960	...	...	89.0	91.4	...	...

[1]Salary has been adjusted to nine-month basis when necessary. The figure has been rounded to the nearest hundred dollars; an entry of $16,600 would stand for an average salary between $16,550 and $16,649.
[2]Includes only those institutions reporting breakdown by sex.
[3]Category I includes institutions which offer the doctorate and which conferred in the most recent three years an annual average of fifteen or more earned doctorates covering a minimum of three nonrelated disciplines.
[4]Category IIA includes institutions awarding degrees above the baccalaureate but not included in Category I.
[5]Insufficient number of cases to compute average salary.
[6]Category IIB includes institutions awarding only the baccalaureate or equivalent degree.
[7]Category III includes two-year institutions with academic ranks.

SOURCE: American Association of University Professors, "An Era of Continuing Decline: Annual Report on the Economic Status of The Profession, 1978-79," *Academe*, Bulletin of the AAUP, Vol. 65, No. 5, September 1979, p. 335.

Table III-C-11. Annual Salaries of Deans of Nursing Programs in American Association of Colleges of Nursing Member Schools, by Type of School, 1978-79

	Number of schools	Annual salary				
		Percentile				
Type of school		10th	25th	50th	75th	90th
Total	171	$24,500	$28,000	$35,700	$41,600	$46,400
University	123	27,800	32,000	38,800	43,700	48,300
Four-year college	44	20,200	22,600	26,000	30,100	38,700
Other	4	...	...	42,600	...	...

SOURCE: American Association of Colleges of Nursing, *Report of Salaries of Nursing Deans in Colleges and Universities, 1978-1979*, p. 10.

Table III-C-12. Annual Salaries of Deans of Nursing Programs in American Association of Colleges of Nursing Member Schools, by Region, 1978-79

	Number of schools	Annual salary				
		Percentile				
Region		10th	25th	50th	75th	90th
United States	171	$24,500	$28,000	$35,700	$41,600	$46,400
Northeast	41	23,000	28,100	35,900	41,000	47,300
Midwest	56	22,400	27,100	33,800	42,100	46,200
South	55	25,200	29,300	35,300	41,300	44,600
West	19	26,800	31,600	40,900	45,000	54,000

SOURCE: American Association of Colleges of Nursing, *Report of Salaries of Nursing Deans in Colleges and Universities, 1978-1979*, pp. 8 and 9.

Table III-C-13. Annual Salaries of Deans of Nursing Programs in American Association of Colleges of Nursing Member Schools, by Highest Earned Degree, 1978-79

	Number of deans	Annual salary				
		Percentile				
Highest earned degree		10th	25th	50th	75th	90th
Total	171	$24,500	$28,000	$35,700	$41,600	$46,400
Ed.D.	72	27,500	31,900	37,600	42,000	46,900
Ph.D.	62	25,000	27,900	36,000	44,100	48,300
D.N.S. or D.N.Sc.	6	...	24,000	31,400	41,000	...
D.P.H. or Dr. P.H.	2	...	...	...	...	...
Master's in nursing	23	22,500	23,800	27,200	35,100	40,200
Master's in other field	6	...	22,400	25,900	36,300	...

SOURCE: American Association of Colleges of Nursing, *Report of Salaries of Nursing Deans in Colleges and Universities, 1978-1979*, p. 12.

Table III-C-14. Annual Salaries of Deans of Nursing Programs in American Association of Colleges of Nursing Member Schools, by Institutional Control, 1978-79

	Number of schools	Annual salary				
		Percentile				
Control		10th	25th	50th	75th	90th
Total	171	$24,500	$28,000	$35,700	$41,600	$46,400
Public	106	27,400	32,000	39,000	42,500	45,600
Secular private	25	23,100	28,900	36,000	42,700	47,700
Religious private	40	20,800	22,500	27,000	32,000	46,600

SOURCE: American Association of Colleges of Nursing, *Report of Salaries of Nursing Deans in Colleges and Universities, 1978-1979*, p. 9.

Table III-C-15. Annual Salaries of Deans of Nursing Programs in American Association of Colleges of Nursing Member Schools, by Type of Program, 1978-79

	Number of schools	Annual salary				
		Percentile				
Type of program		10th	25th	50th	75th	90th
Total	171	$24,500	$28,000	$35,700	$41,600	$46,400
Baccalaureate	90	22,100	25,900	30,000	35,000	40,000
Master's	1	...	...	...	...	...
Baccalaureate and master's	64	27,900	35,800	40,800	44,000	47,200
Baccalaureate, master's and doctoral	16	40,700	42,500	48,900	50,000	54,300

SOURCE: American Association of Colleges of Nursing, *Report of Salaries of Nursing Deans in Colleges and Universities, 1978-1979*, p. 11.

Chapter III, Section D
EARNINGS OF NURSES IN EXPANDED ROLES

Data on a cohort of graduates of nurse practitioner programs between March
and September 1977 were gathered in a special longitudinal study conducted
by the State University of New York at Buffalo under contract with the
Division of Nursing. Details of this study are represented in Chapter I, Section
C. Income data for those graduates who were employed full-time at least 6
months after graduation, when the survey was conducted, are included here.
The average annual income of those employed as nurse practitioners was
$14,452. Graduates from master's programs earned more than their counter-
parts from certificate programs, $15,735 versus $14,244. There was a $454
salary differential among the regions, with nurses in the Western and Southern
states reporting the highest annual incomes, $14,631 and $14,554, respectively.

Nurse practitioners working in rural settings reported lower earnings ($13,698)
than those in other locations. Comparisons of income before and after nurse
practitioner preparation depicted an average gain of $2,138 for certificate
graduates and $2,761 for graduates from master's programs.

The 1977 national sample survey of registered nurses conducted by the
American Nurses' Association under contract with the Division of Nursing
showed the estimated annual salary of the nurse practitioner/midwife to be
$14,220, or $1,185 per month; the clinical nursing specialist averaged
$14,784, or $1,232 per month; and the nurse anesthetist, $19,896.

Data on the earnings of nurse-midwives were reported by the American
College of Nurse-Midwives. In 1976 the mean income for nurse-midwives in
clinical practice was $16,171. The incomes of nurse-midwives varied by major
function, basis of income, and highest educational preparation. The mean
annual salary of nurse-midwives paid on a "fee-for-service" basis was
$21,600, 34 percent higher than that for those who had a fixed annual salary.
The data showed a strong association between the annual salary of the nurse-
midwife and highest educational preparation. Salaries ranged from $14,696 for
nurses without a college degree to $20,500 for nurses with doctorates. Those
whose major function was supervision or administration earned $18,291, while
nurse-midwives functioning in direct patient care averaged $15,944. Nurses
working in the Pacific Coast states showed the highest mean annual income
($18,230), while those working in the Mountain states reported the least
($12,000).

Table III-D-1. Average Hourly Earnings[1] and Number of Full-time Clinical Specialists and Nurse Anesthetists in Nongovernment Hospitals by Metropolitan Area,[2] August 1975 and January 1976

	Clinical specialists		Nurse anesthetists	
Metropolitan area	Number	Average hourly earnings	Number	Average hourly earnings
Atlanta, GA	10	$6.43	...	...
Baltimore, MD	69	7.41	67	$8.76
Boston, MA	174	6.76	95	7.75
Buffalo, NY	...	...	...	...
Chicago, IL.....................	95	6.92	217	7.99
Cleveland, OH	22	6.81	...	...
Dallas-Fort Worth, TX	...	...	89	7.89
Denver-Boulder, CO	12	6.98	20	7.20
Detroit, MI	34	6.69	111	8.53
Houston, TX	...	...	35	7.55
Kansas City, MO-KS	12	5.94	...	...
Los Angeles-Long Beach, CA	46	7.78	28	9.57
Memphis, TN-AR-MS	...	...	...	...
Miami, FL	...	...	43	7.41
Milwaukee, WI	38	6.60	35	7.52
Minneapolis-St. Paul, MN-WI	...	...	177	7.31
New York, NY-NJ	61	9.01	214	9.15
Philadelphia, PA-NJ	96	6.50	218	7.47
Portland, OR-WA	15	7.56	67	7.40
St. Louis, MO-IL................	19	6.40	105	8.29
San Francisco-Oakland, CA	...	...	90	8.68
Seattle-Everett, WA	...	...	...	...
Washington, DC-MD-VA	74	6.82	30	8.52

[1]Excludes premium pay for overtime, work on weekends, holidays and late shifts.
[2]Standard Metropolitan Statistical Areas as defined by the U.S. Office of Management and Budget through February 1974. All metropolitan areas consist of one or more counties.
SOURCE: U.S. Department of Labor, Bureau of Labor Statistics, *Industry Wage Survey: Hospitals, August 1975 and January 1976*, pp. 13-36, 1977.

Table III-D-2. Estimated Number[1] and Mean Monthly Salary of Registered Nurses[2] Employed Full-time in Nursing by Location of Employment, Selected Position Types and Field of Employment, September 1977

Type of position and field of employment	Total			Location of employment					
				SMSA			Non-SMSA		
	(n)	N	Mean salary	(n)	N	Mean salary	(n)	N	Mean salary
Nurse practitioner/midwife									
Hospital	100	7,249	$1,185	62	5,506	$1,196	38	1,743	$1,151
Nursing home	28	2,315	1,238	26	2,196	1,231	2	119	(3)
Nursing education	1	16	(3)	...	...	...	1	16	(3)
Public health	36	2,477	1,114	21	1,789	(3)	15	688	(3)
Student health	10	990	(3)	6	719	(3)	4	272	(3)
Occupational health	1	58	(3)	...	...	...	1	58	(3)
Physician's office	20	1,119	(3)	8	661	(3)	12	458	(3)
Self-employed	4	272	(3)	1	141	(3)	3	131	(3)
Clinical nursing specialist									
Hospital	62	5,382	1,232	51	4,739	1,237	11	643	(3)
Nursing home	45	4,039	1,206	37	3,580	1,210	8	459	(3)
Nursing education	2	207	(3)	2	207	(3)	...	...	...
Public health	1	76	(3)	1	76	(3)	...	...	...
Student health	11	926	(3)	8	742	(3)	3	184	(3)
Occupational health	...	...	...	...	...	...	...	...	...
Physician's office	2	93	(3)	2	93	(3)	...	...	...
Self-employed	1	41	(3)	1	41	(3)	...	...	...
Nurse anesthetist									
Hospital	146	11,167	1,658	100	8,464	1,641	46	2,703	1,712
Nursing home	117	9,431	1,647	84	7,224	1,639	33	2,208	1,672
Nursing education	...	...	...	...	...	...	...	...	...
Public health	...	...	...	...	...	...	...	...	...
Student health	...	...	...	...	...	...	...	...	...
Occupational health	...	...	...	...	...	...	...	...	...
Physician's office	16	1,087	(3)	12	941	(3)	4	146	(3)
Self-employed	13	649	(3)	4	299	(3)	9	350	(3)

[1] Excludes nurses who did not report salary.

[2] Includes only registered nurses actively licensed and working in the United States in September 1977.

[3] Insufficient number of cases to compute mean.

NOTE: "N" corresponds to the weighted population estimate derived from the sample and "n" refers to the actual number of surveys upon which the estimate was based. Because of rounding, sums of estimated numbers (N) and estimated percents may not add to totals.

SOURCE: Roth, Aleda V. et al. *1977 National Sample Survey of Registered Nurses: A Report on the Nurse Population and Factors Affecting their Supply*, final report on Contract No. (HRA 231-76-0085) between the American Nurses' Association and the Division of Nursing, U.S. Department of Health and Human Services, NTIS Publication No. HRP-0900603, 1979.

Table III-D-3. Number[1] and Average Annual Income of Registered Nurses Employed Full-time Who Graduated from Nurse Practitioner Programs by Employment Status, Specialty and Type of Program, 1977

			Employed full-time			
	Total		Employed as nurse practitioner[2]		Not employed as nurse practitioner	
Type of program and specialty	Number of graduates	Average income	Number of graduates	Average income	Number of graduates	Average income
Total	287	$14,415	243	$14,452	44	$14,204
Pediatric	29	14,241	22	14,546	7	13,286
Midwifery	10	15,900	10	15,900	...	...
Maternity	34	13,647	31	13,774	3	12,333
Family	116	14,457	106	14,434	10	14,700
Adult	84	14,702	65	14,677	19	14,790
Psychiatric	5	13,000	2	14,500	3	12,000
Emergency	9	13,778	7	13,286	2	15,500
Certificate	235	14,230	209	14,244	26	14,115
Pediatric	15	14,067	11	14,182	4	13,750
Midwifery	9	15,222	9	15,222	...	...
Maternity	33	13,606	30	13,733	3	12,333
Family	101	14,228	95	14,200	6	14,667
Adult	66	14,515	56	14,590	10	14,100
Psychiatric	2	14,000	1	13,000	1	15,000
Emergency	9	13,778	7	14,244	2	15,500
Master's	52	15,250	34	15,735	18	14,333
Pediatric	14	14,429	11	14,909	3	12,667
Midwifery	1	22,000	1	22,000	...	...
Maternity	1	15,000	1	15,000	...	...
Family	15	16,000	11	16,454	4	14,750
Adult	18	15,389	9	15,222	9	15,556
Psychiatric	3	12,333	1	16,000	2	10,500
Emergency	...	...	...	...	...	...

[1]Includes only those graduates who supplied information on income and specialty. Excludes one foreign-employed graduate.
[2]Includes graduates who are functioning wholly or in part as a nurse practitioner.
SOURCE: U.S. Department of Health, Education, and Welfare, Public Health Service, Health Resources Administration, Division of Nursing, *Longitudinal Study of Nurse Practitioners, Phase III,* DHEW Publication No. HRA 80-2, May, 1980, p. 99.

Table III-D-4. Average, Anticipated, and Actual Increase in Income,
and Average Annual Nursing Income after Nurse Practitioner
Preparation of Graduates Employed Full-time,[1]
by Specialty and Type of Program, 1977

Type of program and specialty	Number of graduates	Average anticipated increase	Average actual increase	Average income
Total	170	$2,197	$2,388	$14,853
Pediatric	19	1,526	2,579	14,737
Midwifery	6	2,833	4,167	16,667
Maternity	21	1,524	1,857	14,238
Family	68	2,581	3,103	14,927
Adult	46	2,152	1,609	15,217
Psychiatric	3	2,000	−1,000	12,333
Emergency	7	2,143	1,429	13,429
Certificate	136	2,092	2,353	14,713
Pediatric	9	2,278	3,111	14,778
Midwifery	5	3,400	4,600	15,600
Maternity	20	1,275	1,650	14,200
Family	57	2,395	2,895	14,667
Adult	38	1,842	1,605	15,158
Psychiatric	...	...	...	...
Emergency	7	2,143	1,429	13,429
Master's	34	2,618	2,529	15,412
Pediatric	10	850	2,100	14,700
Midwifery	1	...	2,000	22,000
Maternity	1	6,500	6,000	15,000
Family	11	3,545	4,182	16,273
Adult	8	3,625	1,625	15,500
Psychiatric	3	2,000	−1,000	12,333
Emergency	...	...	...	...

[1] Based on graduates employed full-time before and after nurse practitioner preparation and on those who could specify their expectations.

SOURCE: U.S. Department of Health, Education, and Welfare, Public Health Service, Health Resources Administration, Division of Nursing, *Longitudinal Study of Nurse Practitioners, Phase III*, DHEW Publication No. HRA 80-2, May, 1980, p. 102.

Table III-D-5. Average Annual Income of Registered Nurses Employed Full-time Before and After Graduation from a Nurse Practitioner Program, by Type of Program, 1977

	Total	Type of program	
		Certificate	Master's
Average income	*N = 248*	*N = 202*	*N = 46*
Before nurse practitioner preparation	$12,306	$12,223	$12,674
After nurse practitioner preparation	14,560	14,361	15,435
Increase	2,254	2,138	2,761

SOURCE: U.S. Department of Health, Education, and Welfare, Public Health Service, Health Resources Administration, Division of Nursing, *Longitudinal Study of Nurse Practitioners, Phase III,* DHEW Publication No. HRA 80-2, May, 1980, p. 100.

Table III-D-6. Number[1] and Average Annual Income of Registered Nurses Employed Full-time Who Graduated from Nurse Practitioner Programs by Type of Program and Region,[2] 1977

	Total		Type of program			
			Certificate		Master's	
Region	*Number*	*Average income*	*Number*	*Average income*	*Number*	*Average income*
Total	287	*$14,415*	235	*$14,230*	52	*$15,250*
Northeast	79	14,177	61	14,000	18	14,778
South	101	14,554	92	14,272	9	17,444
Midwest	42	14,190	35	14,086	7	14,714
West	65	14,631	47	14,553	18	14,833

[1]Includes only those graduates who supplied information on income and region. Excludes one foreign-employed graduate.
[2]For states included in each region, see Table I-C-3.
SOURCE: U.S. Department of Health, Education, and Welfare, Public Health Service, Health Resources Administration, Division of Nursing, *Longitudinal Study of Nurse Practitioners, Phase III,* DHEW Publication No. HRA 80-2, May, 1980, p. 100.

Table III-D-7. Number[1] and Average Annual Income of Registered Nurses Employed Full-time as Nurse Practitioners, Who Graduated from Nurse Practitioner Programs, by Type of Program and Practice Setting Location, 1977

| Practice setting location | Total | | Type of program | | | |
| | | | Certificate | | Master's | |
	Number	Average income	Number	Average income	Number	Average income
Total	239	$14,423	205	$14,205	34	$15,735
Inner city	54	14,352	48	14,167	6	15,833
Other urban	42	14,619	32	14,250	10	15,800
Suburban	37	14,108	31	14,194	6	13,667
Rural	53	13,698	49	13,653	4	14,250
Combination[2]	19	14,316	14	13,929	5	15,400
Other[3]	34	15,824	31	15,226	3	22,000

[1] Includes only graduates who supplied information on income and practice setting location.
[2] Includes two or more of the selected practice setting locations.
[3] Includes various institutional settings.

SOURCE: U.S. Department of Health, Education, and Welfare, Public Health Service, Health Resources Administration, Division of Nursing, *Longitudinal Study of Nurse Practitioners, Phase III,* DHEW Publication No. HRA 80-2, May, 1980, p. 100.

Table III-D-8. Annual Income of American College of Nurse-Midwives Study Participants in Clinical Practice in the United States, 1976-1977

Item	Number[1]	Mean annual income	Percentage distribution by income					
			Total	Less than $10,000	$10,000-15,000	$15,001-20,000	$20,001-25,000	More than $25,000
Nurse-midwives in clinical practice ...	436	$16,171	100	2	37	53	6	2
Nurse-midwives managing deliveries								
Nurse-midwives who manage deliveries	373	16,290	100	2	37	52	7	2
Nurse-midwives who manage deliveries in nonhospital settings	27	15,789	100	15	41	26	11	7
Basis of income								
Fixed annual	430	16,111	100	2	38	53	6	1
Based on patient fees	5	21,600	100	20	...	40	...	40
Highest educational preparation								
Nurse-midwife certificate	122	14,696	100	7	48	44	1	...
Baccalaureate	86	15,257	100	2	49	47	1	1
Master's degree	220	17,242	100	...	27	59	11	3
Doctorate	4	20,500	100	...	25	25	50	...
Major function								
Direct patient care	273	15,944	100	2	40	52	4	2
Teaching	41	15,668	100	5	39	49	7	...
Supervision/administration	19	18,291	100	5	11	58	26	...

[1]Excludes nurse-midwives who are members of the U.S. military or U.S. Public Health Service Commissioned Corps, are members of a religious order, are employed outside of the United States, work less than 11 months per year and 35 hours per week, or did not provide data on annual income.

SOURCE: American College of Nurse-Midwives, *Nurse-Midwifery in the United States: 1976-1977*, p. 27.

**Table III-D-9. Mean Annual Income of American College of
Nurse-Midwives Study Participants in Clinical Practice,
by Geographical Area, 1976-1977**

Geographical area	Number	Mean annual income[1]
Maine, Massachusetts, New Hampshire, Rhode Island and Vermont	17	$15,106
New Jersey, New York, Pennsylvania and Connecticut ...	163	17,385
Delaware, District of Columbia, Maryland and Virginia	52	16,111
Alabama, Florida, Georgia, Mississippi, North Carolina and South Carolina	108	14,842
Kentucky, West Virginia and Tennessee	54	14,601
Illinois, Indiana, Michigan, Minnesota, Ohio and Wisconsin	80	16,417
Arkansas, Louisiana, Oklahoma and Texas	23	14,400
Iowa, Kansas, Missouri, Nebraska, North Dakota and South Dakota	18	14,894
New Mexico, Arizona, Nevada and Utah	48	15,348
Idaho, Colorado, Montana and Wyoming	2	12,000
Alaska, Washington, Oregon, California and Hawaii ...	58	18,230
U.S. territories	11	11,732
Other countries	31	9,497

[1] Excludes nurse-midwives who are members of the U.S. military or U.S. Public Health Service Commissioned Corps, are members of a religious order, work less than 11 months per year and 35 hours per week, or did not provide data on annual income.

SOURCE: American College of Nurse-Midwives, *Nurse-Midwifery in the United States: 1976-1977*, p. 28.

**Table III-D-10. Malpractice Insurance Coverage for U.S. Resident
American College of Nurse-Midwives Study Participants in Clinical
Practice, 1976-1977**

Malpractice insurance coverage	Nurse-midwives in clinical practice	
	Number	Percent
Total	623	100.0
Not insured	43	6.9
Insured	579	92.9
Personal policy only	320	51.4
Personal policy and employer's policy	204	32.7
Employer's policy only	55	8.8
Coverage unknown	1	0.2

SOURCE: American College of Nurse-Midwives, *Nurse-Midwifery in the United States: 1976-1977*, p. 26.

Chapter III, Section E
EARNINGS OF OCCUPATIONAL HEALTH NURSES

Under the annual occupational wage survey program, the Bureau of Labor Statistics canvassed industries with 50 or more employees (100 or more employees in the 13 largest areas) in a sample from the 262 standard metropolitan statistical areas (SMSAs) in the country. Data for the 1977 and 1978 studies were collected throughout each respective year, with a reference date of July for the regional and national summaries. These estimates were derived from 73 sample SMSAs. Excluding supervisory positions, the weekly earnings of industrial registered nurses in metropolitan areas averaged $280.50 in 1978. This amount was an 8.7 percent increase over the average weekly earnings of the previous year.

The earnings of registered nurses in industrial settings showed marked regional differences. The average weekly earnings of those in the Northeast were the lowest, while their counterparts in the West averaged the highest salaries. The Western metropolitan areas have traditionally paid higher salaries than other regions. On the other hand, only in the past few years has the Northeast become the lowest paying region for industrial nurses. The year 1976 marked the turning point between the Southern and the Northeastern regions in terms of lowest average earnings. Calculations of the proportion of change between 1977 and 1978 in the average weekly earnings of industrial nurses showed increases of 10.1 percent, 9.1 percent, 8.4 percent, and 7.6 percent for the Western, North Central, Northeastern, and Southern metropolitan areas, respectively.

More recent data, collected between July 1978 and June 1979 by the BLS, on the individual metropolitan areas is presented in this section. Included here are the average weekly earnings of nurses in 20 Northeastern, 15 Southern, 18 North Central, and 8 Western metropolitan areas. Out of these 61 SMSAs, the highest average weekly earnings ($372.50) were recorded in Detroit, Michigan, (March 1979), while the lower bound in this reporting period was $227.50, shown for Utica-Rome, New York (July 1978). Percentage annual changes in earnings between the 1977-78 and 1978-79 surveys ranged from 2.0 percent for Columbus, Ohio, to 14.1 percent for Wichita, Kansas.

Table III-E-1. Average Weekly Earnings[1] of Industrial Registered Nurses[2] in Metropolitan Areas,[3] by Region,[4] 1972-1978[5]

| Year[6] | United States | Region ||||
		North-east	South	North Central	West
1978	$280.50	$266.00	$269.00	$293.00	$301.00
1977	258.00	245.50	250.00	268.50	273.50
1976	238.00	227.50	227.50	248.00	251.50
1975	220.50	211.50	210.50	228.50	235.50
1974	192.00	186.00	184.50	197.50	200.50
1973	179.00	174.00	171.50	184.00	188.50
1972	169.00	164.50	161.50	173.50	179.00

[1] Earnings relate to straight-time salaries paid for standard workweeks.
[2] Excludes supervisory nurses.
[3] 229 Standard Metropolitan Statistical Areas in the United States (excluding Alaska and Hawaii) as established by the Office of Management and Budget for 1974 and prior years, and 262 SMSAs for 1975 through 1978.
[4] The states included in each region are: *Northeast*—Connecticut, Maine, Massachusetts, New Hampshire, New Jersey, New York, Pennsylvania, Rhode Island, and Vermont; *South*—Alabama, Arkansas, Delaware, District of Columbia, Florida, Georgia, Kentucky, Louisiana, Maryland, Mississippi, North Carolina, Oklahoma, South Carolina, Tennessee, Texas, Virginia and West Virginia; *North Central*—Illinois, Indiana, Iowa, Kansas, Michigan, Minnesota, Missouri, Nebraska, North Dakota, Ohio, South Dakota, and Wisconsin; *West*—Arizona, California, Colorado, Idaho, Montana, Nevada, New Mexico, Oregon, Utah, Washington, and Wyoming.
[5] Data were collected during each calendar year from 1975 through 1978 with July as an average month of reference. In previous years data were collected on a fiscal year basis, with an average month of reference of February.
[6] Since 1973, earnings reflect men and women combined. The 1972 earnings reflect women only.
SOURCE: U.S. Department of Labor, Bureau of Labor Statistics, *Occupational Earnings in All Metropolitan Areas, 1978*, and previous years.

CHART 12. AVERAGE WEEKLY EARNINGS OF INDUSTRIAL REGISTERED NURSES IN METROPOLITAN AREAS, BY REGION, 1972-1978

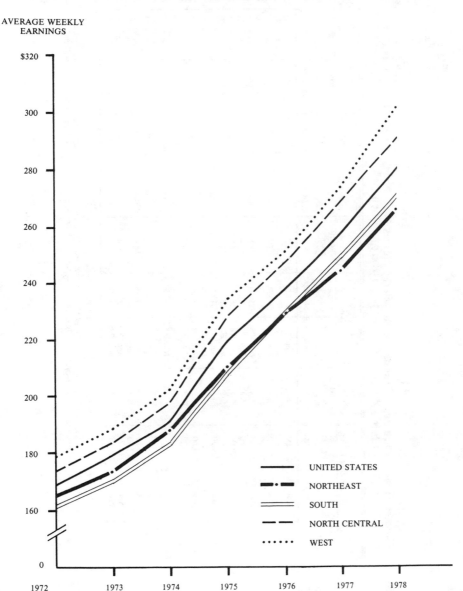

SOURCE: U.S. Department of Labor, Bureau of Labor Statistics, *Occupational Earnings in All Metropolitan Areas, 1978*, and previous years.

Prepared by American Nurses' Association, Research and Policy Analysis Department, Statistics Unit, 1980.

Table III-E-2. Average Weekly Earnings[1] of Industrial Registered Nurses in 20 Northeastern Metropolitan Areas, July 1975-June 1976 to July 1978-June 1979

Northeastern metropolitan areas	July 1978 through June 1979			July 1977 through June 1978			July 1976 through June 1977			July 1975 through June 1976	
	Date of survey	Average weekly earnings	Percent change 1977-78 to 1978-79	Date of survey	Average weekly earnings	Percent change 1976-77 to 1977-78	Date of survey	Average weekly earnings	Percent change 1975-76 to 1976-77	Date of survey	Average weekly earnings
Albany-Schenectady-Troy, NY	Sept. '78	$281.00	8.7	Sept. '77	$258.50	6.2	Sept. '76	$243.50	10.4	Sept. '75	$220.50
Binghamton, NY-PA	...	...	...	...	...	...	July '76	220.00	6.5	July '75	206.50
Boston, MA	Aug. '78	269.00	8.9	Aug. '77	247.00	5.8	Aug. '76	233.50	7.9	Aug. '75	216.50
Buffalo, NY	Oct. '78	294.00	7.3	Oct. '77	274.00	8.7	Oct. '76	252.00	6.8	Oct. '75	236.00
Hartford, CT	Mar. '79	271.00	8.4	Mar. '78	250.00	8.5	Mar. '77	230.50	7.5	Mar. '76	214.50
Nassau-Suffolk, NY	June '79	284.00	8.4	June '78	262.00	12.4	June '77	233.00	9.9	June '76	212.00
Newark, NJ	Jan. '79	286.00	8.5	Jan. '78	263.50	6.9	Jan. '77	246.50	8.1	Jan. '76	228.00
New York, NY-NJ	...	...	...	May '78	287.50	12.5	May '77	255.50	6.7	May '76	239.50
Northeast Pennsylvania	Aug. '78	229.50	4.6	Aug. '77	219.50	17.1	Aug. '76	187.50	...	...	...
Paterson-Clifton-Passaic, NJ	...	...	...	June '78	256.50	5.8	June '77	242.50	6.6	June '76	227.50
Philadelphia, PA-NJ	Nov. '78	274.00	8.3	Nov. '77	253.00	7.4	Nov. '76	235.50	7.5	Nov. '75	219.00
Pittsburgh, PA	Jan. '79	299.50	10.9	Jan. '78	270.00	10.4	Jan. '77	244.50	8.2	Jan. '76	226.00
Poughkeepsie, NY	...	...	...	...	...	...	June '77	242.50	...	...	...
Providence-Warwick-Pawtucket, RI-MA	...	...	...	June '78	233.50	13.9	June '77	205.00	7.6	June '76	190.50
Stamford, CT	...	...	...	...	...	...	...	...	...	May '76	231.50
Syracuse, NY	...	...	...	...	...	...	July '76	222.50	9.6	July '75	203.00
Trenton, NJ	Sept. '78	274.50	11.6	Sept. '77	246.00	11.1	Sept. '76	221.50	6.5	Sept. '75	208.00
Utica-Rome, NY	July '78	227.50	4.8	July '77	217.00	...	...	...	...	July '75	186.00
Worcester, MA	Apr. '79	273.00	8.3	Apr. '78	252.00	6.8	Apr. '77	236.00	7.0	Apr. '76	220.50
York, PA	Feb. '79	260.50	5.9	Feb. '78	246.00	8.8	Feb. '77	226.00	7.6	Feb. '76	210.00

[1]Earnings are for men and women combined and relate to straight-time salaries paid for standard workweeks.

SOURCES: U.S. Department of Labor, Bureau of Labor Statistics, Area Wage Surveys: Selected Metropolitan Areas, 1976, pp. 27-32; Area Wage Surveys: Selected Metropolitan Areas, 1977, pp. 23-27; Occupational Earnings and Wage Trends in Metropolitan Areas, 1978, No. 1, p. 4; No. 2, p. 4; No. 3, p. 4; Occupational Earnings and Wage Trends in Metropolitan Areas, 1979, No. 1, pp. 4-5, and individual releases.

Table III-E-3. Average Weekly Earnings[1] of Industrial Registered Nurses in 15 Southern Metropolitan Areas, July 1975-June 1976 to July 1978-June 1979

Southern metropolitan areas	July 1978 through June 1979			July 1977 through June 1978			July 1976 through June 1977			July 1975 through June 1976	
	Date of survey	Average weekly earnings	Percent change 1977-78 to 1978-79	Date of survey	Average weekly earnings	Percent change 1976-77 to 1977-78	Date of survey	Average weekly earnings	Percent change 1975-76 to 1976-77	Date of survey	Average weekly earnings
Atlanta, GA	May '79	$317.00	7.6	May '78	$294.50	11.3	May '77	$264.50	7.7	May '76	$245.50
Baltimore, MD	Aug. '78	297.00	7.2	Aug. '77	277.00	6.7	Aug. '76	259.50	9.5	Aug. '75	237.00
Birmingham, AL	Sept. '78	253.00	...	Mar. '78	240.00	5.7	Mar. '77	227.00	8.1	Mar. '76	210.00
Chattanooga, TN-GA	...	...	...	...	...	...	...	...	...	...	...
Dallas-Fort Worth, TX	Oct. '78	289.50	13.3	Oct. '77	255.50	8.3	Oct. '76	236.00	6.8	Oct. '75	221.00
Greensboro-Winston-Salem-High Point, NC	Aug. '78	264.00	6.9	Aug. '77	247.00	10.0	Aug. '76	224.50	9.5	Aug. '75	205.00
Greenville-Spartanburg, SC	...	...	...	June '78	207.50	5.3	June '77	197.00	8.5	June '76	181.50
Houston, TX	Apr. '79	295.00	8.9	Apr. '78	271.00	6.9	Aug. '77	253.50	11.7	Apr. '76	227.00
Jacksonville, FL	Dec. '78	277.00	9.9	Dec. '77	252.00	13.5	Dec. '76	222.00	7.5	Dec. '75	206.50
Louisville, KY-IN	Nov. '78	275.00	7.0	Nov. '77	257.00	11.5	Nov. '76	230.50	8.0	Nov. '75	213.50
Memphis, TN-AR-MS	Nov. '78	263.50	4.9	Nov. '77	250.50	8.4	Nov. '76	231.00	7.4	Nov. '75	215.00
Norfolk-Virginia Beach-Portsmouth-Newport News-Hampton, VA-NC	...	...	...	...	...	...	...	...	...	May '76	194.00
Raleigh-Durham, NC	...	...	...	...	...	...	...	...	...	Feb. '76	214.50
Richmond, VA	June '79	265.50	6.6	June '78	249.00	7.3	June '77	232.00	5.5	June '76	220.00
Washington, DC-MD-VA	Mar. '79	290.00	8.6	Mar. '78	267.00	10.1	Mar. '77	242.50	3.4	Mar. '76	234.50

[1]Earnings are for men and women combined and relate to straight-time salaries paid for standard workweeks.

SOURCES: U.S. Department of Labor, Bureau of Labor Statistics, *Area Wage Surveys: Selected Metropolitan Areas, 1976*, pp. 27-32; *Area Wage Surveys: Selected Metropolitan Areas, 1977*, pp.23-27; *Occupational Earnings and Wage Trends in Metropolitan Areas*; No. 1, p. 4; No. 2, p. 4; No. 3, p. 4; *Occupational Earnings and Wage Trends in Metropolitan Areas, 1979*, No. 1, pp. 4-5, and individual releases.

Table III-E-4. Average Weekly Earnings¹ of Industrial Registered Nurses in 18 North Central Metropolitan Areas, July 1975-June 1976 to July 1978-June 1979

North Central metropolitan areas	July 1978 through June 1979 Date of survey	July 1978 through June 1979 Average weekly earnings	Percent change 1977-78 to 1978-79	July 1977 through June 1978 Date of survey	July 1977 through June 1978 Average weekly earnings	Percent change 1976-77 to 1977-78	July 1976 through June 1977 Date of survey	July 1976 through June 1977 Average weekly earnings	Percent change 1975-76 to 1976-77	July 1975 through June 1976 Date of survey	July 1975 through June 1976 Average weekly earnings
Akron, OH	Dec. '78	$294.50	4.6	Dec. '77	$281.50	9.5	Dec. '76	$257.00	11.5	Dec. '75	$230.50
Canton, OH	.....	.....	.....	May '78	278.50	6.3 •	May '77	262.00	14.4	May '76	229.00
Chicago, IL	May '79	296.50	8.8	May '78	272.50	9.7	May '77	248.50	7.6	May '76	231.00
Cincinnati, OH-KY-IN	July '78	273.50	9.8	July '77	249.00	.....	.....	.....	.....	Mar. '76	229.50
Cleveland, OH-KY-IN	Sept. '78	298.00	9.6	Sept. '77	272.00	6.7	Sept. '76	255.00	8.1	Sept. '75	236.00
Columbus, OH	Oct. '78	249.00	2.0	Oct. '77	244.00	11.4	Oct. '76	219.00	7.9	Oct. '75	203.00
Davenport-Rock Island-Moline, IA-IL	Feb. '79	305.50	5.3	Feb. '78	290.00	8.6	May '77	267.00	8.8	Feb. '76	245.50
Dayton, OH	Dec. '78	322.00	9.5	Dec. '77	294.00	9.1	Dec. '77	269.50	5.3	Dec. '75	256.00
Detroit, MI	Mar. '79	372.50	11.2	Mar. '78	335.00	7.7	Mar. '77	311.00	8.7	Mar. '76	286.00
Indianapolis, IN	Oct. '78	319.50	10.2	Oct. '77	290.00	12.0	Oct. '76	259.00	4.0	Oct. '75	249.00
Kansas City, MO-KS	Sept. '78	298.50	8.2	Sept. '77	276.00	11.1	Sept. '76	248.50	5.5	Sept. '75	235.50
Milwaukee, WI	Apr. '79	285.50	7.5	Apr. '78	265.50	8.1	Apr. '77	245.50	4.9	Apr. '76	234.00
Minneapolis-St. Paul, MN-WI	Jan. '79	284.50	8.2	Jan. '78	263.00	6.5	Jan. '77	247.00	8.3	Jan. '76	228.00
Omaha, NE-IA	Oct. '78	266.00	13.0	Oct. '78	235.50	.....	.....	.....	.....	.....	.....
St. Louis, MO-IL	Mar. '79	308.00	9.2	Mar. '78	282.00	9.3	Mar. '77	258.00	7.9	Mar. '76	239.00
South Bend, IN	Aug. '78	246.00	9.6	Aug. '77	224.50	.....	.....	.....	.....	Mar. '76	204.50
Toledo, OH-MI	May '79	323.50	9.1	May '78	296.50	13.8	May '77	260.50	8.3	May '76	240.50
Wichita, KS	Apr. '79	271.00	14.1	Apr. '78	237.50	6.5	Apr. '77	223.00	5.4	Apr. '76	211.50

¹Earnings are for men and women combined and relate to straight-time salaries paid for standard workweeks.

SOURCES: U.S. Department of Labor, Bureau of Labor Statistics, *Area Wage Surveys: Selected Metropolitan Areas, 1976*, pp. 27-32; *Area Wage Surveys: Selected Metropolitan Areas, 1977*, pp. 23-27; *Occupational Earnings and Wage Trends in Metropolitan Areas, 1978*, No. 1, p. 4; No. 2, p. 4; No. 3, p. 4; *Occupational Earnings and Wage Trends in Metropolitan Areas, 1979*, No. 1, pp. 4-5, and individual releases.

Table III-E-5. Average Weekly Earnings¹ of Industrial Registered Nurses in 8 Western Metropolitan Areas, July 1975-June 1976 to July 1978-June 1979

Western metropolitan areas	July 1978 through June 1979		Percent change 1977-78 to 1978-79	July 1977 through June 1978		Percent change 1976-77 to 1977-78	July 1976 through June 1977		Percent change 1975-76 to 1976-77	July 1975 through June 1976	
	Date of survey	Average weekly earnings		Date of survey	Average weekly earnings		Date of survey	Average weekly earnings		Date of survey	Average weekly earnings
Anaheim-Garden Grove-Santa Ana, CA	Oct. '78	$285.50	7.7	Oct. '77	$265.00	8.6	Oct. '76	$244.00	...	Dec. '75	$219.00
Denver-Boulder, CO	Dec. '78	279.00	6.7	Dec. '77	261.50	10.8	Dec. '76	236.00	7.8	Oct. '75	241.50
Los Angeles-Long Beach, CA	Oct. '78	312.00	12.6	Oct. '77	277.00	7.6	Oct. '76	257.50	6.6	May '76	243.00
Portland, OR-WA	...	...	...	...	...	...	...	...	...	...	...
San Diego, CA	Nov. '78	294.50	...	...	...	...	...	...	...	...	...
San Francisco-Oakland, CA	Mar. '79	323.00	6.8	Mar. '78	302.50	12.0	Mar. '77	270.00	8.7	Mar. '76	248.50
San Jose, CA	Mar. '79	342.00	...	...	...	...	Mar. '77	278.00	7.1	Mar. '76	259.50
Seattle-Everett, WA	Dec. '78	329.00	6.5	Dec. '77	309.00	14.4	Jan. '77	270.00	6.7	Jan. '76	253.00

¹Earnings are for men and women combined and relate to straight-time salaries paid for standard workweeks.

SOURCES: U.S. Department of Labor, Bureau of Labor Statistics, *Area Wage Surveys: Selected Metropolitan Areas, 1976*, pp. 27-32; *Area Wage Surveys: Selected Metropolitan Areas, 1977*, pp. 23-27; *Occupational Earnings and Wage Trends in Metropolitan Areas, 1978*, No. 1, No. 2, p. 4; No. 3, p. 4; *Occupational Earnings and Wage Trends in Metropolitan Areas, 1979*, No. 1, pp. 4-5, and individual releases.

Chapter III, Section F
FEDERAL AND STATE GOVERNMENT SALARY SCHEDULES

Presented in this section are established salary ranges for civilian and military nurses in federal government positions as well as those for selected registered nurses in state government. Salaries for federal employees are established by the Congress of the United States; however, special civilian salary adjustments, depending upon occupation, are made by the federal administration when federal salaries are lower than private industry in certain regions of the country. Such salary adjustments are necessary to allow the federal government to become competitive in recruiting for certain types of positions and to make adjustments in different geographic areas according to local economic conditions. Evaluation of and increments in nurse grade salaries when conditions warrant such action is the responsibility of the U.S. Office of Personnel Management.

As of October 1979, a beginning staff nurse holding an associate degree with no prior experience would begin in grade 4, at a starting annual salary of $10,049. A staff nurse with higher qualifications could start in grade 5 at $11,243. Beginning federal government nursing salaries increased 7 percent between 1978 and 1979. Nurses already on staff were advanced within the new salary range to the step corresponding to their present position. Other position salary schedules for civilian nurses employed by the federal government are presented in the tables.

Salary ranges for nurses in the Air Force, Army, and Navy nurse corps are listed by rank and position. A nurse with the rank of second lieutenant in the Air Force as of October 1979 or Army as of March 1980 could begin at an annual salary of $12,751 including base pay, subsistence allowance, and quarters allowance. Nurses in the Navy Nurse Corps with the comparable rank of ensign began at approximately the same salary.

Junior grade nurses in the Veterans Administration started at $12,531 as of October 1979, compared to $11,712 in October 1978. New starting salaries are occasionally established by the VA, allowing nurses below the new minimum to advance to the starting rate. Nurses employed by the U.S. Postal Service started at $13,800 as of July 1979.

Salary ranges for staff nurse, nurse supervisor, nurse consultant, and director of nursing positions in state government are also included in this section. In 1979 the minimum average salary of staff nurses employed by state governments was $11,670; for nursing supervisors, it was $13,809; for nurse consultants, $16,205; and for state directors of nursing, $18,528. The minimum salaries represented 6.5 percent, 6.3 percent, 6.0 percent, and 5.0 percent gains, respectively, between 1978 and 1979.

Table III-F-1. Salary Schedules for Nurses Employed by Federal Government Under U.S. Civil Service,[1] October 1978 and 1979

Grade	Position[2]	Annual salary[3]	
		October 1978	October 1979
GS-4[4]	Staff nurse (beginning nurse)	$ 9,391-12,208	$10,049-13,064
GS-5	Staff nurse (beginning nurse)	10,507-13,657	11,243-14,618
GS-7	Clinical nurse (appropriate specialization)	13,014-16,920	13,925-18,101
	Occupational health nurse		
	Operating room nurse		
	Psychiatric nurse		
	Public health nurse		
GS-9	Clinical nurse (appropriate specialization)	15,920-20,699	17,035-22,147
	Head nurse		
	Instructor		
	Nurse anesthetist		
	Occupational health nurse		
	Operating room nurse		
	Psychiatric nurse		
	Public health nurse		
GS-11	Assistant nurse supervisor	19,263-25,041	20,611-26,794
	Clinical nurse specialist		
	Consultant		
	Head nurse		
	Instructor		
	Nurse anesthetist		
	Operating room nurse specialist		
	Psychiatric nurse specialist		
	Public health nurse		
	Supervisory nurse		
GS-12	Nurse supervisor (appropriate specialization)	23,087-30,017	24,703-32,110
GS-13	Consultant	27,453-35,688	29,375-38,186
	Director of nursing		
GS-14	Director of nursing	32,442-42,171	34,713-45,126
GS-15	Director of nursing	[5]38,160-49,608	[5]40,832-53,081

[1]Positions under the federal position classifications system (Title 5, USC, Chapter 51).
[2]Grade levels are assigned to individual positions in accordance with Civil Service Commission position classification standards for the Nurse Series, GS-610, June 1968 and December 1969; Nurse Anesthetist Series, GS-605, June 1965; and Public Health Nurse Series, GS-615, November 1969. Grade levels depend upon responsibilities assigned, not all of which are indicated simply by the title of a position. Therefore above the entrance grades, a position bearing a certain title may be above or below the grade level shown in the table.
[3]Salary deductions come out of every salary check for the retirement fund. A deduction for Federal Group Life Insurance is optional.
[4]For associate degree graduates with no prior experience.
[5]Salary rates are limited by law to $47,500 in 1978 and $50,112.50 in 1979.
SOURCE: U.S. Office of Personnel Management, Intergovernmental Personnel Programs Division, 1980.

Table III-F-2. Salary Schedule for Nurses in the Army Nurse Corps, March 1980

Rank	Position	Annual salary [1,2] Excluding quarters allowance	Including quarters allowance [3]
Second lieutenant	Clinical nurse	$10,735-13,302	$12,751-15,318
First lieutenant	Clinical nurse (clinical specialty)	12,244-16,643	14,829-19,228
	Nurse practitioner (clinical specialty)		
	Assistant clinical head nurse		
Captain	Clinical head nurse	13,929-22,151	16,906-25,128
	Assistant clinical head nurse		
	Nurse practitioner (clinical specialty)		
	Clinical nurse specialist (clinical specialty)		
	Instructor		
Major	Clinical head nurse	14,926-25,492	18,313-28,879
	Nurse practitioner (clinical specialty)		
	Clinical nurse specialist (clinical specialty)		
	Instructor		
	Nursing methods analyst		
	Nursing researcher		
	Educational coordinator		
	Chief, clinical nursing section		
	Assistant chief nurse		
	Staff officers, medical command headquarters		
Lieutenant colonel	Chief, department of nursing, general hospital	17,557-30,323	21,359-34,125
	Assistant chief, evening and night, department of nursing, general hospital		
	Chief, clinical nursing section		
	Nurse practitioner (clinical specialty)		
	Educational coordinator		
	Director, clinical specialty course		
	Staff officer, medical command headquarters		
	Staff officer, Department of Army		
Colonel	Assistant chief, Army Nurse Corps	30,165-36,983	34,290-41,109
	Chief nurse, major command headquarters		
	Chief, department of nursing, medical center or general hospital		
	Director of nursing science division, Academy of Health Sciences		
Brigadier general	Chief, Army Nurse Corps	41,980	46,577

[1] Includes base pay and subsistence allowance.
[2] Excludes additional pay for duty subject to hostile fire.
[3] Quarters allowance without dependents. Quarters allowance is authorized if government quarters are unavailable.
SOURCE: Army Nurse Corps, Office of the Surgeon General, 1980.

Table III-F-3. Salary Schedule for Nurses in the Navy Nurse Corps, October 1978 and 1979

Rank	Annual salary[1],[2]	
	1978	1979
Ensign	$11,900-14,800	$12,700-15,900
Lieutenant, (j.g.)	13,800-18,600	14,800-19,900
Lieutenant	15,800-24,100	16,900-25,800
Lieutenant commander	17,100-27,600	18,300-29,500
Commander	24,500-32,600	20,900-34,900
Captain	28,200-39,200	30,600-42,000
Rear admiral	37,700-44,600	46,500-47,700

[1]Depends on service credit and years in service.
[2]Includes base pay, subsistence and quarters allowance as authorized; however, excludes additional special pay for duty subject to hostile fire.
SOURCE: Navy Nurse Corps, Bureau of Medicine and Surgery, 1980.

Table III-F-4. Salary Schedule for Nurses in the Navy Nurse Corps, October 1977

Rank	Position	Annual salary[1],[2]	
		Excluding quarters allowance	Including quarters allowance[3]
Ensign	Staff nurse	$ 8,795- 9,155	$11,295-11,655
Lieutenant (j.g.)	Charge nurse	10,130-13,741	13,134-16,745
	Nurse practitioner		
Lieutenant	Nurse practitioner	11,621-18,450	14,974-21,803
	Charge nurse		
	Instructor		
	Patient care coordinator		
Lieutenant commander ...	Nurse practitioner	16,538-21,863	20,251-25,576
	Instructor		
	Patient care coordinator		
	Nursing service administrator assistant		
	Nursing service administrator		
Commander[4]	Senior instructor	19,192-26,143	23,276-30,227
	Assistant director of nursing service		
	Director of nursing service		
Captain[5]	Director of nursing service	26,003-32,040	30,371-36,408
Rear admiral[6]	Director of Nurse Corps	36,468	41,254

[1]Includes base pay and subsistence allowance.
[2]Excludes additional special pay for duty subject to hostile fire.
[3]Quarters allowance without dependents. Quarters allowance is authorized if government quarters are unavailable.
[4]Salary level reflects a minimum of 10 years of service.
[5]Salary level reflects a minimum of 16 years of service.
[6]Salary level reflects a minimum of 20 years of service.
SOURCE: Navy Nurse Corps, Bureau of Medicine and Surgery, 1978.

Table III-F-5. Salary Schedule for Nurses in the Air Force Nurse Corps, October 1977 and 1979

Rank	Position	Annual salary[1,2]			
		1977		1979[3]	
		Excluding quarters allowance	Including quarters allowance[4]	Excluding quarters allowance	Including quarters allowance[4]
Second lieutenant ...	Clinical nurse Mental health nurse Operating room nurse	$ 9,509	$11,295	$10,735	$12,751
First lieutenant	Clinical nurse Mental health nurse Operating room nurse Flight nurse Certified nurse midwife OB/GYN nurse practitioner Pediatric nurse practitioner Nurse anesthetist	11,781	14,070	13,302	15,883
Captain	Clinical nurse Mental health nurse Operating room nurse Flight nurse Certified nurse midwife OB/GYN nurse practitioner Pediatric nurse practitioner Community health nurse Nurse anesthetist Environmental health nurse Clinical nurse specialist	16,079	18,718	18,155	21,132
Major	Clinical nurse Mental health nurse Operating room nurse Flight nurse Certified nurse midwife OB/GYN nurse practitioner Pediatric nurse practitioner Community health nurse Nurse anesthetist Environmental health nurse Clinical nurse specialist Nursing service administrator	20,229	23,228	21,640	25,027
Lieutenant colonel ...	Clinical nurse Mental health nurse Operating room nurse Flight nurse Certified nurse midwife OB/GYN nurse practitioner Pediatric nurse practitioner Community health nurse Nurse anesthetist Environmental health nurse Clinical nurse specialist Nursing service administrator	25,236	28,604	26,986	30,787
Colonel	Mental health nurse Operating room nurse Flight nurse Certified nurse midwife OB/GYN nurse practitioner Pediatric nurse practitioner Community health nurse Nurse anesthetist Environmental health nurse Clinical nurse specialist Nursing service administrator	30,260	33,914	32,332	36,457
Brigadier general ...	Administrator	37,282	41,254	42,340	46,937

[1]Includes base pay and subsistence allowance (at approximate year of grade attainment).
[2]Excludes additional special pay for duty subject to hostile fire and for aeromedical evacuation duties.
[3]For individuals appointed in grades higher than Second lieutenant, initial salaries will be lower than amount reflected for that grade.
[4]Quarters allowance without dependents. Quarters allowance is authorized if government quarters are unavailable.
SOURCE: Air Force Nurse Corps, Office of the Surgeon General, 1978 and 1980.

Table III-F-6. Salary Schedules[1] for Nurses Employed by Veterans Administration, October 1978 and 1979

	Annual salary[3]	
Grade[2]	October 1978	October 1979
Junior grade	$11,712-15,222	$12,531-16,293
Associate grade	13,700-17,813	14,659-19,060
Full grade	15,920-20,699	17,035-22,147
Intermediate grade	19,263-25,041	20,611-26,794
Senior grade	23,087-30,017	24,703-32,110
Chief grade	27,453-35,688	29,375-32,186
Assistant director grade	32,442-42,171	34,713-45,126
Director grade	[4]38,160-49,608	[4]40,832-53,081

[1]Excludes certain localities where a special higher entrance rate has been established.
[2]Initial appointment is usually made to one of these grades, depending on the nature and extent of one's education and professional experience. Generally, the new A.A. or diploma graduate enters at the junior grade; the B.S. graduate at the associate, full, intermediate, or senior grade.
[3]Salary deductions are made for retirement fund, Federal Group Life Insurance (optional) and Federal Employees Health Benefits (optional).
[4]Salary rates are limited by law to $47,500 in 1978 and $50,112.50 in 1979.

SOURCE: Veterans Administration, *Veterans Administration Recruitment Bulletin*, November 6, 1978 and November 19, 1979.

Table III-F-7. Salary Schedules for Nurses Employed by the United States Postal Service

		Annual salary[1]		
Grade	Position	July 1979	July 1978	July 1977
EAS-13[2]	Staff nurse	$13,800-19,300	$13,264-16,547	$13,264-16,547
EAS-15[3]	Head nurse	15,400-21,500	16,119-20,214	15,305-19,197

[1]Nurses also earn $125 uniform allowance in addition to basic salary.
[2]Grade for staff nurses in 1977 and 1978 was PTAC-13 (Postal Technical, Administrative and Clerical Schedule).
[3]Grade for head nurse in 1977 and 1978 was PMS-15 (Postal Management Schedule).
SOURCE: U.S. Postal Service, Employee Relations Department, 1980, and previous years.

**Table III-F-8. State Government Salary Ranges for Registered Nurses,[1]
August 1, 1979**

State	Salary range		State	Salary range	
	Minimum	Maximum		Minimum	Maximum
United States, average ...	$11,670	$15,505			
Alabama	13,195	15,964	Missouri[4]	$10,692	$13,824
Alaska[2,3]	17,112	20,268	Montana	11,874	15,686
Arizona[4]	12,244	15,663	Nebraska	10,603	14,479
Arkansas	10,426	15,158	Nevada[2,4]	12,606	17,274
California	15,444	18,575	New Hampshire[2,8]	10,858	12,956
Colorado	12,900	16,464	New Jersey[4]	10,875	14,677
Connecticut[2]	10,835	13,223	New Mexico[4]	10,608	17,304
Delaware	10,757	14,521	New York[8]	10,624	13,555
District of Columbia[5]	...	...	North Carolina[2]	10,836	14,772
Florida[6]	10,466	13,654	North Dakota	10,992	15,456
Georgia[2,7]	11,100	14,898	Ohio[2]	11,107	14,164
Hawaii[2]	10,488	13,068	Oklahoma[2]	10,860	14,460
Idaho[2,8]	11,592	15,540	Oregon	12,996	16,608
Illinois	11,976	15,420	Pennsylvania	12,185	15,585
Indiana	11,986	18,330	Rhode Island[2]	12,345	14,318
Iowa[4]	12,709	16,536	South Carolina	11,612	16,458
Kansas[2]	10,884	14,232	South Dakota	10,877	16,178
Kentucky[2]	9,384	15,288	Tennessee	11,100	14,676
Louisiana[4]	11,244	16,812	Texas[10]	12,000	15,108
Maine	11,544	14,789	Utah	12,012	17,532
Maryland[4]	12,574	16,491	Vermont............	9,100	14,430
Massachusetts[4,8]	10,993	13,086	Virginia	10,992	14,328
Michigan[2,9]	13,133	15,743	Washington[11]	11,892	13,776
Minnesota	13,593	17,915	West Virginia	10,488	17,112
Mississippi	12,000	16,500	Wisconsin	12,570	16,017
			Wyoming[2]	12,204	16,356

[1]Beginning level classification for nursing work in a hospital or clinic; requirements are graduation from an accredited school of nursing and state licensure or certification. Some states permit the license to be acquired during the probationary period.
[2]Longevity payments are authorized but not included in the range reported.
[3]Additional salary for cost-of-living is paid in remote areas.
[4]Appointments are frequently made above the minimum of the range.
[5]Not reported.
[6]Salary rate effective September 1, 1979.
[7]Hiring at advanced steps may be done if nurse has a B.S. in nursing.
[8]Special conditions may affect salary range.
[9]Salaries will be increased by seven percent, effective October 1, 1979.
[10]Salaries will be increased by 5.1 percent, effective September 1, 1979.
[11]Employees will receive a second salary increase, effective October 1, 1979.

SOURCE: U.S. Office of Personnel Management, Intergovernmental Personnel Programs Division, *State Salary Survey, August 1, 1979*, p. 55.

Table III-F-9. State Government Salary Ranges for Nursing Supervisors,[1] August 1, 1979

State	Salary range		State	Salary range	
	Minimum	Maximum		Minimum	Maximum
United States, average ...	*$13,809*	*$18,613*			
Alabama	14,898	18,733	Missouri[7]	$13,236	$17,244
Alaska[2,3]	19,548	23,508	Montana[2]	15,443	20,346
Arizona	14,005	18,440	Nebraska	11,882	16,252
Arkansas	13,884	20,202	Nevada[2]	16,504	22,790
California	19,909	23,980	New Hamsphire[2,6]	12,201	14,559
Colorado	15,672	21,000	New Jersey	13,879	18,740
Connecticut[2]	13,129	15,799	New Mexico[7]	13,560	22,068
Delaware[2]	12,693	17,423	New York[6]	11,904	15,124
District of Columbia[4] ...	...	...	North Carolina[2]	11,796	16,188
Florida[5]	11,022	14,446	North Dakota	13,344	18,780
Georgia[2]	13,680	18,546	Ohio[2]	12,958	17,139
Hawaii[2]	14,292	17,928	Oklahoma[2,7]	13,080	17,340
Idaho[2,6]	14,796	19,824	Oregon	14,940	19,104
Illinois	13,932	20,412	Pennsylvania	15,585	20,175
Indiana	13,156	19,864	Rhode Island[2]	13,853	16,309
Iowa	13,998	17,950	South Carolina	13,062	18,514
Kansas[2]	12,468	16,308	South Dakota	12,858	19,411
Kentucky[2]	12,576	20,484	Tennessee	14,112	18,204
Louisiana[7]	12,048	17,616	Texas[9]	15,624	19,668
Maine	12,480	16,141	Utah	16,680	24,348
Maryland[7]	14,571	19,133	Vermont	12,298	19,448
Massachusetts[6,7]	11,660	13,866	Virginia	12,000	15,000
Michigan[2,8]	13,885	16,683	Washington[10]	12,492	15,936
Minnesota	14,887	20,003	West Virginia	11,568	18,864
Mississippi	13,200	21,060	Wisconsin	15,718	21,701
			Wyoming[2]	13,464	18,048

[1] Requirements for the classification of nursing supervisor are graduation from an accredited school of nursing and considerable professional experience. A bachelor's degree in nursing may be required and may usually substitute for part of the professional experience requirement. State licensure or certification is required.
[2] Longevity payments are authorized but not included in the range reported.
[3] Additional salary for cost-of-living is paid in remote areas.
[4] Not reported.
[5] Salary rate effective September 1, 1979.
[6] Special conditions may affect salary range.
[7] Appointments are frequently made above the minimum of the range.
[8] Salaries will be increased by seven percent, effective October 1, 1979.
[9] Salaries will be increased by 5.1 percent, effective September 1, 1979.
[10] Employees will receive a second salary increase, effective October 1, 1979.
SOURCE: U.S. Office of Personnel Management, Intergovernmental Personnel Programs Division, *State Salary Survey, August 1, 1979*, p. 56.

Table III-F-10. State Government Salary Ranges for Nurse Consultants,[1] August 1, 1979

State	Salary range		State	Salary range	
	Minimum	Maximum		Minimum	Maximum
United States, average ...	$16,205	$21,774			
Alabama[2]	...	...	Missouri[9]	$17,244	$22,620
Alaska[3,4]	28,260	33,960	Montana[2]	...	...
Arizona[2]	...	...	Nebraska[2]	15,036	20,749
Arkansas	13,884	20,202	Nevada[2]	...	...
California	22,885	27,617	New Hampshire[3,8]	13,485	16,217
Colorado	18,144	24,300	New Jersey[2]	...	...
Connecticut[3]	16,348	19,924	New Mexico[9]	16,488	20,844
Delaware[3,5]	15,171	20,754	New York[4]	16,469	20,780
District of Columbia[6] ..	...	...	North Carolina[2]	...	...
Florida[7]	15,495	20,760	North Dakota	14,724	20,712
Georgia[3]	16,242	22,176	Ohio[2]	...	...
Hawaii[3]	14,292	17,928	Oklahoma[2]	...	...
Idaho[3,8]	16,320	21,864	Oregon	17,220	21,960
Illinois	13,920	18,144	Pennsylvania	16,606	21,614
Indiana[2]	...	...	Rhode Island[3]	15,000	17,716
Iowa	16,536	21,403	South Carolina	17,189	24,363
Kansas[3]	18,708	24,552	South Dakota	11,826	17,722
Kentucky[3]	13,860	22,584	Tennessee	16,356	20,772
Louisiana[9]	13,002	20,568	Texas[11]	19,668	27,768
Maine[2]	...	...	Utah	18,516	27,012
Maryland[9]	16,901	22,205	Vermont	11,544	18,252
Massachusetts[2]	...	...	Virginia	15,000	20,500
Michigan[3,10]	18,228	22,842	Washington[12]	15,168	19,380
Minnesota	16,015	21,548	West Virginia[9]	15,516	25,296
Mississippi	10,980	17,340	Wisconsin	16,921	21,765
			Wyoming	16,812	22,524

[1] The classification of nurse consultant usually requires a bachelor's degree in nursing, state licensure or certification, and extensive experience both as a practitioner and supervisor. A master's degree in nursing may be required.
[2] No comparable class within scope of definition.
[3] Longevity payments are authorized but not included in the range reported.
[4] Additional salary for cost-of-living is paid in remote areas.
[5] Minimum qualifications are significantly lower than those defined.
[6] Not reported.
[7] Salary rate effective September 1, 1979.
[8] Special conditions may affect salary range.
[9] Appointments are frequently made above the minimum of the range.
[10] Salaries will be increased by seven percent, effective October 1, 1979.
[11] Salaries will be increased by 5.1 percent, effective September 1, 1979.
[12] Employees will receive a second salary increase, effective October 1, 1979.
SOURCE: U.S. Office of Personnel Management, Intergovernmental Personnel Programs Division, *State Salary Survey, August 1, 1979*, p. 57.

Table III-F-11. State Government Salary Ranges for Directors of Nursing,[1] August 1, 1979

State	Salary range		State	Salary range	
	Minimum	Maximum		Minimum	Maximum
United States, average ...	$18,528	$25,040			
Alabama	16,575	21,073	Missouri[7]	$18,876	$24,792
Alaska[2,3]	28,932	34,800	Montana[2]	20,074	26,391
Arizona	17,752	23,339	Nebraska	16,949	23,485
Arkansas	18,642	27,144	Nevada	19,822	27,481
California	21,846	26,339	New Hampshire[2,4]	18,937	23,012
Colorado	22,656	30,348	New Jersey	20,509	27,690
Connecticut[2,4]	18,488	22,695	New Mexico[7]	17,304	28,164
Delaware[2]	16,648	22,447	New York	21,355	25,000
District of Columbia[5] ...	...	...	North Carolina	15,468	21,396
Florida[6]	18,195	24,597	North Dakota	20,712	29,124
Georgia[2]	17,748	24,246	Ohio[2]	15,579	20,716
Hawaii[2]	17,136	21,540	Oklahoma	17,340	23,100
Idaho[2,4]	18,888	25,308	Oregon	19,608	25,080
Illinois	20,856	31,128	Pennsylvania	20,675	26,739
Indiana	19,136	28,730	Rhode Island[2]	17,716	20,103
Iowa	18,678	24,669	South Carolina	15,892	22,525
Kansas[2]	17,076	22,464	South Dakota	16,524	25,501
Kentucky	15,288	24,888	Tennessee	17,568	22,176
Louisiana[7]	15,228	22,704	Texas[10]	22,428	28,248
Maine	16,827	22,339	Utah	18,516	27,012
Maryland	19,619	25,770	Vermont	14,430	23,322
Massachusetts	17,592	21,879	Virginia	18,700	25,600
Michigan[2,8]	20,003	24,951	Washington[11]	20,340	25,956
Minnesota	19,001	25,682	West Virginia[7,9]	12,756	20,808
Mississippi[5]	14,520	23,220	Wisconsin	21,980	30,785
			Wyoming[2]	19,032	25,488

[1] The classification of director of nursing usually requires a bachelor's degree in nursing and extensive experience in a responsible supervisory position. A master's degree in nursing may be required or may be substituted for part of the professional experience requirement. State licensure or certification is required.
[2] Longevity payments are authorized but not included in the range reported.
[3] Additional salary for cost-of-living is paid in remote areas.
[4] Special conditions may affect salary range.
[5] Not reported.
[6] Salary rate effective September 1, 1979.
[7] Appointments are frequently made above the minimum of the range.
[8] Salaries will be increased by seven percent, effective October 1, 1979.
[9] Minimum qualifications are significantly lower than those defined.
[10] Salaries will be increased by 5.1 percent, effective September 1, 1979.
[11] Employees will receive a second salary increase, effective October 1, 1979.
SOURCE: U.S. Office of Personnel Management, Intergovernmental Personnel Programs Division, *State Salary Survey, August 1, 1979*, p. 58.

Chapter IV, Section A
DISTRIBUTION OF LICENSED PRACTICAL NURSES

The Division of Nursing of the Public Health Service estimated there were 429,600 full-time equivalent licensed practical nurses employed in the United States in 1976. The number of full-time equivalents is calculated by adding to the full-time nurses one-half of the part-time complement. The total number of employed licensed practical nurses in that year was 489,000. This represented an increase of about 22 percent since 1972. (In February 1977 the nation's supply of employed registered nurses was estimated to be 988,050, more than twice the size of the practical nurse complement.)

In 1974 the American Nurses' Association conducted the second inventory of licensed practical nurses. Selected data from the study are presented in this section. There were 533,459 licensed practical nurses in the nation in 1974. Nearly 71 percent (377,889) reported employment in nursing. After adjusting for nonresponse to items on employment status and county and state of employment, it was estimated that 405,546 licensed practical nurses were employed in 1974, a 50.4 percent increase from 1967. Nurse-to-population ratios were calculated for each state and region, using these estimated employed figures. The number of licensed practical nurses per 100,000 population in the United States increased from 135 in 1967 to 191 in 1974. The nurse-to-population ratio declined in only three states—Colorado, Florida, and Pennsylvania—and in each state the decine was negligible (4, 2, and 3 licensed practical nurses, respectively, per 100,000 population). (The remaining tables from the inventory are composed of unadjusted figures).

State-by-state comparisons, as printed in *Facts About Nursing 76-77*, indicated that the states reporting the largest number of licensed practical nurses in 1974 were California (47,725), New York (45,798), Texas (42,913), and Pennsylvania (35,578). In eight states, at least 80 percent of the licensed practical nurses reported being employed in nursing: District of Columbia (86.5 percent), Wisconsin (85.1 percent), Mississippi (83.4 percednt), Missouri (83.0 percent), South Carolina (82.1 percent), Alabama (81.7 percent), Illinois (81.7 percent), and North Dakota (80.0 percent).

The median age of employed licensed practical nurses dropped more than 5 years between 1967 and 1974, from 43.8 years in 1967, to 38.7 years in 1974. In every jurisdiction except Maryland, Minnesota, North Dakota, and South Dakota, the median age of employed licensed practical nurses was lower in 1974 than it had been in 1967.

Nearly 3 percent of the 504,079 licensed practical nurses who reported their sex were male. Among those employed in nursing, male licensed practical nurses were more likely than females to be employed full-time rather than on a part-time basis.

In 1974, a majority of employed licensed practical and vocational nurses (63.1 percent) worked in hospitals, and the second largest group worked in nursing homes (17.3 percent). Private nursing accounted for 7.5 percent, and physicians' or dentists' offices for 6.5 percent. Only 1.5 percent worked in public health and 0.6 percent in industry, while 2.8 percent reported working in "other" fields within the nursing profession. A substantial shift in employment settings for licensed practical nurses occurred between 1967 and 1974. The number of licensed practical nurses employed by nursing homes increased 119 percent in 7 years, and the number of licensed practical nurses employed by industry increased 130 percent. In the same time period, the number of licensed practical nurses employed in private nursing declined 18 percent.

The proportion of employed licensed practical nurses working in nursing homes was twice as high in New England (24.8 percent) as in the South Atlantic (12.2 percent) and East South Central (12.0 percent) regions. The proportion engaged in private nursing in the Middle Atlantic region (12.6 percent) was two-thirds higher than the national average (7.5 percent). The West South Central region reported the highest proportion of employed licensed practical nurses working in physicians' and dentists' offices (9.1 percent).

The National League for Nursing annually surveys newly licensed practical nurses. In 1978 the study showed 87.4 percent of the newly licensed practical nurses were employed in nursing 6 months after graduation; about 2.5 percent were employed in another field; 4.3 percent were not employed in nursing but actively seeking a nursing position; and 5.8 percent were entirely out of the labor force. There was considerable geographic variation in these rates.

The 1976 distribution of full-time employed nurses in selected health care facilities was collected by the National Center for Health Statistics. According to the NCHS data, hospitals accounted for 215,875 full-time licensed practical nurses, yielding a ratio of 156 full-time LPNs per 1,000 beds. The 1976 figures reflected a 7.4 percent increase since 1973 in the full-time complement and a 12.2 percent increase in the ratio of full-time licensed practical nurses to 1,000 beds. American Hospital Association data on licensed practical nurses in hospitals is presented in tables in Chapter I. The AHA reported there were 255,773 full-time equivalent licensed practical nurse positions in hospitals in 1977 and 257,132 FTEs in 1978, an increase of 0.5.

The second-largest employer of licensed practical nurses are nursing homes and personal care facilities. The 1977 National Nursing Home Survey conducted by the National Center for Health Statistics reported 97,500 licensed practical nurses were employed in nursing homes in 1977. Enumeration showed 65,900, or 67.6 percent, were full-time employees. That number had increased 7.0 percent since 1976, when about 61,564 full-time employees were reported in nursing and personal care homes. Characteristics of licensed practical nurses in these settings showed almost 20 percent had minority racial/ethnic backgrounds. The vast majority were females; males represented only 2.4 percent of the total. Other selected demographics are presented in the tables.

The Division of Biometry and Epidemiology of the National Institute of Mental Health reported 14,891 licensed practical nurses were working in federally funded community mental health centers in 1977. This figure represents a 0.8 percent net gain over 1976. The total number of licensed practical nurse staff were converted into 10,934 full-time equivalent nurses, reflecting an average 22.0 licensed practical nurses per community mental health center in 1977.

The Division of Biometry and Epidemiology also presented information on licensed practical nurses in mental health facilities exclusive of federally funded community mental health centers. They numbered 16,323 in January 1976. Of the total positions, 88.4 percent were working full-time; 8.3 percent, part-time; and 3.3 percent were trainees. State and county mental hospitals and nonfederal inpatient psychiatric services accounted for the majority of these pràctical nurses, 46.4 percent and 23.0 percent respectively.

Table IV-A-1. Estimated Number of Licensed Practical Nurses
in Relation to Population, Selected Years, 1964-1976

Year[1]	Resident population (in thousands)	Number of employed LPNs[2]	LPNs per 100,000 population
1976	214,047	489,000	228
1975	212,318	468,000	220
1974	210,674	447,000	212
1973	209,118	423,000	202
1972	207,364	401,000	193
1970	203,145	370,000	172
1968	199,017	320,000	161
1966	194,899	282,000	145
1964	190,169	250,000	131

[1] As of January 1.
[2] Projected from numbers reported by the American Hospital Association; the National Center for Health Statistics, Master Facilities Index; and the Division of Nursing, Public Health Nursing Census and comparative data from the 1967 and 1974 ANA inventory of licensed practical nurses.
SOURCE: U.S. Department of Health, Education, and Welfare, Public Health Service, Health Resources Administration, Bureau of Health Manpower, Division of Nursing, 1977. Unpublished data.

Table IV-A-2. Adjusted Totals for Employed Licensed Practical or Vocational Nurses in Each State and Region and Ratio per 100,000 Population, 1974

State and region	Employed nurses[1] (adjusted figure)	Nurse-population ratio[2]	State and region	Employed nurses[1] (adjusted figure)	Nurse-population ratio[2]
United States	405,546	191			
New England	26,236	215	East North Central ...	71,742	175
Connecticut	5,840	188	Illinois	15,363	137
Maine	1,882	180	Indiana	6,463	121
Massachusetts	13,418	230	Michigan	17,803	196
New Hampshire	1,532	188	Ohio	24,161	225
Rhode Island	2,285	245	Wisconsin	7,952	173
Vermont	1,279	270			
			West North Central ...	33,159	197
Middle Atlantic	72,348	193	Iowa	5,597	194
New Jersey	14,605	198	Kansas	3,185	139
New York	33,162	182	Minnesota	9,534	242
Pennsylvania	24,581	207	Missouri	9,420	196
			Nebraska	2,847	182
South Atlantic	58,068	174	North Dakota	1,392	215
Delaware	838	144	South Dakota	1,184	170
Dist. of Columbia ...	2,352	328			
Florida	12,788	156	Mountain	16,177	169
Georgia	10,818	221	Arizona	3,281	149
Maryland	5,235	127	Colorado	4,498	177
North Carolina	8,927	166	Idaho	1,995	250
South Carolina	4,622	165	Montana	1,415	191
Virginia	8,974	182	Nevada	990	171
West Virginia	3,514	194	New Mexico	1,797	158
			Utah	1,715	144
East South Central ...	30,264	225	Wyoming	486	134
Alabama	8,398	234			
Kentucky	5,229	155	Pacific	47,144	169
Mississippi	4,722	203	Alaska	400	111
Tennessee	11,915	286	California	35,535	169
			Hawaii	1,703	198
West South Central....	50,408	243	Oregon	3,104	136
Arkansas	5,008	240	Washington	6,402	185
Louisiana	7,565	199			
Oklahoma	5,481	202			
Texas	32,354	266			

[1]Adjusted for nonresponse to county not identified and employment status not reported.
[2]Ratios based on December 31, 1974 population from Market Statistics, Survey of Buying Power, New York.
SOURCE: American Nurses' Association, Statistics Department, *LPNs: 1974 Inventory of Licensed Practical Nurses*, 1977.

Table IV-A-3. Percent of Licensed Practical or Vocational Nurses by Age Group, Sex, and Employment Status, 1974

Sex and employment status	Total		Percentage by age group					
	Number	Percent	Under 30	30-39	40-49	50-59	60 and over	Not reported
Total	533,459	...	144,394	106,853	92,120	84,876	61,618	43,598
Female, number	489,231	...	135,546	99,530	86,088	79,919	58,352	29,796
percent		100.0	100.0	100.0	100.0	100.0	100.0	100.0
Employed in nursing	365,373	74.7	78.1	75.2	82.3	79.5	60.0	51.5
Full-time	266,616	54.5	58.5	51.8	63.0	62.3	35.3	37.4
Regular part-time	45,265	9.3	10.1	11.6	9.1	7.6	8.1	4.6
Irregular part-time	41,787	8.5	7.3	9.4	7.4	6.9	14.0	8.5
Full or part-time not reported	11,705	2.4	2.2	2.4	2.8	2.7	2.6	1.0
Not employed in nursing	110,033	22.5	21.5	24.1	16.8	19.3	36.8	18.7
Employment status not reported ...	13,825	2.8	0.4	0.7	0.9	1.2	3.2	29.8
Male, number	14,848	...	4,153	3,298	2,790	2,177	1,213	1,217
percent		100.0	100.0	100.0	100.0	100.0	100.0	100.0
Employed in nursing	11,407	76.8	82.0	81.8	81.4	78.0	58.8	51.2
Full-time	9,504	64.0	67.4	68.6	69.5	67.9	42.7	42.0
Regular part-time	790	5.3	6.8	5.4	4.9	3.9	5.9	3.0
Irregular part-time	823	5.5	6.1	5.8	4.4	4.1	8.5	5.1
Full or part-time not reported	290	2.0	1.7	2.0	2.6	2.1	1.7	1.1
Not employed in nursing	2,834	19.1	17.0	17.3	17.2	20.5	38.4	13.3
Employment status not reported ...	607	4.1	1.0	0.9	1.4	1.5	2.8	35.5
Sex not reported, number	29,380	...	4,695	4,025	3,242	2,780	2,053	12,585
percent		100.0	100.0	100.0	100.0	100.0	100.0	100.0
Employed in nursing	1,109	3.8	2.1	3.3	6.6	9.3	11.4	1.3
Full-time	827	2.8	1.6	2.2	5.5	7.7	7.0	1.0
Regular part-time	103	0.4	0.3	0.6	0.5	0.7	0.9	0.1
Irregular part-time	165	0.6	0.2	0.5	0.6	0.8	3.3	0.2
Full or part-time not reported	14	(1)	...	(1)	(1)	0.1	0.2	(1)
Not reported in nursing	822	2.8	0.9	1.6	2.0	3.6	14.5	2.1
Employment status not reported ...	27,449	93.4	97.0	95.1	91.4	87.1	74.1	96.6

¹Less than 0.1 percent.

SOURCE: American Nurses' Association, Statistics Department, LPNs: 1974 Inventory of Licensed Practical Nurses, 1977.

**Table IV-A-4. Employed Licensed Practical or Vocational Nurses,
by Field of Employment and Sex, 1974**

| Field of employment | Total | | Sex | | | | | |
| | | | Male | | Female | | Not reported | |
	Number	Percent	Number	Percent	Number	Percent	Number	Percent
Total	377,889	100.0	11,407	100.0	365,373	100.0	1,109	100.0
Hospital	238,467	63.1	7,791	68.3	230,017	63.0	659	59.4
Nursing home	65,351	17.3	1,433	12.6	63,729	17.4	189	17.1
Private nursing ...	28,210	7.5	826	7.2	27,288	7.5	96	8.7
Public health	5,863	1.5	184	1.6	5,651	1.6	28	2.5
Industry	2,320	0.6	178	1.6	2,133	0.6	9	0.8
Physician's or dentist's office ..	24,497	6.5	173	1.5	24,255	6.6	69	6.2
Other	10,708	2.8	739	6.5	9,941	2.7	28	2.5
Not reported	2,473	0.7	83	0.7	2,359	0.6	31	2.8

SOURCE: American Nurses' Association, Statistics Department, *LPNs: 1974 Inventory of Licensed Practical Nurses*, 1977.

**Table IV-A-5. Percent of Licensed Practical or Vocational Nurses,
Employed in Nursing, by Marital Status and Age Group, 1974**

| Age group | Total | | Marital status | | | | |
	Number	Percent	Single	Married	Widowed	Divorced or separated	Not reported
Total, number	377,889	...	59,022	229,642	30,888	52,471	5,866
percent	...	100.0	100.0	100.0	100.0	100.0	100.0
Under 25	54,394	14.4	42.0	11.7	0.3	4.7	4.8
25-29	54,985	14.5	21.1	15.5	1.0	12.0	7.4
30-34	41,437	11.0	9.4	12.1	1.6	13.6	9.0
35-39	36,205	9.6	5.1	10.9	2.5	13.2	8.6
40-44	36,956	9.8	3.9	11.1	4.6	13.4	10.3
45-49	36,341	9.6	3.5	10.8	8.3	12.0	10.6
50-54	35,149	9.3	3.1	10.0	13.5	10.4	10.6
55-59	30,312	8.0	3.2	7.7	19.4	7.8	10.2
60-64	21,630	5.7	3.0	4.6	20.3	5.0	8.4
65 and over	14,336	3.8	2.6	1.9	21.0	2.8	7.1
Not reported	16,144	4.3	3.1	3.7	7.5	5.1	13.0

SOURCE: American Nurses' Association, Statistics Department, *LPNs: 1974 Inventory of Licensed Practical Nurses*, 1977.

Table IV-A-6. Percent of Licensed Practical or Vocational Nurses, Not Employed in Nursing, by Marital Status and Age Group, 1974

| | Total | | Marital status | | | | |
Age group	Number	Percent	Single	Married	Widowed	Divorced or separated	Not reported
Total, number	113,689	...	7,362	85,140	11,136	7,895	2,156
percent	...	100.0	100.0	100.0	100.0	100.0	100.0
Under 25	10,409	9.2	27.9	9.4	0.3	3.7	2.1
25-29	19,447	17.1	16.8	20.0	0.8	12.2	5.1
30-34	15,621	13.7	8.7	16.1	1.3	12.4	5.5
35-39	8,989	7.9	4.8	8.9	1.5	10.2	5.0
40-44	7,584	6.7	3.3	7.3	2.2	9.2	6.0
45-49	7,421	6.5	3.6	7.0	3.6	8.6	5.7
50-54	7,864	6.9	3.5	7.2	5.4	8.4	8.0
55-59	8,112	7.1	4.2	7.2	8.7	7.4	6.8
60-64	8,588	7.6	6.0	6.4	16.8	8.1	10.5
65 and over	13,668	12.0	16.3	6.3	49.7	13.5	23.4
Not reported	5,986	5.3	4.9	4.2	9.7	6.3	21.9

SOURCE: American Nurses' Association, Statistics Department, *LPNs: 1974 Inventory of Licensed Practical Nurses,* 1977.

Table IV-A-7. Estimated Number and Percent of Licensed Practical Nurses Employed in Nursing Homes, by Selected Nursing Home Characteristics, 1977

Nursing home characteristics[1]	Licensed practical nurse					
	Total		Full-time		Part-time	
	Number	Percent	Number	Percent	Number	Percent
Total	97,500	100.0	65,900	100.0	31,600	100.0
Ownership						
Proprietary ...	63,400	65.0	42,500	64.5	20,900	66.1
Voluntary nonprofit ...	22,600	23.2	15,000	22.8	7,600	24.1
Government	11,500	11.8	8,400	12.7	3,100	9.8
Certification						
Skilled nursing facility	22,600	23.2	14,700	22.3	7,900	25.0
Skilled nursing facility and intermediate care facility	40,600	41.6	27,900	42.3	12,700	40.2
Intermediate care facility	28,400	29.1	19,700	29.9	8,700	27.5
Not certified	5,900	6.1	3,600	5.5	2,300	7.3
Bed size						
Less than 50 beds	15,000	15.4	8,200	12.4	6,800	21.5
50-99	28,900	29.6	19,600	29.7	9,300	29.4
100-199	37,700	38.7	25,900	39.3	11,800	37.3
200 beds or more	15,900	16.3	12,200	18.5	3,700	11.7
Location						
Region						
Northeast	23,400	24.0	15,000	22.8	8,400	26.6
North Central	30,900	31.7	19,400	29.4	11,500	36.4
South	30,100	30.9	22,300	33.8	7,800	24.7
West	13,000	13.3	9,200	14.0	3,800	12.0
Standard federal administrative region						
Region I ...	6,500	6.7	3,100	4.7	3,400	10.8
Region II ...	11,000	11.3	7,300	11.1	3,700	11.7
Region III	9,000	9.2	6,600	10.0	2,400	7.6
Region IV	15,400	15.8	11,400	17.3	4,000	12.7
Region V ...	22,800	23.4	13,800	20.9	9,000	28.5
Region VI	11,700	12.0	9,000	13.7	2,700	8.5
Region VII	7,400	7.6	5,300	8.0	2,100	6.6
Region VIII	2,600	2.7	1,600	2.4	1,000	3.2
Region IX	8,300	8.5	6,000	9.1	2,300	7.3
Region X ...	2,700	2.8	1,800	2.7	900	2.8
Type of facility						
Nursing care	90,900	93.2	62,200	94.4	28,700	90.8
Other	6,600	6.8	3,700	5.6	2,900	9.2

[1] Detail in each nursing home characteristic may not add to total due to rounding.

SOURCE: U.S. Department of Health, Education, and Welfare, Public Health Service, Office of Health Research, Statistics, and Technology, National Center for Health Statistics, *The National Nursing Home Survey: 1977 Summary for the United States*, Vital and Health Statistics, Series 13, No. 43, DHEW Publication No. (PHS) 79-1794, 1979, p. 17.

**Table IV-A-8. Estimated Number and Percent of Licensed Practical
Nurses Employed in Nursing Homes, by Selected Employee
Characteristics, 1977**

| Employee characteristics[1] | Licensed practical nurse | | | | | |
| | Total | | Full-time | | Part-time | |
	Number	Percent	Number	Percent	Number	Percent
Total	97,500	100.0	65,900	100.0	31,600	100.0
Racial/ethnic background						
White (not Hispanic)..	78,300	80.3	51,800	78.6	26,500	83.9
Black (not Hispanic)..	15,900	16.3	11,800	17.9	4,100	13.0
Hispanic	900	0.9	900	1.4	(2)	(2)
Other	1,900	1.9	1,400	2.1	500	1.6
Sex						
Male	2,300	2.4	1,500	2.3	800	2.5
Female	95,200	97.6	64.400	97.7	30,800	97.5
Age group						
Under 35 years	40,000	41.0	25,600	38.8	14,400	45.6
35-44	22,100	22.7	15,800	24.0	6,300	19.9
45-54	18,500	19.0	13,500	20.5	5,000	15.8
55 years and over ...	16,800	17.2	11,000	16.7	5,800	18.4
Years of education						
Less than 12 years	8,800	9.0	6,200	9.4	2,600	8.2
12	15,500	15.9	10,900	16.5	4,600	14.6
13-14	64,600	66.3	43,700	66.3	20,900	66.1
15-16	7,800	8.0	4,700	7.1	3,100	9.8
17 years or more	(2)	(2)	(2)	(2)	(2)	(2)
Years of current employment						
Less than 2 years	45,800	47.0	30,800	46.7	15,000	47.5
2-4	27,400	28.1	17,700	26.9	9,700	30.7
5-9	15,400	15.8	11,000	16.7	4,400	13.9
10-14	5,600	5.7	3,900	5.9	1,700	5.4
15 years or more	3,200	3.3	2,400	3.6	800	2.5
Years of total experience						
Less than 5 years	36,000	36.9	24,300	36.9	11,700	37.0
5-9	28,300	29.0	19,000	28.8	9,300	29.4
10-14	15,300	15.7	10,300	15.6	5,000	15.8
15 years or more	18,000	18.5	12,400	18.8	5,600	17.7

[1]Detail in each employee characteristic may not add to total due to rounding.
[2]Figure does not meet standards of reliability or precision (more than 30 percent relative standard error).

SOURCE: U.S. Department of Health, Education, and Welfare, Public Health Service, Office of Health
Research, Statistics, and Technology, National Center for Health Statistics, *The National
Nursing Home Survey: 1977 Summary for the United States*, Vital and Health Statistics, Series
13, No. 43, DHEW Publication No. (PHS) 79-1794, 1979, p. 20.

Table IV-A-9. Distribution of Agencies and Licensed Practical Nurses Employed in Community Health Work, January, 1974

Type of agency	Number of agencies	Number of licensed practical nurses		
		Total	Full-time	Part-time
Total[1]	11,516	4,069	3,606	463
National agency	10	1	11	...
University	303	...	...	...
State agency	207	266	255	11
Local agency	10,996	3,802	3,350	452
Official	2,867	1,678	1,487	191
Health department	1,810	1,132	1,051	81
Other official	1,057	546	436	110
Organized categorical program	412	542	479	63
Mental health	116	125	119	6
Neighborhood health center	156	135	108	27
Other categorical	140	282	252	30
Combination	51	179	164	15
Nonofficial	620	674	576	98
Visiting nurse association	567	663	567	96
Other nonofficial	53	11	9	2
Organized home health ...	399	389	314	75
Hospital based program .	239	97	78	19
Other home health	160	292	236	56
Board of education	6,647	340	330	10

[1] Includes Guam, Puerto Rico, and Virgin Islands.

SOURCE: U.S. Department of Health, Education, and Welfare, Public Health Service, Health Resources Administration, Bureau of Health Manpower, Division of Nursing, *1974 Survey of Community Health Nursing*, 1976. Prepublication data.

Table IV-A-10. Distribution of Full-time Licensed Practical Nurses Employed in Hospitals, Nursing Care and Related Homes, and Other Inpatient Health Facilities,[1] by State, 1976

State	Hospitals			Nursing care and related homes			Other inpatient health facilities		
	Beds	LPNs (full-time)	LPNs per 1,000 beds	Beds	LPNs (full-time)	LPNs per 1,000 beds	Beds	LPNs (full-time)	LPNs per 1,000 beds
Total	1,381,267	215,875	156	[2]1,406,778	61,326	44	[2]412,875	9,360	23
Alabama	23,482	5,395	230	19,281	1,339	69	7,172	115	16
Alaska	1,629	248	152	782	44	56	461	10	22
Arizona[3]	11,198	1,692	151	5,914	218	37	2,957	20	7
Arkansas	13,625	3,236	238	18,722	977	52	4,811	233	48
California	111,176	18,171	163	139,054	5,208	37	37,698	2,270	60
Colorado[3]	15,123	2,392	158	22,708	810	36	5,025	57	11
Connecticut	17,941	2,324	130	24,374	820	34	8,060	72	9
Delaware	4,073	607	149	2,228	60	27	1,491	42	28
District of Columbia	10,541	1,304	124	2,872	119	41	1,166	45	39
Florida	54,798	8,800	161	32,859	1,819	55	13,487	188	14
Georgia	32,391	6,094	188	29,641	1,834	62	6,273	121	19
Hawaii	3,877	1,104	285	3,172	193	61	1,340	80	60
Idaho[3]	3,610	939	260	4,823	219	45	1,887	37	20
Illinois	71,776	9,003	125	87,805	2,957	34	22,380	577	26
Indiana	32,610	3,823	117	35,935	1,121	31	9,501	90	9
Iowa	19,892	2,662	134	32,856	1,028	31	5,539	114	21
Kansas	17,003	2,441	144	22,502	564	25	5,550	56	10
Kentucky	19,473	3,150	162	20,543	741	36	4,310	67	16
Louisiana	25,128	4,371	174	19,070	1,111	58	7,494	151	20
Maine	6,699	967	144	8,644	263	30	2,619	73	28
Maryland	25,322	3,018	119	18,874	942	50	6,952	110	16
Massachusetts[3]	44,827	5,903	132	50,940	2,022	40	15,262	465	30
Michigan[3]	50,581	9,205	182	66,416	2,219	33	14,109	414	29
Minnesota[3]	29,468	3,901	132	43,036	1,222	28	9,036	98	11
Mississippi	17,660	3,144	178	8,939	791	88	3,698	33	9

Missouri[3]	35,869	5,291	148	33,628	1,268	38	5,936	58	10
Montana	5,426	713	131	5,299	269	51	920	24	26
Nebraska[3]	11,539	1,507	131	23,022	595	26	2,629	74	28
Nevada	3,358	618	184	1,574	127	81	583	11	19
New Hampshire	5,082	631	124	6,256	234	37	1,710	22	13
New Jersey	45,041	6,537	145	34,463	1,248	36	12,439	204	16
New Mexico	6,239	1,116	179	3,042	165	54	2,604	76	29
New York	137,488	16,213	118	102,591	5,523	54	43,681	725	17
North Carolina[3]	32,438	5,255	162	24,432	937	38	9,926	167	17
North Dakota	5,470	844	154	6,753	173	26	2,341	21	9
Ohio	65,432	11,961	183	64,096	3,700	58	22,277	592	27
Oklahoma	17,005	3,216	189	26,103	1,089	42	7,621	108	14
Oregon	12,076	1,586	131	15,906	442	28	4,954	67	14
Pennsylvania[3]	89,645	12,360	138	64,090	3,911	61	24,565	421	17
Rhode Island[3]	7,017	931	133	7,330	252	34	1,699	16	9
South Carolina	17,405	2,862	164	8,642	445	51	5,918	87	15
South Dakota	5,884	716	122	7,840	176	22	2,596	13	5
Tennessee[3]	32,402	6,397	197	20,074	1,281	64	6,262	125	20
Texas[3]	76,861	16,708	217	101,418	6,442	64	22,894	577	25
Utah	5,105	784	154	4,569	249	54	1,941	48	25
Vermont[3]	3,134	575	183	5,130	207	40	1,744	4	2
Virginia[3]	32,409	5,298	163	28,479	1,251	44	9,091	128	14
Washington	16,290	3,553	218	30,079	939	31	7,111	318	45
West Virginia	16,029	2,478	155	5,575	259	46	2,308	36	16
Wisconsin[3]	30,081	3,559	118	52,606	1,436	27	9,759	164	17
Wyoming	2,639	272	103	1,791	67	37	1,088	6	6

[1]Included are residential schools or homes for the deaf, blind, and physically handicapped; homes for alcoholics and drug abusers; schools or homes for the emotionally disturbed; homes for unwed mothers; orphanages; homes for dependent children; and facilities for the mentally retarded including hospitals and homes or resident schools.

[2]Preliminary data.

[3]States reporting data for nursing care and related homes, and other inpatient health facilities through the Cooperative Health Statistics System. Data may not always agree with individual State reports, usually because of variations in imputation procedures or in time period over which data were collected.

SOURCE: U.S. Department of Health, Education, and Welfare, Public Health Service, Office of Health Research, Statistics, and Technology, National Center for Health Statistics, *Health Resources Statistics: Health Manpower and Health Facilities, 1976–77 ed.*, DHEW Publication No. (PHS) 79-1509, pp. 179-181.

Table IV-A-11. Licensed Practical Nurses Employed in Nursing and Personal Care Homes, by State, 1976

State	Licensed practical nurses		State	Licensed practical nurses	
	Full-time	Part-time		Full-time	Part-time
Total	61,564	27,711			
Alabama	1,358	412	Missouri	1,271	483
Alaska	44	5	Montana	272	117
Arizona	218	100	Nebraska	630	315
Arkansas	989	264	Nevada	127	24
California	5,206	2,235	New Hampshire	236	147
Colorado	810	484	New Jersey	1,244	641
Connecticut	822	869	New Mexico	187	52
Delaware	60	37	New York	5,590	2,350
Dist. of Columbia	117	35	North Carolina	941	402
Florida	1,819	562	North Dakota	173	167
Georgia	1,825	435	Ohio	3,726	1,722
Hawaii	193	41	Oklahoma	1,102	266
Idaho	219	142	Oregon	456	171
Illinois	2,971	1,224	Pennsylvania	3,853	1,266
Indiana	1,127	465	Rhode Island	252	202
Iowa	1,077	587	South Carolina	445	146
Kansas	583	279	South Dakota	167	134
Kentucky	738	262	Tennessee	1,281	395
Louisiana	1,114	349	Texas	6,467	1,646
Maine	275	193	Utah	250	101
Maryland	952	418	Vermont	207	107
Massachusetts	2,022	2,137	Virginia	1,230	394
Michigan	2,190	1,430	Washington	946	500
Minnesota	1,222	1,275	West Virginia	262	92
Mississippi	793	175	Wisconsin	1,436	1,413
			Wyoming	69	43

SOURCE: U.S. Department of Health and Human Services, Public Health Service, Health Resources Administration, National Center for Health Statistics, Division of Health Manpower and Facilities Statistics, 1976 Master Facility Inventory. Unpublished data.

Table IV-A-12. Licensed Practical Nurses Employed in Nursing and
Personal Care Homes, by Type of Ownership, Home Size, and
Type of Care Provided, 1976

Type of ownership and number of beds	All types of care		Nursing care		Personal care and other homes[1]	
	Full-time	Part-time	Full-time	Part-time	Full-time	Part-time
Total	61,564	27,711	57,809	25,422	3,755	2,289
1-24 beds	2,171	1,350	1,697	983	474	367
25-49 beds	6,526	3,810	5,947	3,313	579	497
50-99 beds	18,364	9,226	17,421	8,530	943	696
100 or more beds ...	34,503	13,325	32,744	12,596	1,759	729
Government	8,309	1,988	7,825	1,860	484	128
1-24 beds	193	95	181	88	12	7
25-49 beds	760	319	733	303	27	16
50-99 beds	1,459	584	1,390	538	69	46
100 or more beds	5,897	990	5,521	931	376	59
Church and other nonprofit	12,637	6,162	11,470	5,387	1,167	775
1-24 beds	550	396	473	321	77	75
25-49 beds	1,490	936	1,311	761	179	175
50-99 beds	3,616	2,058	3,306	1,807	310	251
100 or more beds	6,981	2,772	6,380	2,498	601	274
Proprietary	40,618	19,561	38,514	18,175	2,104	1,386
1-24 beds	1,428	859	1,043	574	385	285
25-49 beds	4,276	2,555	3,903	2,249	373	306
50-99 beds	13,289	6,584	12,725	6,185	564	399
100 or more beds	21,625	9,563	20,843	9,167	782	396

[1] Includes personal care homes with nursing, personal care homes without nursing, and domiciliary care homes.

SOURCE: U.S. Department of Health and Human Services, Public Health Service, Health Resources Administration, National Center for Health Statistics, Division of Health Manpower and Facilities Statistics, 1976 Master Facility Inventory. Unpublished data.

Table IV-A-13. Number of Licensed Practical Nurses Employed in Mental Health Facilities, January 1976

Type of facility	Number of facilities		Number of licensed practical nurses employed			
	Total	Report-ing	Total	Full-time	Part-time	Trainee
Total	3,791	3,231	16,323	14,430	1,362	531
Psychiatric hospital ...	487	464	8,904	8,301	388	215
State and county mental hospitals...	304	297	7,576	7,317	100	159
Private mental hospitals	183	167	1,328	984	288	56
VA psychiatric services	198	189	1,622	1,479	25	118
Neuropsychiatric hospitals	24	24	899	862	14	23
General hospital in-patient psychiatric unit	89	85	703	599	9	95
General hospital out-patient psychiatric unit	85	80	20	18	2	...
Non-federal general hospital psychiatric service	1,094	849	3,807	3,009	658	140
Inpatient psychiatric service	791	612	3,762	2,973	649	140
Outpatient psychiatric service	303	237	45	36	9	...
Residential treatment center for emotionally disturbed children...	331	278	145	106	37	2
Freestanding outpatient clinics	1,076	904	221	160	38	23
Community mental health centers	528	486	1,421	1,188	200	33
Other	77	61	203	187	16	...
Freestanding day/ night facilities	38	29	1	1	...	...
Other multi-service facilities	39	32	202	186	16	...

SOURCE: U.S. Department of Health, Education, and Welfare, Public Health Service, Alcohol, Drug Abuse, and Mental Health Administration, *Staffing of Mental Health Facilities, United States, 1976*, National Institute of Mental Health, Series B, No. 14, DHEW Publication No. (ADM) 78-522, p. 2 and p. 48.

**Table IV-A-14. Licensed Practical Nurses in Federally Funded
Community Mental Health Centers, 1973-1977**

Year	Licensed practical nurse		
	Total	Full-time equivalent	Average FTE per CMHC
1977	14,891	10,934	20.0
1976	14,776	10,561	20.0
1975	13,538	9,564	22.0
1974	12,325	8,972	22.4
1973	10,342	7,331	22.5

SOURCE: U.S. Department of Health, Education, and Welfare, Public Health Service, National Institute of
Mental Health, Division of Biometry and Epidemiology, Survey and Reports Branch, *Provisional
Data on Federally Funded Community Mental Health Centers, 1976-77*, May 1978, p. 30.

**Table IV-A-15. Licensed Practical Nurse Positions in Federally
Funded Community Mental Health Centers, by Employment Status
and Number of Years Facility has been in Operation, February 1977**

Number of years in operation	Total	Employment status			
		Full-time	Part-time	Trainee	Volunteer
Total	55,367	50,840	3,782	712	33
1-2 years	6,562	6,211	277	74	...
3-5	15,621	14,121	1,375	114	11
6-7	13,719	13,064	655	...	...
8 years or more	19,465	17,444	1,475	524	22

SOURCE: U.S. Department of Health, Education, and Welfare, Public Health Service, National Institute of
Mental Health, Division of Biometry and Epidemiology, Survey and Reports Branch, *Provisional
Data on Federally Funded Community Mental Health Centers, 1976-77*, May 1978, pp. 12-14.

Table IV-A-16. Employment Status of Newly Licensed Practical Nurses, Six Months After Licensure, by State of Residence, 1978

		Employment status			
			Not employed in nursing		
		Employed in nursing	Employed in other field	Looking for work	Not looking for work
State	Total number	Percent	Percent	Percent	Percent
Total	¹27,146	87.4	2.5	4.3	5.8
Alabama	690	90.4	1.6	3.8	4.2
Alaska	17	82.4	5.9	...	11.8
Arizona	298	82.6	2.0	6.7	8.7
Arkansas	491	88.0	2.9	2.2	6.9
California²	...	...	...	...	...
Colorado	358	87.4	2.5	4.5	5.6
Connecticut	361	91.7	2.2	3.0	3.0
Delaware	81	84.0	6.2	6.2	3.7
District of Columbia	37	91.9	2.7	2.7	2.7
Florida	1,472	88.9	2.2	2.9	6.0
Georgia	704	87.6	3.6	5.5	3.3
Hawaii	127	83.5	4.7	4.7	7.1
Idaho	128	89.1	2.3	2.3	6.3
Illinois	988	89.5	1.8	3.0	5.7
Indiana	615	90.6	1.3	2.8	5.4
Iowa²	...	...	...	...	...
Kansas	255	87.1	3.1	3.9	5.9
Kentucky	342	90.1	2.0	4.7	3.2
Louisiana	623	86.0	1.8	4.2	8.0
Maine	186	89.2	2.2	4.3	4.3
Maryland	331	89.7	2.4	3.6	4.2
Massachusetts	673	93.8	1.0	2.1	3.1
Michigan	1,249	93.2	1.0	2.8	3.0
Minnesota	819	91.7	2.2	1.8	4.3
Mississippi	429	91.8	0.9	3.0	4.2
Missouri	666	92.6	1.5	1.7	4.2
Montana	116	85.3	3.4	3.4	7.8
Nebraska	271	91.9	3.0	2.2	3.0
Nevada	64	78.1	6.3	3.1	12.5
New Hampshire ...	101	90.1	2.0	3.0	5.0
New Jersey	1,288	86.0	2.8	5.0	6.2
New Mexico	174	78.7	4.0	6.3	10.9
New York	3,031	76.2	5.8	9.5	8.5
North Carolina	701	83.0	3.7	5.1	8.1
North Dakota	161	91.3	1.9	3.7	3.1
Ohio	1,432	92.2	1.5	2.5	3.7
Oklahoma²	...	...	...	...	...
Oregon	296	79.4	2.0	8.1	10.5
Pennsylvania	1,647	89.8	2.1	2.9	5.2
Rhode Island	73	95.9	1.4	1.4	1.4
South Carolina	392	91.1	1.8	2.8	4.3
South Dakota	171	90.6	1.2	4.1	4.1
Tennessee	646	92.4	1.7	2.9	2.9
Texas	2,102	87.2	1.8	4.1	6.9
Utah	259	81.9	1.2	5.4	11.6
Vermont	103	85.4	1.9	5.8	6.8
Virginia	705	87.8	2.6	3.4	6.2
Washington	536	83.2	3.5	4.9	8.4
West Virginia	293	83.3	2.0	7.8	6.8
Wisconsin	455	92.7	1.5	2.0	3.7
Wyoming	54	70.4	7.4	5.6	16.7

¹Includes 135 California nurses who took the SBTP examination in another state.
²Did not participate in survey.

SOURCE: National League for Nursing, *Employment, Mobility, and Personal Characteristics of Nurses Newly Licensed in 1978*, State Summaries, Volume 1, Publication No. 19-2050 (DS 8001), 1980.

Chapter IV, Section B
DISTRIBUTION OF OTHER ALLIED NURSING PERSONNEL

In 1976, the Division of Nursing of the Public Health Service estimated there were 936,800 full-time equivalent nurses' aides, orderlies and attendants, other nursing assistants, and home health aides in the United States. This group is generally considered to constitute the category "allied nursing personnel."

The 1977 National Nursing Home survey conducted by the National Center for Health Statistics provided detailed information on nurses' aides within nursing homes. In that year, there were 424,900 full-time equivalent nurses' aides in the nation's nursing homes, yielding a ratio of 30.3 nurses' aides per 100 beds. The total number of aides in these facilities was 462,900, of whom 74.5 percent were full-time employees. According to their demographic characteristics, nurses' aides were predominantly white (74.9 percent), female (93.4 percent), under 35 years of age (55.6 percent) and had 12 years or less education (77.0 percent). Information on registered nurses from this same study appears in Chapter I, "Nurses Functioning in Institutions"; for practical nurses, see Chapter IV, Section A.

Table IV-B-1. Estimated Number and Percent of Nurses' Aides Employed in Nursing Homes, by Selected Nursing Home Characteristics, 1977

Nursing home characteristics[1]	Nurses' aide					
	Total		Full-time		Part-time	
	Number	Percent	Number	Percent	Number	Percent
Total	462,900	100.0	345,000	100.0	117,900	100.0
Ownership						
Proprietary	307,500	66.4	227,700	66.0	79,800	67.7
Voluntary nonprofit	110,900	24.0	79,400	23.0	31,500	26.7
Government	44,400	9.6	37,900	11.0	6,500	5.5
Certification						
Skilled nursing facility ...	105,700	22.8	79,500	23.0	26,200	22.2
Skilled nursing facility and intermediate care facility	207,700	44.9	154,700	44.8	53,000	45.0
Intermediate care facility	115,300	24.9	86,200	25.0	29,100	24.7
Not certified	34,200	7.4	24,600	7.1	9,600	8.1
Bed size						
Less than 50 beds	54,600	11.8	35,100	10.2	19,500	16.5
50-99	147,100	31.8	108,100	31.3	39,000	33.1
100-199	187,500	40.5	144,000	41.7	43,500	36.9
200 beds or more	73,600	15.9	57,700	16.7	15,900	13.5
Location						
Region						
Northeast	108,800	23.5	75,700	21.9	33,100	28.1
North Central	170,600	36.9	123,500	35.8	47,100	39.9
South	116,200	25.1	93,800	27.2	22,400	19.0
West	67,200	14.5	51,900	15.0	15,300	13.0
Standard federal administrative region						
Region I	33,300	7.2	18,700	5.4	14,600	12.4
Region II	46,800	10.1	34,800	10.1	12,000	10.2
Region III	44,100	9.5	33,700	9.8	10,400	8.8
Region IV	66,800	14.4	56,700	16.4	10,100	8.6
Region V	126,100	27.2	91,400	26.5	34,700	29.4
Region VI	34,700	7.5	26,200	7.6	8,500	7.2
Region VII	39,400	8.5	28,400	8.2	11,000	9.3
Region VIII	15,900	3.4	10,600	3.1	5,300	4.5
Region IX	41,300	8.9	33,000	9.6	8,300	7.0
Region X	14,500	3.1	11,400	3.3	3,100	2.6
Type of facility						
Nursing care	423,200	91.4	315,800	91.5	107,400	91.1
Other	39,800	8.6	29,200	8.5	10,600	9.0

[1] Detail in each nursing home characteristic may not add to total due to rounding.

SOURCE: U.S. Department of Health, Education, and Welfare, Public Health Service, Office of Health Research, Statistics, and Technology, National Center for Health Statistics, *The National Nursing Home Survey: 1977 Summary for the United States*, Vital and Health Statistics, Series 13, No. 43, DHEW Publication No. (PHS) 79-1794, 1979, p. 17.

Table IV-B-2. Estimated Number and Percent of Nurses' Aides Employed in Nursing Homes, by Selected Employee Characteristics, 1977

Employee characteristics[1]	Nurses' aide					
	Total		Full-time		Part-time	
	Number	Percent	Number	Percent	Number	Percent
Total	462,900	100.0	345,000	100.0	117,900	100.0
Racial/ethnic background						
White (not Hispanic) ...	346,900	74.9	248,900	72.1	98,000	83.1
Black (not Hispanic)	95,100	20.5	77,900	22.6	17,200	14.6
Hispanic	5,300	1.1	5,300	1.5	(2)	(2)
Other ....:..	12,800	2.8	12,800	3.7	(2)	(2)
Sex						
Male	30,600	6.6	25,400	7.4	5,200	4.4
Female	432,400	93.4	319,600	92.6	112,800	95.7
Age group						
Under 35 years	257,500	55.6	189,600	55.0	67,900	57.6
35-44	78,100	16.9	61,400	17.8	16,700	14.2
45-54	61,800	13.4	49,000	14.2	12,800	10.9
55 years and over	65,700	14.2	45,100	13.1	20,600	17.5
Years of education						
Less than 12 years	154,000	33.3	117,400	34.0	36,600	31.0
12	202,200	43.7	148,900	43.2	53,300	45.2
13-14	80,600	17.4	59,100	17.1	21,500	18.2
15-16	20,500	4.4	15,500	4.5	5,000	4.2
17 years or more	4,000	0.9	4,000	1.2	(2)	(2)
Years of current employment						
Less than 2 years	257,300	55.6	188,100	54.5	69,200	58.7
2-4	108,800	23.5	81,800	23.7	27,000	22.9
5-9	63,200	13.7	49,300	14.3	13,900	11.8
10-14	24,900	5.4	18,200	5.3	6,700	5.7
15 years or more	7,600	1.6	7,600	2.2	(2)	(2)
Years of total experience						
Less than 5 years	299,300	64.7	218,000	63.2	81,300	69.0
5-9	87,900	19.0	70,500	20.4	17,400	14.8
10-14	44,100	9.5	32,800	9.5	11,300	9.6
15 years or more	31,700	6.8	23,700	6.9	8,000	6.8

[1]Detail in each employee characteristic may not add to total due to rounding.
[2]Figure does not meet standards of reliability or precision (more than 30 percent relative standard error).
SOURCE: U.S. Department of Health, Education, and Welfare, Public Health Service, Office of Health Research, Statistics, and Technology, National Center for Health Statistics, *The National Nursing Home Survey: 1977 Summary for the United States*, Vital and Health Statistics, Series 13, No. 43, DHEW Publication No. (PHS) 79-1794, 1979, p. 20.

Chapter IV, Section C
PRACTICAL NURSING EDUCATION

While the educational route preparing for licensure as a practical or vocational nurse may take place in a variety of settings, the most common are trade, technical, or vocational schools. Additionally, community colleges, universities, independent agencies, government agencies, and some high schools, as well as hospitals, offer training in practical nursing skills. Practical nursing programs vary in length from 8 to 36 months, although, most programs are 12 months.

In 1978, there were 1,329 state-approved programs of practical and vocational nursing reported by the National League for Nursing's annual survey. The number of practical nursing programs declined by a total of 10 (0.7 percent) since 1977, marking the first annual decline in the number of these programs since 1973. States varied in the number of practical/vocational nursing programs, ranging from one each in Alaska, Rhode Island, American Samoa, and Guam to 157 in Texas.

Slightly over half of the programs in 1978 were administratively controlled by trade, technical, or vocational schools. In terms of control, programs in junior colleges, colleges and universities ranked second (30.0 percent), followed by 8.6 percent in hospitals, 5.7 percent in secondary schools, 1.7 percent under other government agencies, and 0.5 percent in independent agencies.

Enrollments in practical nursing programs in 1977-78 decreased 4.1 percent to 55,620, continuing a downward climb since the 1974-75 peak. Also on the decline, 2.8 percent from the previous year, were the graduations from practical nursing programs. In 1977-78 graduations totaled 45,991. Admissions (61,586) in the same year were up slightly (1.0 percent) over 1976-77, however.

NLN periodically collects data on minorities in nursing educational programs. In the 1978 study, 84.5 percent of the 1,296 practical nursing programs responded to the survey. Out of these responding programs, 73 percent reported having admitted at least one minority student that year; 70 percent had enrolled at least one minority student, while 62 percent had graduated at least one. In the reporting programs, 15.6 percent of the admissions, 15.0 percent of the enrollments, and 12.5 percent of the graduations in 1978 were minority students. Male students constituted 4.5 percent of the admissions, 3.9 percent of the enrollments, and 3.5 percent of the graduates from these same programs.

Table IV-C-1. Number of State-Approved Programs of Practical and Vocational Nursing in the United States and Outlying Areas,[1] October 15, 1969-1978

Year, as of October 15	Total programs		Number of programs reporting
	Number	Percent change	
1978	1,329	−0.7	1,329
1977	1,339	0.0	1,339
1976	1,339	0.1	1,339
1975	1,337	1.7	1,337
1974	1,315	0.7	1,315
1973	1,306	−0.3	1,306
1972	1,310	1.5	1,310
1971	1,291	3.0	1,291
1970	1,253	0.1	1,253
1969	1,252	5.1	1,252

[1] Includes American Samoa and Puerto Rico for all years, Virgin Islands for 1969-1972, and Guam beginning in 1972.

SOURCE: National League for Nursing, *State-Approved Schools of Nursing—L.P.N./L.V.N., 1979*, and previous years.

Table IV-C-2. Number of State-Approved Programs
of Practical and Vocational Nursing, October 15, 1976,
1977 and 1978

State or area	Number of programs		
	1978	1977	1976
Total	1,329	1,339	1,339
United States, total	1,310	1,319	1,318
Alabama	25	25	26
Alaska	1	1	1
Arizona	14	14	13
Arkansas	29	30	29
California	97	96	100
Colorado	18	17	17
Connecticut	10	10	10
Delaware	5	5	5
District of Columbia	3	3	5
Florida	35	35	33
Georgia	53	53	52
Hawaii	4	4	4
Idaho	11	11	11
Illinois	43	42	42
Indiana	17	17	18
Iowa	25	25	25
Kansas	17	16	16
Kentucky	16	15	15
Louisiana	36	35	31
Maine	5	5	5
Maryland	20	22	22
Massachusetts	31	32	32
Michigan	36	37	37
Minnesota	27	27	27
Mississippi	14	13	13
Missouri	33	33	32
Montana	6	6	7
Nebraska	9	9	9
Nevada	7	7	6
New Hampshire	4	4	4
New Jersey	34	37	38
New Mexico	11	11	11
New York	99	106	111
North Carolina	42	41	41
North Dakota	5	5	3
Ohio	42	42	42
Oklahoma	29	27	26
Oregon	12	12	12
Pennsylvania	53	53	53
Rhode Island	1	1	2
South Carolina	31	34	33
South Dakota	6	6	6
Tennessee	7	7	7
Texas	157	158	157
Utah	5	5	5
Vermont	3	3	3
Virginia	58	59	59
Washington	29	28	27
West Virginia	18	18	18
Wisconsin	14	14	14
Wyoming	3	3	3
Outlying areas, total	19	20	21
American Samoa	1	1	1
Guam	1	1	1
Puerto Rico	17	18	19

SOURCE: National League for Nursing, *State-Approved Schools of Nursing—*
L.P.N./L.V.N., 1979, and previous years.

Table IV-C-3. Number of State-Approved Programs of Practical and Vocational Nursing in the United States and Outlying Areas,[1] by Type of Administrative Control, October 15, 1976-1978

	Number of programs		
Administrative control	1978	1977	1976
Total	1,329	1,339	1,339
Trade, technical or vocational school	710	708	699
University, college or junior college	399	392	380
Hospital	115	123	137
Government agency other than hospital	22	23	27
Other independent agency	7	7	9
Secondary school	76	86	87

[1] Includes American Samoa, Guam, and Puerto Rico.

SOURCES: National League for Nursing, *State-Approved Schools of Nursing—L.P.N./L.V.N., 1977, State-Approved Schools of Nursing—L.P.N./L.V.N., 1978*; and unpublished data, 1980.

Table IV-C-4. Enrollments, Admissions, and Graduations in State-Approved Programs of Practical and Vocational Nursing in the United States and Outlying Areas,[1] Academic Years 1968-69 to 1977-78

Academic year[2]	Enrollments[3]	Admissions	Graduations
1977-78	55,620	61,586	45,991
1976-77	58,003	60,975	47,297
1975-76	59,370	62,272	48,081
1974-75	59,453	61,557	46,080
1973-74	58,872	60,249	45,863
1972-73	57,085	60,475	46,456
1971-72	58,186	61,680	44,446
1970-71	57,890	60,057	38,556
1969-70	53,080	55,635	37,128
1968-69	48,342	49,107	34,864

[1] Includes American Samoa and Puerto Rico for all years, Virgin Islands for 1968-69 thru 1971-72, and Guam beginning in 1971-72.
[2] Prior to 1970-71, reporting dates for academic year are September 1 to August 31. Beginning with the 1970-71 period, the reporting dates were changed to August 1 to July 31.
[3] As of October 15, following close of academic year.

SOURCE: National League for Nursing, *State-Approved Schools of Nursing—L.P.N./L.V.N., 1979*, and previous years.

Table IV-C-5. Enrollments, Admissions, and Graduations in State-Approved Programs of Practical and Vocational Nursing, 1978[1]

State or area	Number of programs	Enrollments	Admissions[2]	Graduations[2]
Total	1,329	55,620	61,586	45,991
United States, total ...	1,310	54,543	60,610	45,350
Alabama	25	1,373	1,641	959
Alaska	1	23	35	31
Arizona	14	488	589	415
Arkansas	29	849	1,347	824
California	97	4,449	4,582	3,276
Colorado	18	555	762	665
Connecticut	10	485	506	463
Delaware	5	164	170	153
District of Columbia	3	203	190	85
Florida	35	2,135	2,505	1,978
Georgia	53	1,664	2,052	1,378
Hawaii	4	135	165	116
Idaho	11	197	196	172
Illinois	43	2,548	2,764	2,223
Indiana	17	934	1,056	958
Iowa	25	979	1,087	808
Kansas	17	518	583	568
Kentucky	16	638	707	439
Louisiana	36	1,428	1,775	962
Maine	5	211	235	194
Maryland	20	703	660	498
Massachusetts	31	1,289	1,356	1,129
Michigan	36	1,898	2,203	1,664
Minnesota	27	1,300	1,419	1,133
Mississippi	14	859	1,033	700
Missouri	33	1,106	1,268	1,085
Montana	6	186	286	185
Nebraska	9	437	525	432
Nevada	7	118	126	70
New Hampshire ...	4	184	203	142
New Jersey	34	1,628	1,870	1,490
New Mexico	11	349	406	281
New York	99	5,531	4,958	3,591
North Carolina	42	1,208	1,411	1,064
North Dakota	5	202	372	305
Ohio	42	2,398	2,585	2,081
Oklahoma	29	867	928	703
Oregon	12	264	360	362
Pennsylvania	53	2,679	2,996	2,435
Rhode Island	1	114	118	108
South Carolina	31	891	866	624
South Dakota	6	288	274	234
Tennessee	7	1,048	1,474	953
Texas	157	4,116	4,883	3,715
Utah	5	287	438	230
Vermont	3	178	206	170
Virginia	58	1,962	1,553	982
Washington	29	823	965	810
West Virginia	18	469	535	433
Wisconsin	14	1,121	1,307	1,016
Wyoming	3	64	79	58
Outlying areas, total	19	1,077	976	641
American Samoa...	1	34	23	...
Guam	1	47	53	41
Puerto Rico	17	996	900	600

[1] Admissions and graduations are based on academic year August 1, 1977-July 31, 1978, enrollments and number of programs are as of October 15, 1978.
[2] Admissions and graduations include programs which closed during the academic year.

SOURCE: National League for Nursing, *State-Approved Schools of Nursing— L.P.N./L.V.N., 1979*, p. 65.

Table IV-C-6. Minority Student Admissions, Enrollments, and Graduations in State-Approved Programs of Practical or Vocational Nursing,[1] in the United States and Outlying Areas, 1978

| | | Programs returning questionnaire | | | |
| | | | | Minority students | |
Item	Number	Percent reporting at least one minority student	Total students	Number	Percent
Minority, total					
Admissions	1,095	73	53,002	8,279	15.6
Enrollments[2]	1,095	70	48,453	7,292	15.0
Graduations	1,095	62	39,396	4,942	12.5
Blacks					
Admissions	1,095	59	53,002	5,883	11.1
Enrollments[2]	1,095	56	48,453	5,141	10.6
Graduations	1,095	50	39,396	3,515	8.9
Hispanic					
Admissions	1,095	31	53,002	1,655	3.1
Enrollments[2]	1,095	30	48,453	1,543	3.2
Graduations	1,095	24	39,396	1,012	2.6
American Indians/Orientals					
Admissions	1,095	26	53,002	741	1.4
Enrollments[2]	1,095	23	48,453	608	1.3
Graduations	1,095	18	39,396	415	1.1

[1]Total number of programs receiving questionnaire was 1,296 as of October 15, 1978.
[2]Enrollments are as of October 15, 1978.
SOURCE: National League for Nursing, "Educational Preparation for Nursing—1978," *Nursing Outlook*, Vol. 27, No. 9, September 1979, pp. 612-613.

Table IV-C-7. Male Student Admissions, Enrollments, and Graduations in State-Approved Programs of Practical or Vocational Nursing,[1] in the United States and Outlying Areas, 1978

| | | Programs returning questionnaire | | | |
| | | | | Male students | |
Item	Number	Percent reporting at least one male student	Total students	Number	Percent
Admissions	1,095	57	53,002	2,365	4.5
Enrollments[2]	1,095	54	48,453	1,901	3.9
Graduations	1,095	44	39,396	1,395	3.5

[1]Total number of programs receiving questionnaire was 1,296 as of October 15, 1978.
[2]Enrollments are as of October 15, 1978.
SOURCE: National League for Nursing, "Educational Preparation for Nursing—1978," *Nursing Outlook*, Vol. 27, No. 9, September 1979, pp. 612-613.

Chapter IV, Section D
EARNINGS OF LICENSED PRACTICAL NURSES
AND ALLIED NURSING PERSONNEL

Various periodic studies provide information on salaries paid to persons in allied nursing positions. Survey data from the Bureau of Labor Statistics, the National League for Nursing, the University of Texas Medical Branch at Galveston, and the American Nurses' Association are included in this section. Since these same resources also provided salary data on registered nurses, the reader is referred to Chapter III for comparative statistics.

The average hourly earnings of licensed practical nurses and nurses' aides in nonfederal hospitals and nongovernment nursing homes and related facilities was available from the latest periodic surveys conducted by the Bureau of Labor Statistics of the U.S. Department of Labor. For hospitals, the 1978 survey data represented the earnings of auxiliary nursing personnel in 23 sample standard metropolitan statistical areas (SMSAs) included in the study; for the nursing home sector, 21 SMSAs constituted the original sample. All institutions meeting the BLS criteria within each of the sample SMSAs were covered. Average salaries of licensed practical nurses working full-time in nongovernmental hospitals in 1978 ranged from $4.10 per hour in Atlanta to $6.45 per hour in the San Francisco-Oakland area. Their counterparts in nongovernment nursing homes and related facilities commanded generally lower average hourly salaries within the sample metropolitan areas, ranging from $3.88 in Atlanta to $7.16 in the New York area. Average hourly earnings of nurses' aides holding full-time positions in nongovernment hospitals ranged from $3.26 in Dallas-Fort Worth to $5.73 in the New York City area, while those in nursing homes had salaries ranging from $2.75 in Atlanta and Dallas-Fort Worth to $5.61 in the New York City area.

The 1979 University of Texas study showed that the average monthly starting salary of licensed practical nurses in hospitals and medical schools was $775, an increase of 6.0 percent since 1978. This salary generally reflected the amount normally paid to fill a vacant licensed practical nurse position in 1979. The maximum monthly salary earned by licensed practical nurses in the sample facilities increased 8.4 percent to $1,011 in 1979. The American Nurses' Association 1976 study of nursing salaries in nonfederal short-term hospitals indicated that the starting salaries of licensed practical nurses and nurses' aides rose with the size of the hospital and were greater in metropolitan areas than in non-metropolitan areas.

In the survey of nursing personnel engaged in community health work, the National League for Nursing Division of Home Health Agencies and Community Health Services reported salaries of auxiliary nursing personnel. The 1979 study showed full-time licensed practical nurses in nonofficial agencies, official state and local health agencies, and combination services had a median annual salary of $10,344 in 1979. Public health assistants and home health aides in those agencies earned $9,502 and $7,205, respectively, in that same year. Between 1978 and 1979 the median annual salaries of licensed practical nurses, public health assistants, and home health aides increased 8.1 percent, 8.3 percent, and 7.9 percent, respectively.

Table IV-D-1. Average Hourly Earnings and Number of Licensed Practical Nurses in Nonfederal Hospitals, by Metropolitan Area,[1] September 1978

Metropolitan area	Full-time		Part-time[2]	
	Number	Average hourly earnings	Number	Average hourly earnings
Atlanta, Ga.	1,205	$4.20	175	$4.15
Baltimore, Md.	1,684	5.77	362	5.48
Boston, Ma.	2,344	5.35	881	5.32
Buffalo, N.Y.	1,129	4.73	455	4.67
Chicago, Il.	4,087	5.63	692	5.45
Cleveland, Oh.	2,229	5.14	881	4.97
Dallas-Fort Worth, Tx.	2,206	4.37	418	4.19
Denver-Boulder, Co.	902	4.66	319	4.47
Detroit, Mi.	2,918	5.93	975	5.88
Houston, Tx.	2,504	4.60	493	4.37
Kansas City, Mo.-Ks.	1,204	4.58	280	4.52
Los Angeles-Long Beach, Ca.	5,517	5.63	1,425	5.73
Memphis, Tn.-Ar.-Ms.	...	...	...	...
Miami, Fl.	1,319	5.08	134	5.08
Milwaukee, Wi.	785	5.11	585	4.94
Minneapolis-St. Paul, Mn.-Wi.	1,007	5.05	588	4.90
New York, N.Y.-N.J.	6,083	6.21	704	5.69
Philadelphia, Pa.-N.J.	4,394	5.30	1,198	5.01
Portland, Or.-Wa.	834	5.26	1,425	5.73
St. Louis, Mo.-Il.	2,591	4.80	332	4.86
San Francisco-Oakland, Ca.	1,887	6.34	755	6.35
Seattle-Everett, Wa.	788	4.95	835	4.86
Washington, D.C.-Md.-Va.	1,625	5.12	309	4.89

[1] Standard Metropolitan Statistical Areas as defined by the U.S. Office of Management and Budget through February 1974. All metropolitan areas consist of one or more counties.
[2] Part-time employees are those working a schedule regularly calling for fewer weekly hours than those of full-time employees.

SOURCE: U.S. Department of Labor, Bureau of Labor Statistics, *Industry Wage Survey: Hospitals, September 1978*. Individual releases.

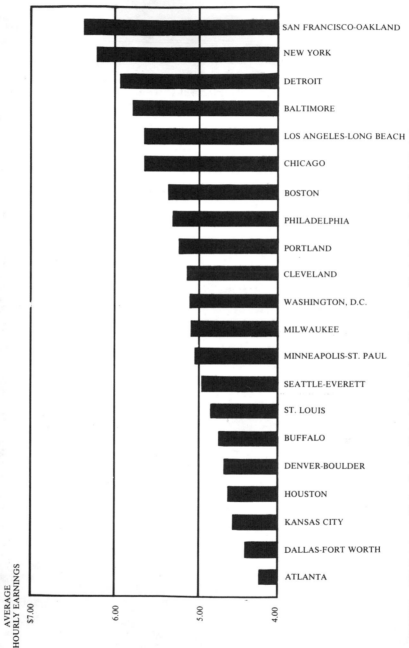

CHART 13. AVERAGE HOURLY EARNINGS OF FULL-TIME LICENSED PRACTICAL NURSES IN NONFEDERAL HOSPITALS IN TWENTY-ONE METROPOLITAN AREAS, SEPTEMBER 1978

AVERAGE HOURLY EARNINGS

SAN FRANCISCO-OAKLAND
NEW YORK
DETROIT
BALTIMORE
LOS ANGELES-LONG BEACH
CHICAGO
BOSTON
PHILADELPHIA
PORTLAND
CLEVELAND
WASHINGTON, D.C.
MILWAUKEE
MINNEAPOLIS-ST. PAUL
SEATTLE-EVERETT
ST. LOUIS
BUFFALO
DENVER-BOULDER
HOUSTON
KANSAS CITY
DALLAS-FORT WORTH
ATLANTA

$7.00   6.00   5.00   4.00

SOURCE: U.S. Department of Labor, Bureau of Labor Statistics, *Industry Wage Survey: Hospitals, September 1978.* Individual releases. Prepared by American Nurses' Association, Research and Policy Analysis Department, Statistics Unit, 1980.

Table IV-D-2. Average Hourly Earnings and Number of Licensed Practical Nurses in Nongovernment Hospitals, by Metropolitan Area,[1] September 1978

Metropolitan area	Full-time		Part-time[2]	
	Number	Average hourly earnings	Number	Average hourly earnings
Atlanta, Ga.	435	$4.10	34	$4.05
Baltimore, Md.	835	5.59	305	5.47
Boston, Ma.	1,662	5.42	694	5.42
Buffalo, N.Y.	846	4.69	441	4.67
Chicago, Il.	3,388	5.61	641	5.44
Cleveland, Oh.	1,893	5.18	691	5.04
Dallas-Fort Worth, Tx.	1,648	4.39	310	4.23
Denver-Boulder, Co.	715	4.63	208	4.58
Detroit, Mi.	2,485	5.94	817	5.91
Houston, Tx.	2,118	4.57	452	4.35
Kansas City, Mo.-Ks.	849	4.62	237	4.56
Los Angeles-Long Beach, Ca.	4,513	5.63	1,374	5.74
Memphis, Tn.-Ar.-Ms.	...	...	...	...
Miami, Fl.	1,022	5.11	126	5.13
Milwaukee, Wi.	662	4.98	585	4.94
Minneapolis-St. Paul, Mn.-Wi.	756	4.91	574	4.89
New York, N.Y.-N.J.	3,751	6.31	590	5.64
Philadelphia, Pa.-N.J.	4,124	5.26	1,195	5.01
Portland, Or.-Wa.	729	5.27	348	5.14
St. Louis, Mo.-Il.	2,346	4.79	309	4.85
San Francisco-Oakland, Ca.	1,123	6.45	558	6.41
Seattle-Everett, Wa.	539	4.98	590	4.88
Washington, D.C.-Md.-Va.	1,218	4.96	276	4.87

[1] Standard Metropolitan Statistical Areas as defined by the U.S. Office of Management and Budget through February 1974. All metropolitan areas consist of one or more counties.
[2] Part-time employees are those working a schedule regularly calling for fewer weekly hours than those of full-time employees.

SOURCE: U.S. Department of Labor, Bureau of Labor Statistics, *Industry Wage Survey: Hospitals, September 1978.* Individual releases.

Table IV-D-3. Average Hourly Earnings and Number of Licensed
Practical Nurses in State and Local Government Hospitals,
by Metropolitan Area,[1] September 1978

Metropolitan area	Full-time		Part-time[2]	
	Number	Average hourly earnings	Number	Average hourly earnings
Atlanta, Ga.	770	$4.26	141	$4.18
Baltimore, Md.	849	5.94	...	...
Boston, Ma.	682	5.16	...	...
Buffalo, N.Y.	283	4.85	...	...
Chicago, Il.	699	5.71	...	...
Cleveland, Oh.	336	4.93	190	4.75
Dallas-Fort Worth, Tx.	558	4.30	108	4.07
Denver-Boulder, Co.	187	4.77	...	...
Detroit, Mi.	433	5.87	158	5.77
Houston, Tx.	...	...	42	4.50
Kansas City, Mo.-Ks.	355	4.48	43	4.28
Los Angeles-Long Beach, Ca.	1,004	5.65	51	5.52
Memphis, Tn.-Ar.-Ms.	...	...	...	...
Miami, Fl.	...	...	...	...
Milwaukee, Wi.	...	...	...	...
Minneapolis-St. Paul, Mn.-Wi.	...	...	...	...
New York, N.Y.-N.J.	...	...	114	5.97
Philadelphia, Pa.-N.J.	270	5.94	...	...
Portland, Or.-Wa.	...	...	...	...
St. Louis, Mo.-Il.	245	4.88	...	...
San Francisco-Oakland, Ca.	801	6.20	211	6.16
Seattle-Everett, Wa.	...	...	...	...
Washington, D.C.-Md.-Va.	407	5.58	...	...

[1] Standard Metropolitan Statistical Areas as defined by the U.S. Office of Budget and Management through February 1974. All metropolitan areas consist of one or more counties.
[2] Part-time employees are those working a schedule regularly calling for fewer weekly hours than those of full-time employees.

SOURCE: U.S. Department of Labor, Bureau of Labor Statistics, *Industry Wage Survey: Hospitals, September 1978.* Individual releases.

Table IV-D-4. Salaries of Licensed Practical or Vocational Nurses in Hospitals and Medical Schools in the United States, by Type of Institution

Date and type of institution	Starting monthly salary[1]				Maximum monthly salary[2]			
	Lowest	Highest	Midpoint	Average	Lowest	Highest	Midpoint	Average
July 1979								
Institutions combined	$579	$1,183	$757	$775	$748	$1,594	$986	$1,011
Hospitals	643	1,183	760	789	816	1,594	986	1,016
Medical schools	579	1,030	680	741	748	1,393	888	972
Medical centers	624	993	757	769	787	1,475	996	1,017
July 1978								
Institutions combined	563	1,095	704	731	667	1,505	920	933
Hospitals	606	1,095	707	746	667	1,505	920	943
Medical schools	563	952	695	714	703	1,169	831	870
Medical centers	569	969	700	718	704	1,175	938	942
July 1977								
Institutions combined	523	1,010	767	681	658	1,421	1,040	874
Hospitals	536	1,010	774	691	664	1,421	1,042	885
Medical schools	595	912	753	699	658	1,124	892	851
Medical centers	523	969	747	665	704	1,111	908	868

[1] Salaries normally paid in order to fill vacancies in a particular job class.
[2] Highest reported salaries actually paid to employees in a particular job class.
SOURCE: University of Texas Medical Branch at Galveston, *1979 National Survey of Hospital and Medical School Salaries*, and previous years.

Table IV-D-5. Median Monthly Salaries of Licensed Practical Nurses and Aides Employed in Nonfederal, Short-term, General Hospitals According to Location, Hospital Size, Region, and Type of Control, July 1976

Type of position	Location			Size (beds)					
	Non-SMSA¹	SMSA¹	Unknown	Under 50	50-99	100-199	200-399	400 and over	Unknown
Licensed practical nurse Starting salary									
No experience	$528	$597	$563	$520	$540	$560	$610	$613	$564
With experience	555	626	572	550	568	589	639	652	573
Nurses' aide Starting salary—no experience	398	459	407	390	399	420	475	488	399

Type of position	Region²					Type of control			
	North-east	South	North Central	West	Unknown	Government nonfederal	Non-government nonprofit	Non-government for profit	Unknown
Licensed practical nurse Starting salary									
No experience	$600	$523	$554	$626	$564	$533	$570	$536	$564
With experience	633	551	575	647	573	561	598	566	573
Nurses' aide Starting salary—no experience	469	398	400	479	399	398	425	400	399

¹Standard Metropolitan Statistical Area.
²The states included in each region are: *Northeast*—Connecticut, Maine, Massachusetts, New Hampshire, New Jersey, New York, Pennsylvania, Rhode Island, Vermont; *South*—Alabama, Arkansas, Delaware, District of Columbia, Florida, Georgia, Kentucky, Louisiana, Maryland, Mississippi, North Carolina, Oklahoma, South Carolina, Tennessee, Texas, Virginia, West Virginia; *North Central*—Illinois, Indiana, Iowa, Kansas, Michigan, Minnesota, Missouri, Nebraska, North Dakota, Ohio, South Dakota, Wisconsin; *West*—Alaska, Arizona, California, Colorado, Hawaii, Idaho, Montana, Nevada, New Mexico, Oregon, Utah, Washington, Wyoming.
SOURCE: American Nurses' Association, Statistics Department, "Survey of Economic Factors Related to Nurse Manpower in Nonfederal, Short-term, General Hospitals, July 1976."

Table IV-D-6. Average Hourly Earnings and Number of Licensed Practical Nurses in Nongovernment Nursing Homes and Related Facilities, by Metropolitan Area,[1] September 1978

Metropolitan area	Total		Full-time		Part-time[2]	
	Number	Average hourly earnings	Number	Average hourly earnings	Number	Average hourly earnings
Atlanta, Ga.	478	$3.86	386	$3.88	92	$3.76
Baltimore, Md.	556	4.76	298	4.80	258	4.72
Boston, Ma.	1,349	4.72	642	4.76	707	4.69
Buffalo, N.Y.	465	3.93	271	4.00	194	3.82
Chicago, Il.	833	4.73	584	4.75	249	4.69
Cleveland, Oh.	779	4.46	549	4.44	230	4.52
Dallas-Fort Worth, Tx. ..	1,620	4.50	1,412	4.52	208	4.40
Denver-Boulder, Co. ...	466	4.32	308	4.33	158	4.30
Detroit, Mi.	1,026	4.93	566	4.97	460	4.87
Houston, Tx.	774	4.56	679	4.56	95	4.54
Kansas City, Mo.-Ks. ...	290	4.27	201	4.30	89	4.20
Los Angeles-Long Beach, Ca. ...	3,721	5.77	2,717	5.78	1,004	5.76
Miami, Fl.	297	4.38	251	4.39	46	4.33
Minneapolis-St Paul, Mn.-Wi.	979	4.91	492	4.97	487	4.84
Milwaukee, Wi.	788	5.40	321	5.38	467	5.42
New York, N.Y.-N.J.	3,972	7.22	2,750	7.16	1,222	7.35
Philadelphia, Pa.-N.J.	1,286	4.68	819	4.78	467	4.49
St Louis, Mo.-Il.	742	4.43	474	4.43	268	4.42
San Francisco-Oakland, Ca.	1,032	5.25	709	5.30	323	5.16
Seattle-Everett, Wa.	538	4.66	330	4.74	208	4.54
Washington, D.C.-Md.-Va. ...	436	4.71	305	4.70	131	4.73

[1] Standard Metropolitan Statistical Areas as defined by the U.S. Office of Management and Budget through February 1974. All metropolitan areas consist of one or more counties.
[2] Part-time employees are those working on a schedule regularly calling for fewer weekly hours than those of full-time employees.

SOURCE: U.S. Department of Labor, Bureau of Labor Statistics, *Industry Wage Survey: Nursing and Personal Care Facilities, September 1978*. Individual releases.

Table IV-D-7. Average Hourly Earnings and Number of Licensed Practical Nurses in Nongovernment Nursing Homes and Related Facilities, by Metropolitan Area,[1] May 1976

Metropolitan area	Total		Full-time		Part-time[2]	
	Number	Average hourly earnings	Number	Average hourly earnings	Number	Average hourly earnings
Atlanta, Ga.	458	$3.43	387	$3.42	71	$3.49
Baltimore, Md.	593	4.25	412	4.32	181	4.08
Boston, Ma.	1,684	4.15	783	4.23	901	4.07
Buffalo, N.Y.	414	3.58	252	3.63	162	3.49
Chicago, Il.	1,090	4.10	747	4.14	343	4.03
Cincinnati, Oh.-Ky.-In.	632	3.90	402	3.95	230	3.82
Cleveland, Oh.	766	3.66	519	3.71	247	3.54
Dallas-Fort Worth, Tx.	1,078	3.70	827	3.73	251	3.63
Denver-Boulder, Co.	409	3.48	260	3.51	149	3.44
Detroit, Mi.	1,033	4.24	615	4.29	418	4.17
Kansas City, Mo.-Ks.	241	3.57	176	3.60	65	3.46
Los Angeles-Long Beach, Ca.	2,880	4.48	1,986	4.50	894	4.43
Miami, Fl.	387	4.04	316	4.05	71	4.00
Milwaukee, Wi.	780	4.45	327	4.51	453	4.41
Minneapolis-St. Paul, Mn.-Wi.	815	4.04	411	4.07	404	4.01
New York, N.Y.-N.J.	2,520	6.37	1,805	6.31	715	6.53
Philadelphia, Pa.-N.J.	1,448	3.73	1,007	3.79	441	3.58
St Louis, Mo.-Il.	626	3.67	431	3.68	195	3.65
San Francisco-Oakland, Ca.	851	3.91	520	3.98	331	3.81
Seattle-Everett, Wa.	507	3.69	324	3.75	183	3.58
Washington, D.C.-Md.-Va.	318	4.08	192	4.07	126	4.11

[1]Standard Metropolitan Statistical Areas as defined by the U.S. Office of Management and Budget through February 1974. All metropolitan areas consist of one or more counties.
[2]Part-time employees are those working a schedule regularly calling for fewer weekly hours than those of full-time employees.

SOURCE: U.S. Department of Labor, Bureau of Labor Statistics, Industry Wage Survey: Nursing Homes and Related Facilities, May 1976, and individual releases, 1977.

Table IV-D-8. Average Hourly Earnings[1] of Licensed Practical Nurses Employed Full-time and Part-time in Nursing Homes, by Selected Nursing Home Characteristics, 1977

| | Licensed practical nurse | |
| | Full-time | Part-time |
Nursing home characteristics	Average hourly earnings	Average hourly earnings
Total	$4.04	$4.02
Ownership		
Proprietary	4.01	4.05
Voluntary nonprofit	4.07	3.92
Government	4.13	4.03
Certification		
Skilled nursing facility	4.36	4.20
Skilled nursing facility and		
intermediate care facility	4.08	4.10
Intermediate care facility	3.78	3.80
Not certified	3.90	(2)
Bed size		
Less than 50 beds	3.88	3.84
50-99	3.88	3.77
100-199	3.97	4.12
200 beds or more	4.55	4.62
Location		
Region		
Northeast	4.49	4.16
North Central	3.95	4.09
South	3.71	3.71
West	4.30	4.12
Standard federal administrative region		
Region I	4.31	4.09
Region II	4.91	(2)
Region III	3.95	3.84
Region IV	3.59	3.59
Region V	4.13	4.24
Region VI	3.82	3.81
Region VII.....................	3.50	(2)
Region VIII....................	(2)	(2)
Region IX	4.52	(2)
Region X	(2)	(2)
Type of facility		
Nursing care	4.03	4.02
Other	4.22	4.01

[1] Includes only nurses who reported salary.
[2] Insufficient number of cases to compute average hourly earnings.

SOURCE: U.S. Department of Health, Education, and Welfare, Public Health Service, Office of Health Research, Statistics, and Technology, National Center for Health Statistics, *The National Nursing Home Survey: 1977 Summary for the United States*, Vital and Health Statistics, Series 13, No. 43, DHEW Publication No. (PHS) 79-1794, 1979, p. 19.

Table IV-D-9. Average Hourly Earnings[1] of Licensed Practical Nurses Employed Full-time and Part-time in Nursing Homes, by Selected Employee Characteristics, 1977

	Licensed practical nurse	
	Full-time	Part-time
Employee characteristics	Average hourly earnings	Average hourly earnings
Total	$4.04	$4.02
Racial/ethnic background		
White (not Hispanic)	3.97	3.93
Black (not Hispanic)	4.34	4.61
Hispanic	(2)	(2)
Other	(2)	(2)
Sex		
Male	(2)	(2)
Female	4.04	4.02
Age group		
Under 35 years	3.89	3.91
35-44	4.08	4.12
45-54	4.15	4.35
55 years and over	4.19	3.89
Years of education		
Less than 12 years	3.89	(2)
12	3.91	4.06
13-14	4.06	4.03
15-16	4.25	3.86
17 years or more	(2)	(2)
Years of current employment		
Less than 2 years	3.91	3.87
2-4	4.08	4.29
5-9	4.20	3.87
10 years or more	4.31	(2)
Years of total experience		
Less than 5 years	3.87	3.94
5-9	4.07	3.98
10-14	4.12	3.94
15 years or more	4.26	4.32
Benefits		
Paid vacation, sick leave	4.07	4.11
Other leave[3]	4.09	3.99
Pension	4.29	4.28
Health, life insurance	4.18	4.46
Direct medical benefits	4.39	(2)
Meals	4.09	3.96
Employment arrangements		
Contract	(2)	(2)
On staff	4.04	3.95

[1] Includes only nurses who reported salary.
[2] Insufficient number of cases to compute average hourly earnings.
[3] Includes civil and personal leave (jury duty, military reserves, voting, funerals) and release time for attending training institutes.

SOURCE: U.S. Department of Health, Education, and Welfare, Public Health Service, Office of Health Research, Statistics, and Technology, National Center for Health Statistics, *The National Nursing Home Survey: 1977 Summary for the United States*, Vital and Health Statistics, Series 13, No. 43, DHEW Publication No. (PHS) 79-1794, 1979, p. 22.

Table IV-D-10. Employment and Median Annual Salaries of Full-time Licensed Practical Nurses and Auxiliary Nursing Personnel in Selected Community Health Nursing Agencies,[1] April 1976-1979

Item	Licensed practical nurse	Auxiliary nursing personnel			Nonnurse specialist		Nonnurse executive director
		Public health assistant	Home health aide	Other auxiliary personnel	Physical therapist	Other	
April 1976							
Number of agencies with position	260	50	214	188	[2]116	121	(3)
Number of full-time employees ...	1,483	787	2,142	1,650	285	394	(3)
Median annual salary	$8,371	$7,615	$6,366	$7,162	$13,029	$12,675	(3)
April 1977							
Number of agencies with position	218	43	234	140	145	85	46
Number of full-time employees ...	1,290	627	2,376	1,520	368	281	46
Median annual salary	$8,995	$8,544	$6,522	$7,532	$14,100	$13,007	$30,033
April 1978							
Number of agencies with position	228	52	263	155	141	47	24
Number of full-time employees ...	1,419	823	2,898	1,535	356	120	24
Median annual salary	$9,572	$8,775	$6,675	$7,303	$14,517	$13,567	$28,750
April 1979							
Number of agencies with position	226	52	246	152	135	67	27
Number of full-time employees ...	1,201	674	3,025	1,368	384	245	27
Median annual salary	$10,344	$9,502	$7,205	$8,323	$15,231	$13,179	$27,250

[1] Includes nonofficial agencies, official state and local health agencies, and combination services.
[2] Some physical therapists are also RNs.
(3) No such classification listed in 1976.

SOURCE: National League for Nursing, "Salaries in Community Health Agencies—1979," *Nursing Outlook*, Vol. 27, No. 12, December 1979, p. 799, and previous years.

Table IV-D-11. Average Hourly Earnings and Number of Nurses' Aides in Nonfederal Hospitals by Metropolitan Area,[1] September 1978

Metropolitan area	Full-time		Part-time[2]	
	Number	Average hourly earnings	Number	Average hourly earnings
Atlanta, Ga.	2,303	$3.39	461	$3.23
Baltimore, Md.	3,771	4.54	1,197	4.28
Boston, Ma.	4,195	4.32	957	4.05
Buffalo, N.Y.	1,466	3.81	528	3.65
Chicago, Il.	6,915	4.61	1,576	4.22
Cleveland, Oh.	2,302	4.34	722	4.11
Dallas-Fort Worth, Tx.	2,091	3.28	286	3.03
Denver-Boulder, Co.	1,483	3.80	397	3.64
Detroit, Mi.	5,750	4.45	946	4.25
Houston, Tx.	2,310	3.56	581	3.27
Kansas City, Mo.-Ks.	1,868	3.50	361	3.29
Los Angeles-Long Beach, Ca.	8,274	4.30	1,322	4.22
Memphis, Tn.-Ar.-Ms.	...	...	...	...
Miami, Fl.	2,469	3.70	177	3.31
Milwaukee, Wi.	1,189	4.32	806	3.85
Minneapolis-St. Paul, Mn.-Wi.	1,159	4.08	1,064	3.98
New York, N.Y.-N.J.	16,102	5.65	535	4.72
Philadelphia, Pa.-N.J.	3,886	4.61	1,535	4.30
Portland, Or.-Wa.	799	4.41	626	4.35
St. Louis, Mo.-Il.	4,760	3.78	1,298	3.50
San Francisco-Oakland, Ca.	2,464	5.81	564	5.76
Seattle-Everett, Wa.	696	4.18	405	4.05
Washington, D.C.-Md.-Va.	2,339	4.36	315	4.11

[1] Standard Metropolitan Statistical Areas as defined by the U.S. Office of Management and Budget through February 1974. All metropolitan areas consist of one or more counties.
[2] Part-time employees are those working a schedule regularly calling for fewer weekly hours than those of full-time employees.
SOURCE: U.S. Department of Labor, Bureau of Labor Statistics, *Industry Wage Survey: Hospitals, September 1978*. Individual releases.

Table IV-D-12. Average Hourly Earnings and Number of Nurses' Aides in Nongovernment Hospitals by Metropolitan Area,[1] September 1978

Metropolitan area	Full-time		Part-time[2]	
	Number	Average hourly earnings	Number	Average hourly earnings
Atlanta, Ga.	969	$3.36	156	$3.17
Baltimore, Md.	2,931	4.50	1,192	4.28
Boston, Ma.	2,570	4.37	846	4.02
Buffalo, N.Y.	1,170	3.66	509	3.67
Chicago, Il.	6,303	4.60	1,562	4.22
Cleveland, Oh.	1,887	4.38	640	4.12
Dallas-Fort Worth, Tx.	1,473	3.26	173	3.16
Denver-Boulder, Co.	1,241	3.76	295	3.69
Detroit, Mi.	5,287	4.44	847	4.25
Houston, Tx.	1,790	3.53	561	3.27
Kansas City, Mo.-Ks.	1,440	3.49	321	3.26
Los Angeles-Long Beach, Ca.	6,876	4.26	1,294	4.21
Memphis, Tn.-Ar.-Ms.	...	...	...	...
Miami, Fl.	2,011	3.68	177	3.31
Milwaukee, Wi.	906	4.02	795	3.84
Minneapolis-St. Paul, Mn.-Wi.	868	3.98	750	3.92
New York, N.Y.-N.J.	11,332	5.73	535	4.72
Philadelphia, Pa.-N.J.	3,733	4.62	1,535	4.30
Portland, Or.-Wa.	637	4.39	596	4.34
St. Louis, Mo.-Il.	3,594	3.78	1,298	3.50
San Francisco-Oakland, Ca.	1,391	5.93	410	5.86
Seattle-Everett, Wa.	481	4.13	282	4.04
Washington, D.C.-Md.-Va.	2,143	4.31	310	4.11

[1] Standard Metropolitan Statistical Areas as defined by the U.S. Office of Budget and Management through February 1974. All metropolitan areas consist of one or more counties.
[2] Part-time employees are those working a schedule regularly calling for fewer weekly hours than those of full-time employees.

SOURCE: U.S. Department of Labor, Bureau of Labor Statistics, *Industry Wage Survey: Hospitals, September 1978*. Individual releases.

Table IV-D-13. Average Hourly Earnings and Number of Nurses' Aides in State and Local Government Hospitals by Metropolitan Area,[1] September 1978

Metropolitan area	Full-time		Part-time[2]	
	Number	Average hourly earnings	Number	Average hourly earnings
Atlanta, Ga.	1,334	$3.42	305	$3.27
Baltimore, Md.	840	4.68	...	...
Boston, Ma.	1,625	4.24	111	4.23
Buffalo, N.Y.	296	4.40	...	...
Chicago, Il.	...	...	...	...
Cleveland, Oh.	415	4.15	82	4.00
Dallas-Fort Worth, Tx.	618	3.34	...	...
Denver-Boulder, Co.	242	4.00	...	...
Detroit, Mi.	463	4.52	99	4.27
Houston, Tx.	520	3.68	20	3.24
Kansas City, Mo.-Ks.	428	3.55	40	3.45
Los Angeles-Long Beach, Ca.	1,398	4.51	28	4.33
Memphis, Tn.-Ar.-Ms.	295	3.79	...	...
Miami, Fl.	...	...	...	...
Milwaukee, Wi.	...	...	...	...
Minneapolis-St. Paul, Mn.-Wi.	291	4.37	...	...
New York, N.Y.-N.J.	...	...	...	...
Philadelphia, Pa.-N.J.	...	...	...	...
Portland, Or.-Wa.	...	...	...	...
St. Louis, Mo.-Il.	1,166	3.77	...	...
San Francisco-Oakland, Ca.	1,259	5.64	178	5.54
Seattle-Everett, Wa.	215	4.29	...	...
Washington, D.C.-Md.-Va.	196	4.97	...	...

[1] Standard Metropolitan Statistical Areas as defined by the U.S. Office of Budget and Management through February 1974. All metropolitan areas consist of one of more counties.
[2] Part-time employees are those working a schedule regularly calling for fewer weekly hours than those of full-time employees.

SOURCE: U.S. Department of Labor, Bureau of Labor Statistics, *Industry Wage Survey: Hospitals, September 1978.* Individual releases.

Table IV-D-14. Average Hourly Earnings and Number of Nurses' Aides in Nongovernment Nursing Homes and Related Facilities, by Metropolitan Area,[1] September 1978

Metropolitan area	Total		Full-time		Part-time[2]	
	Number	Average hourly earnings	Number	Average hourly earnings	Number	Average hourly earnings
Atlanta, Ga.	1,969	$2.74	1,732	$2.75	237	$2.72
Baltimore, Md.	3,278	3.37	2,654	3.40	624	3.23
Boston, Ma.	8,728	3.13	4,710	3.14	4,018	3.11
Buffalo, N.Y.	1,958	2.99	1,183	3.03	775	2.95
Chicago, Il.	6,676	3.04	5,258	3.07	1,418	2.91
Cleveland, Oh.	3,269	2.97	2,368	3.01	901	2.87
Dallas-Fort Worth, Tx.	5,562	2.75	5,148	2.75	414	2.73
Denver-Boulder, Co.	2,497	2.85	1,581	2.87	916	2.81
Detroit, Mi.	7,491	2.92	5,461	2.95	2,030	2.85
Houston, Tx.	2,628	2.80	2,363	2.81	265	2.74
Kansas City, Mo.-Ks.	2,025	2.82	1,802	2.82	223	2.83
Los Angeles-Long Beach, Ca.	17,003	3.11	14,383	3.12	2,620	3.08
Miami, Fl.	1,632	2.90	1,543	2.91	89	2.71
Minneapolis-St. Paul, Mn.-Wi.	6,938	3.46	2,798	3.55	4,140	3.40
Milwaukee, Wi.	4,124	3.21	1,983	3.23	2,141	3.19
New York, N.Y.-N.J.	16,597	5.53	13,984	5.61	2,613	5.08
Philadelphia, Pa.-N.J.	8,642	3.12	6,507	3.16	2,135	3.00
St. Louis, Mo.-Il.	4,863	2.90	3,972	2.91	891	2.87
San Francisco-Oakland, Ca.	6,059	3.40	4,539	3.44	1.520	3.30
Seattle-Everett, Wa.	3,806	3.18	2,231	3.22	1,575	3.14
Washington, D.C.-Md.-Va.	3,055	3.09	2,463	3.10	592	3.06

[1] Standard Metropolitan Statistical Areas as defined by the U.S. Office of Management and Budget through February 1974. All metropolitan areas consist of one or more counties.
[2] Part-time employees are those working a schedule regularly calling for fewer weekly hours than those of full-time employees.

SOURCE: U.S. Department of Labor, Bureau of Labor Statistics, *Industry Wage Survey: Nursing and Personal Care Facilities, September 1978.* Individual releases.

Table IV-D-15. Average Hourly Earnings and Number of Nurses' Aides[1] in Nongovernment Nursing Homes and Related Facilities,[2] by Metropolitan Area,[2] May 1976

Metropolitan area	Total		Full-time		Part-time[3]	
	Number	Average hourly earnings	Number	Average hourly earnings	Number	Average hourly earnings
Atlanta, Ga.	2,124	$2.33	1,897	$2.33	227	$2.35
Baltimore, Md.	2,901	2.95	2,419	2.97	482	2.81
Boston, Ma.	7,873	2.72	4,230	2.78	3,643	2.66
Buffalo, N.Y.	1,893	2.63	1,252	2.66	641	2.57
Chicago, Il.	8,033	2.67	5,906	2.71	2,127	2.55
Cincinnati, Oh.-Ky.-In.	2,763	2.40	1,830	2.43	933	2.34
Cleveland, Oh.	3,237	2.40	2,518	2.43	719	2.31
Dallas-Fort Worth, Tx.	3,768	2.28	3,305	2.29	463	2.24
Denver-Boulder, Co.	2,473	2.31	1,614	2.32	859	2.29
Detroit, Mi.	6,452	2.46	5,316	2.47	1,136	2.41
Kansas City, Mo.-Ks.	1,925	2.33	1,636	2.33	289	2.30
Los Angeles-Long Beach, Ca.	13,757	2.37	10,809	2.38	2,948	2.31
Miami, Fl.	1,810	2.57	1,746	2.57	64	2.55
Milwaukee, Wi.	4,614	2.64	2,421	2.63	2,193	2.64
Minneapolis-St. Paul, Mn.-Wi.	6,637	2.80	3,273	2.85	3,364	2.75
New York, N.Y.-N.J.	11,610	4.80	9,780	4.83	1,830	4.62
Philadelphia, Pa.-N.J.	6,734	2.65	5,115	2.68	1,619	2.54
St. Louis, Mo.-Il.	4,597	2.40	3,783	2.41	814	2.34
San Francisco-Oakland, Ca.	5,579	2.60	3,934	2.65	1,645	2.49
Seattle-Everett, Wa.	4,146	2.40	2,558	2.42	1,588	2.36
Washington, D.C.-Md.-Va.	2,635	2.65	2,100	2.66	535	2.59

[1]Includes orderlies.
[2]Standard Metropolitan Statistical Areas as defined by the U.S. Office of Management and Budget through February 1974. All metropolitan areas consist of one or more counties.
[3]Part-time employees are those working a schedule regularly calling for fewer weekly hours than those of full-time employees.
SOURCE: U.S. Department of Labor, Bureau of Labor Statistics, *Industry Wage Survey: Nursing Homes and Related Facilities, May 1976*, and individual releases, 1977.

Table IV-D-16. Average Hourly Earnings[1] of Nurses' Aides Employed Full-time and Part-time in Nursing Homes, by Selected Nursing Home Characteristics, 1977

| | Nurses' aide | |
| | Full-time | Part-time |
Nursing home characteristics	Average hourly earnings	Average hourly earnings
Total	$2.76	$2.78
Ownership		
Proprietary	2.64	2.74
Voluntary nonprofit	2.91	2.84
Government	3.15	3.06
Certification		
Skilled nursing facility	3.00	2.83
Skilled nursing facility and		
intermediate care facility	2.80	2.90
Intermediate care facility	2.50	2.56
Not certified	2.66	2.67
Bed size		
Less than 50 beds	2.54	2.62
50-99	2.60	2.67
100-199	2.74	2.78
200 beds or more	3.26	3.25
Location		
Region		
Northeast	3.22	3.04
North Central	2.66	2.72
South	2.49	2.61
West	2.82	2.68
Standard federal administrative region		
Region I	2.77	2.78
Region II	3.64	3.41
Region III	2.90	2.85
Region IV	2.45	2.48
Region V	2.72	2.79
Region VI	2.44	2.73
Region VII	2.49	2.47
Region VIII	2.54	(2)
Region IX	2.95	2.74
Region X	2.63	(2)
Type of facility		
Nursing care	2.77	2.80
Other	2.65	2.62

[1] Includes only nurses' aides who reported salary.
[2] Insufficient number of cases to compute average hourly earnings.

SOURCE: U.S. Department of Health, Education, and Welfare, Public Health Service, Office of Health Research, Statistics, and Technology, National Center for Health Statistics, *The National Nursing Home Survey: 1977 Summary for the United States*, Vital and Health Statistics, Series 13, No. 43, DHEW Publication No. (PHS) 79-1794, 1979, p. 19.

Table IV-D-17. Average Hourly Earnings[1] of Nurses' Aides Employed Full-time and Part-time in Nursing Homes, by Selected Employee Characteristics, 1977

Employee characteristics	Nurses' aide	
	Full-time	Part-time
	Average hourly earnings	Average hourly earnings
Total	$2.76	$2.78
Racial/ethnic background		
White (not Hispanic)	2.71	2.79
Black (not Hispanic)	2.91	2.75
Hispanic	(2)	(2)
Other	2.79	(2)
Sex		
Male	3.08	(2)
Female	2.74	2.78
Age group		
Under 35 years	2.64	2.70
35-44	2.90	2.98
45-54	2.91	2.94
55 years and over	2.91	2.79
Years of education		
Less than 12 years	2.76	2.76
12	2.73	2.78
13-14	2.77	2.82
15-16	3.07	(2)
17 years or more	(2)	(2)
Years of current employment		
Less than 2 years	2.58	2.66
2-4	2.91	2.95
5-9	3.03	3.07
10 years or more	3.13	2.77
Years of total experience		
Less than 5 years	2.64	2.70
5-9	2.90	2.90
10-14	3.00	3.08
15 years or more	3.13	2.98
Benefits		
Paid vacation, sick leave	2.80	2.85
Other leave[3]	2.81	2.80
Pension	3.31	3.25
Health, life insurance	2.96	2.92
Direct medical benefits	3.10	2.90
Meals	2.83	2.68
Employment arrangement		
Contract	3.02	2.78
On staff	2.75	2.78

[1]Includes only nurses' aides who reported salary.
[2]Insufficient number of cases to compute average hourly earnings.
[3]Includes civil and personal leave (jury duty, military reserves, voting, funerals) and release time for attending training institutes.

SOURCE: U.S. Department of Health, Education, and Welfare, Public Health Service, Office of Health Research, Statistics, and Technology, National Center for Health Statistics, The National Nursing Home Survey: 1977 Summary for the United States, Vital and Health Statistics, Series 13, No. 43, DHEW Publication No. (PHS) 79-1794, 1979, p. 22.

Chapter IV, Section E
LICENSURE FOR PRACTICE OF PRACTICAL NURSES

Practical nurses or vocational nurses are licensed under the nursing practice act legislation in each state. The term "licensed vocational nurse" rather than "licensed practical nurse" is used in California and Texas. Within this section, vocational nurses are included in the counts of practical nurses.

While the majority of the jurisdictions have practice acts that include both registered nurses and licensed practical nurses, 12 states have separate regulations. In all but nine states, the nursing practice acts are administered by a board having jurisdiction over both registered nurse licensure and practical nurse licensure. California, Colorado, Delaware, Georgia, Louisiana, New York, Texas, Washington, and West Virginia have separate boards administering the registered nurse and practical nurse licensure.

The state boards of nursing are surveyed annually by the American Nurses' Association for up-to-date information on licensure within the state. In 1979, 44 states supplied the requested data. Aggregate data reflects the responding states only. In these states, 90.8 percent of the first-time practical nurse candidates who were graduates of schools located within the same state in which they were seeking a license passed the written licensing examination in 1979. Similarly, more than two-fifths (43.4 percent) of this same group passed the exam after retaking it.

There were 464,092 license renewals issued in 1979 from the states reporting licensure renewals. Licenses issued to practical nurses for the first time on the basis of examination totalled 40,700 in 1979. As with the registered nurse licenses, (reported in Chapter I), the total number of current practical nurse licenses is not equivalent to the number of licensed practical nurses in the nation since the licensure figures include multiple licenses held by one nurse. It is for this reason that the American Nurses' Association periodically conducts inventories of licensed practical nurses. In the ANA inventory, the nurse is counted only once, regardless of the number of licenses held. The inventory is the sole source of data on the numbers and characteristics of licensed practical nurses. Selected data from the last study, conducted in 1974, are presented in Chapter IV, Section A.

In 1979, 17 jurisdictions reported having a minimum age requirement, and 6 had citizenship requirements for obtaining a license. Licensing fees for practical nurses in 1980 were also reported by the state boards of nursing. Fees charged for renewal of licenses ranged from $1.00 to $25.00. For practical nurse candidates applying for licensure by examination, the fees varied from $5.00 to $60.00.

Table IV-E-1. Licenses Renewed for Practical Nurses, 1976-1979

State or territory	Type of renewal and licensing period	Number of licenses renewed during			
		1976	1977	1978	1979
Total		597,984	427,394	509,496	464,092
Alabama	Annual	10,589	12,680	...	...
	Biennial (1/1/even year-12/31/odd year)	...	...	[1]12,797	107
Alaska	Biennial (7/1/even year-6/30/even year)	513	...	706	5
Arizona	Annual (calendar)	4,716	4,581	5,289	5,654
Arkansas	Biennial (5/1/even year-4/30/even year)	8,033	...	(2)	(2)
California	Biennial (birthdate)	41,183	(3)	(3)	(3)
Colorado	Biennial (7/1/even year-6/30/even year)	[1]6,269	(2)	(3)	(3)
Connecticut	Annual (calendar)	[4]7,970	[4]8,287	[4]8,288	[4]9,898
Delaware	Biennial (1/1/odd year-12/31/even year)	1,661	60	1,232	320
District of Columbia .	Annual (fiscal)	(3)	(3)	(3)	(3)
Florida	Annual	22,517	24,203	25,789	25,960
Georgia	Biennial (1/1/odd year-12/31/even year)	16,904	(3)	(2)	[4]19,028
Guam	Annual (fiscal)	67	70	81	101
Hawaii	Annual (fiscal)	[1]2,518	...	...	...
	Biennial (7/1/odd year-6/30/odd year)	...	2,713	...	[5]3,275
Idaho	Annual (fiscal)	[1]3,046	[1]3,276	...	...
	Biennial (7/1/even year-6/30/even year)	...	...	[1]3,207	...
Illinois	Annual	25,326	(3)	...	...
	Biennial (5/1/even year-4/30/even year)	...	...	[1]27,270	[1]3,412
Indiana	Biennial (1/1/even year-12/31/even year)	[1]8,913	[1]9,721	[1]10,019	[1]11,038
Iowa	Annual (fiscal)	[1]8,218	[1]8,772	[1]9,382	[1]10,052
Kansas	Biennial (birthdate-even or odd year)	[1]5,756	[1]6,434	[6]6,785	[6]6,753
Kentucky	Annual	8,631	9,013	9,377	9,387
Louisiana	Annual (calendar)	[1]10,900	[1]11,418	[1]12,278	[1]12,852
Maine	Annual (fiscal)	2,995	3,483	3,549	3,573
Maryland	Biennial (2/1/odd year-1/31/even year)	[4]4,563	4,866	5,044	5,232
Massachusetts	Biennial (birthdate-odd year)	[1]2,258	[1]23,232	(3)	(3)
Michigan	Annual	[1]29,043	(3)	[1]33,899	[1]35,859
Minnesota	Annual (calendar)	[1]13,526	12,613	(3)	(3)
Mississippi	Annual (fiscal)	6,579	6,576	...	...
	Biennial (1/1/odd year-12/31/even year)	...	...	6,755	...
Missouri	Annual (fiscal)	[1]13,153	[1]14,023	(2)	[1]13,761
Montana	Annual (calendar)	[4]2,230	2,547	2,626	2,598
Nebraska	Annual (calendar)	[1]5,193	[1]5,667	[1]6,062	[1]5,946
Nevada	Biennial (3/1/even year-2/28/even year)	1,644	...	1,761	...
New Hampshire	Biennial (birthdate)	1,678	1,069	2,097	853
New Jersey	Biennial (1/1/even or odd year-12/31/odd or even year)	[8]21,805	[1]4,457	[1]16,192	[1]7,539
New Mexico	Biennial (birthdate-even year)	3,178	61	3,352	137
New York	Biennial (9/1/even year-8/31/even year)	[9]63,765	[4]67,339	67,084	71,013
North Carolina	Biennial (1/1/even or odd year-12/31/odd or even year)	7,307	[1]3,292	[1]9,375	[1]6,043
North Dakota	Annual (calendar)	2,143	2,398	2,469	2,630
Ohio	Annual (calendar)	[4]35,538	[4]37,270	37,970	39,098
Oklahoma	Annual (fiscal)	8,420	8,721	9,177	9,620
Oregon	Biennial (4/1/even year-3/31/even year)	4,918	(3)	5,214	...
Pennsylvania	Biennial (7/1/even year-6/30/even year)	[1]44,118	[1]923	[1]44,998	1,130
Rhode Island	Annual	[10]3,517	[1]3,494	[5]3,494	[5]3,534
South Carolina	Annual (calendar)	6,430	5,962	7,382	8,455
South Dakota	Annual (calendar)	2,796	(3)	...	...
	Biennial (birthdate-even or odd year)	...	...	280	2,012
Tennessee	Biennial (1/1/even year-12/31/odd year)	16,033	[11]15,956	[1]16,892	[1]18,120
Texas	Annual	[1]50,981	53,600	55,918	57,749
Utah	Annual (calendar)	3,558	[12]3,772	(3)	(3)
Vermont	Biennial (5/1/even year-4/30/even year)	2,174	...	2,244	...
Virgin Islands	Annual (fiscal)	[4]184	192	184	182
Virginia	Annual (birthdate)	[13]14,490	[4]13,309	[9]14,732	[14]16,427
Washington	Annual (birthdate)	12,257	12,684	12,635	16,017
West Virginia	Annual (fiscal)	5,162	5,339	5,611	5,870
Wisconsin	Annual (fiscal)	[1]11,955	...	...	...
	Biennial (7/1/odd year-6/30/odd year)	...	[1]12,538	...	[1]12,852
Wyoming	Annual (fiscal)	663	783	(3)	(3)

[1]Includes reinstatements.
[2]Information not available.
[3]Not reported.
[4]Current registration as of December 31.
[5]Current registration as of June 30.
[6]Current registration as of April 30.
[7]Even or odd year based on last digit of registration number.
[8]Current registration for licensing period of 1/1/75-12/31/76.
[9]Estimated.
[10]Current registration as of July 1.
[11]Current registration as of June 1.
[12]Current registration as of May 1978.
[13]Current registration as of January 31.
[14]Current registration as of November 1.

SOURCE: American Nurses' Association, Research and Policy Analysis Department, Statistics Unit, special tabulations from licensure table update sheets, 1980.

Table IV-E-2. Licenses Issued to Practical Nurses Previously Licensed in the U.S.,[1] by Method of Licensure and State Issuing License, 1978 and 1979

State or territory	1978			1979		
	Endorse-ment	Exami-nation	Reinstate-ment	Endorse-ment	Exami-nation	Reinstate-ment
Total	12,524	315	2,833	13,837	368	1,568
Alabama	259	4	(2)	240	5	(2)
Alaska	101	3	...	124	3	10
Arizona	527	30	...	578	37	...
Arkansas	(3)	(3)	(3)	(3)	(3)	(3)
California	(4)	(4)	(4)	(4)	(4)	(4)
Colorado	(4)	(4)	(4)	(4)	(4)	(4)
Connecticut	223	...	1	215	...	...
Delaware	69	...	17	46	...	33
District of Columbia	(4)	(4)	(4)	(4)	(4)	(4)
Florida	1,774	...	...	1,930	...	...
Georgia	381	...	(2)	444	...	(2)
Guam	8	...	3	5	...	1
Hawaii	184	4	(2)	...	7	(2)
Idaho	131	8	(2)	140	8	(2)
Illinois	504	...	(2)	456	...	(2)
Indiana	307	...	(2)	354	...	(2)
Iowa	239	...	(2)	210	...	(2)
Kansas	259	...	(2)	244	...	(2)
Kentucky	273	...	147	273	...	171
Louisiana	288	...	(2)	307	...	(2)
Maine	124	...	208	149	...	190
Maryland	376	...	...	351	...	...
Massachusetts	(4)	(4)	(4)	(4)	(4)	(4)
Michigan	314	6	(2)	406	2	(2)
Minnesota	(4)	(4)	(4)	(4)	(4)	(4)
Mississippi	172	...	563	210	...	88
Missouri	(3)	(3)	(3)	424	4	(2)
Montana	123	...	...	92	...	...
Nebraska	139	...	(2)	122	2	(2)
Nevada	173	...	129	136	...	21
New Hampshire	202	1	148	163	2	71
New Jersey	308	...	(2)	317	...	(2)
New Mexico	209	...	119	192	...	...
New York	...	247	...	...	293	...
North Carolina	325	...	(2)	402	...	(2)
North Dakota	71	...	...	79	...	...
Ohio	406	...	...	422	...	...
Oklahoma	362	...	260	317	...	222
Oregon	349	...	204	322	...	76
Pennsylvania	291	2	(2)	297	...	(2)
Rhode Island	64	...	(2)	94	...	(2)
South Carolina	220	...	(2)	253	...	(2)
South Dakota	65	...	...	86	...	...
Tennessee	300	...	...	362	...	...
Texas	1,003	...	(2)	1,217	...	(2)
Utah	(4)	(4)	(4)	(4)	(4)	(4)
Vermont	82	1	105	73	...	...
Virgin Islands	10	...	...	15	...	...
Virginia	488	9	(2)	469	5	(2)
Washington	360	...	684	880	...	425
West Virginia	208	...	245	182	...	260
Wisconsin	253	...	...	239	...	...
Wyoming	(4)	(4)	(4)	(4)	(4)	(4)

[1]Includes foreign nurses previously licensed in the U.S. or territories.
[2]Reinstatements included in renewals, see Table IV-E-1.
[3]Information not available.
[4]Not reported.

SOURCE: American Nurses' Association, Research and Policy Analysis Department, Statistics Unit, special tabulations from licensure table update sheets, 1980.

Table IV-E-3. Licenses Issued to Practical Nurses for the First Time in the U.S., by Method of Licensure and State Issuing License, 1978 and 1979

State or territory	1978				1979			
	Total	Waiver	Examination[1]	Endorsement[2]	Total	Waiver	Examination[1]	Endorsement[2]
Total	[3]39,771	26	[3]39,558	187	[3]40,915	26	[3]40,700	189
Alabama	1,069	...	1,069	...	1,018	...	1,018	...
Alaska	27	...	27	...	25	...	25	...
Arizona	468	...	468	...	497	...	497	...
Arkansas	(4)	(4)	(4)	(4)	(4)	(4)	(4)	(4)
California	(5)	(5)	(5)	(5)	(5)	(5)	(5)	(5)
Colorado	(5)	(5)	(5)	(5)	(5)	(5)	(5)	(5)
Connecticut	492	...	492	...	424	...	424	...
Delaware	116	...	116	...	71	...	71	...
District of Columbia	(5)	(5)	(5)	(5)	(5)	(5)	(5)	(5)
Florida	2,403	...	2,403	...	2,565	...	2,565	...
Georgia	1,553	...	1,553	...	1,925	...	1,925	...
Guam	39	...	39	...	29	...	29	...
Hawaii	190	...	190	...	160	...	160	...
Idaho	186	...	186	...	203	...	203	...
Illinois	2,187	...	2,187	...	2,093	...	2,093	...
Indiana	850	...	850	...	758	...	758	...
Iowa	1,094	...	1,094	...	1,092	...	1,092	...
Kansas	(4)	(4)	(4)	(4)	(4)	(4)	(4)	(4)
Kentucky	480	...	480	...	491	...	491	...
Louisiana	858	...	858	...	1,028	...	1,028	...
Maine	280	...	269	11	301	...	296	5
Maryland	444	...	444	...	375	...	375	...
Massachusetts	(5)	(5)	(5)	(5)	(5)	(5)	(5)	(5)
Michigan	1,775	...	1,775	...	1,606	...	1,606	...
Minnesota	(5)	(5)	(5)	(5)	(5)	(5)	(5)	(5)

Mississippi	687		687		619		619	
Missouri	(4)	(4)	(4)	(4)	1,025		1,025	
Montana	204		204		176		176	
Nebraska	421		421		392		392	
Nevada	304		130	174	311		132	179
New Hampshire	132		132		151		151	
New Jersey	2,052		2,052		1,883		1,883	
New Mexico	290		290		332		329	3
New York	5,586		5,586		5,623		5,623	
North Carolina	992		991	1	1,049		1,049	1
North Dakota	307		307		298		297	
Ohio	2,027	1	2,026		2,039	2	2,037	1
Oklahoma	653		653		712		712	
Oregon	475		475		384		384	
Pennsylvania	2,226		2,225	1	2,728		2,727	1
Rhode Island	146		146		106		106	
South Carolina	617		617		516		516	
South Dakota	280	25	255		252	24	228	
Tennessee	992		992		974		974	
Texas	3,312		3,312		3,400		3,400	
Utah	(5)	(5)	(5)	(5)	(5)	(5)	(5)	(5)
Vermont	163		163		135		135	
Virgin Islands	2		2		10		10	
Virginia	1,033		1,033		1,003		1,003	
Washington	849		849		757		757	
West Virginia	427		427		400		400	
Wisconsin	1,083		1,083		979		979	
Wyoming	(5)	(5)	(5)	(5)	(5)	(5)	(5)	(5)

[1] Includes some foreign nurses required to write the SBTP examination but licensed through the endorsement procedure.
[2] License issued on the basis of license or certificate issued by foreign country.
[3] Includes some foreign nurses previously licensed in the U.S.
[4] Information not available.
[5] Not reported.

SOURCE: American Nurses' Association, Research and Policy Analysis Department, Statistics Unit, special tabulations from licensure table update sheets, 1980.

Table IV-E-4. Practical Nurse Licensing Examination

| | State graduates | | | | | | Out-of-state | | |
| | First time candidates | | | Retakes | | | First time candidates | | |
State or territory	Number written	Number passed	Percent passed	Number written	Number passed	Percent passed	Number written	Number passed	Percent passed
Alabama	1,070	952	89.0	140	48	34.3	16	16	100.0
Alaska	12	12	100.0	2	...	...	12	11	91.7
Arizona	439	427	97.3	10	6	60.0	25	23	92.0
Arkansas	(1)	(1)	(1)	(1)	(1)	(1)	(1)	(1)	(1)
California	(2)	(2)	(2)	(2)	(2)	(2)	(2)	(2)	(2)
Colorado	(2)	(2)	(2)	(2)	(2)	(2)	(2)	(2)	(2)
Connecticut	387	386	99.7	1	...	...	32	28	87.5
Delaware	67	63	94.0	12	5	41.7	3	3	100.0
District of Columbia	(2)	(2)	(2)	(2)	(2)	(2)	(2)	(2)	(2)
Florida	1,682	1,612	95.8	801	593	74.0	51	50	98.0
Georgia	[1]1,890	[1]1,190	[1]63.0	...	...	...	...	...	...
Guam	25	21	84.0	7	4	57.1	...	...	...
Hawaii	115	113	98.3	7	4	57.1	25	21	84.0
Idaho	168	165	98.2	3	2	66.7	25	21	84.0
Illinois	2,114	1,961	92.8	219	112	51.1	12	12	100.0
Indiana	734	717	97.7	17	13	76.5	29	26	89.7
Iowa	[5]1,066	[5]1,054	[5]98.9	[5]28	[5]13	[5]46.4	18	17	94.4
Kansas	[3]498	[3]477	[3]95.8	[3]40	[3]16	[3]40.0	...	...	...
Kentucky	481	439	91.3	56	18	32.1	20	17	85.0
Louisiana	1,051	955	90.9	107	42	39.3	14	12	85.7
Maine	[6]325	[6]308	[6]94.8	[6]11	[6]5	[6]45.5	14	14	100.0
Maryland	378	347	91.8	43	26	60.5	37	30	81.1
Massachusetts	(2)	(2)	(2)	(2)	(2)	(2)	(2)	(2)	(2)
Michigan	1,546	1,527	98.8	56	31	55.4	46	44	95.7
Minnesota	(2)	(2)	(2)	(2)	(2)	(2)	(2)	(2)	(2)
Mississippi	658	569	86.5	109	46	42.2	3	3	100.0
Missouri	1,021	989	96.9	57	25	43.9	6	6	100.0
Montana	141	135	95.7	9	5	55.6	11	10	90.9
Nebraska	346	343	99.1	5	4	80.0	5	4	80.0
Nevada	91	87	95.6	1	1	100.0	51	43	84.3
New Hampshire	135	132	97.8	1	1	100.0	18	18	100.0
New Jersey	[5]1,887	[5]1,570	[5]83.2	363	88	24.2	13	12	92.3
New Mexico	298	290	97.3	21	8	38.1	22	17	77.3
New York	2,810	2,250	80.1	974	302	31.0	59	52	88.1
North Carolina	1,059	976	92.2	133	53	39.8	13	13	100.0
North Dakota	266	256	96.2	15	10	66.7	23	22	95.7
Ohio	1,981	1,943	98.1	39	24	61.5	69	64	92.8
Oklahoma	(7)	(7)	(7)	(7)	(7)	(7)	(7)	(7)	(7)
Oregon	309	300	97.1	81	67	82.7	14	14	100.0
Pennsylvania	2,744	2,620	95.5	293	88	30.0	32	29	90.6
Rhode Island	92	87	94.6	6	1	16.7	4	4	100.0
South Carolina	515	468	90.9	70	31	44.3	9	9	100.0
South Dakota	180	176	97.8	7	4	57.1	12	11	91.7
Tennessee	1,022	898	87.9	217	60	27.6	32	30	93.8
Texas	3,346	3,008	89.9	550	219	39.8	45	40	88.9
Utah	(2)	(2)	(2)	(2)	(2)	(2)	(2)	(2)	(2)
Vermont	[5]132	[5]129	[5]97.7	2	2	100.0	4	4	100.0
Virgin Islands	11	9	81.8	1	...	...	...	...	...
Virginia	972	900	92.6	168	56	33.3	46	41	89.1
Washington	732	684	93.4	37	12	32.4	86	67	77.9
West Virginia	405	380	95.9	19	5	26.3	14	13	92.9
Wisconsin	[3]942	[5]885	[5]93.9	44	25	56.8	65	60	92.3
Wyoming	(2)	(2)	(2)	(2)	(2)	(2)	(2)	(2)	(2)

[1] Information not available.
[2] Not reported.
[3] Includes out-of-state and foreign nurse candidates.
[4] Includes foreign nurse graduates who repeated the examination.

SOURCE: American Nurses' Association, Research and Policy Analysis Department, Statistics Unit, special

Given by State and Territorial Boards, 1979

graduates			Foreign nurse graduates					
	Retakes		First time candidates			Retakes		
Number written	Number passed	Percent passed	Number written	Number passed	Percent passed	Number written	Number passed	Percent passed
2	2	100.0	1	...	...	1	...	...
1	...	...	5	2	40.0	2	...	...
8	1	12.5	47	30	63.8	...	...	...
(1)	(1)	(1)	(1)	(1)	(1)	(1)	(1)	(1)
(2)	(2)	(2)	(2)	(2)	(2)	(2)	(2)	(2)
(2)	(2)	(2)	(2)	(2)	(2)	(2)	(2)	(2)
1	...	...	16	6	37.5	5	1	20.0
1	...	...	...	...	...	...	...	...
(2)	(2)	(2)	(2)	(2)	(2)	(2)	(2)	(2)
32	14	43.8	296	234	79.1	205	115	56.1
...	...	...	...	...	...	...	...	...
...	...	...	12	4	33.3	4	...	...
12	6	50.0	41	17	41.5	42	6	14.3
9	9	100.0	2	2	100.0	...	...	...
7	4	57.1	⁴14	⁴4	⁴28.6	...	...	...
3	2	66.7	...	...	...	...	...	...
...	...	...	⁵13	⁵5	⁵38.5	⁵6	⁵3	⁵50.0
...	...	...	...	...	...	...	...	...
9	3	33.3	...	...	...	...	...	...
31	19	61.3	...	...	...	...	...	...
...	...	...	...	...	...	3	2	66.7
8	4	50.0	2	...	...	6	2	33.3
(2)	(2)	(2)	(2)	(2)	(2)	(2)	(2)	(2)
2	2	100.0	1	...	...	...	...	...
(2)	(2)	(2)	(2)	(2)	(2)	(2)	(2)	(2)
1	1	100.0	...	...	...	...	...	...
2	1	50.0	1	1	100.0	...	...	...
...	...	...	1	...	...	...	...	...
1	...	...	...	...	...	...	...	...
1	1	100.0	...	...	...	...	...	...
2	1	50.0	...	...	...	2	1	50.0
36	12	33.3	201	131	65.2	141	70	49.6
18	12	66.7	2	1	50.0	1	1	100.0
10	4	40.0	707	356	50.4	1,267	351	27.7
...	...	...	2	1	50.0	...	...	...
1	...	...	10	8	80.0	1	1	100.0
7	4	57.1	2	2	100.0	...	...	...
(7)	(7)	(7)	(7)	(7)	(7)	(7)	(7)	(7)
2	1	50.0	...	...	...	...	...	...
6	5	83.3	1	...	...	2	...	...
1	...	...	...	...	...	...	...	...
6	4	66.7	7	2	28.6	5	2	40.0
3	2	66.7	...	...	...	...	...	...
15	3	20.0	2	1	50.0	...	...	...
15	11	73.3	135	104	77.0	36	18	50.0
(2)	(2)	(2)	(2)	(2)	(2)	(2)	(2)	(2)
...	...	...	...	...	...	...	...	...
...	...	...	8	2	25.0	5	5	100.0
6	3	50.0	5	3	60.0	...	...	...
15	5	33.3	21	6	28.6	7	...	...
3	2	66.7	...	...	...	...	...	...
10	5	50.0	4	3	75.0	2	1	50.0
(2)	(2)	(2)	(2)	(2)	(2)	(2)	(2)	(2)

⁵Includes candidates who qualified on basis of equivalency.
⁶Includes candidates who qualified on basis of equivalency and by armed service qualifications.
⁷Permission to publish withheld.

tabulations from licensure table update sheets, 1980.

Table IV-E-5. Licenses Issued to Practical Nurses from Foreign Countries,[1] by Method of Licensure and State Issuing Licenses, 1978 and 1979

	1978			1979		
State or territory	Total	Exami-nation[2]	Endorse-ment	Total	Exami-nation[2]	Endorse-ment
Total	1,460	1,449	11	1,040	1,028	12
Alabama	...	...	...	...	...	...
Alaska	2	2	...	2	2	...
Arizona	1	1	...	30	30	...
Arkansas	(3)	(3)	(3)	(3)	(3)	(3)
California	(4)	(4)	(4)	(4)	(4)	(4)
Colorado	(4)	(4)	(4)	(4)	(4)	(4)
Connecticut	9	9	...	7	7	...
Delaware	...	...	...	...	...	...
District of Columbia	(4)	(4)	(4)	(4)	(4)	(4)
Florida	642	642	...	349	349	...
Georgia	(3)	(3)	(3)	(3)	(3)	(3)
Guam	4	4	...	4	4	...
Hawaii	23	23	...	23	23	...
Idaho	...	...	...	2	2	...
Illinois	2	2	...	4	4	...
Indiana	...	...	...	...	...	...
Iowa	7	7	...	8	8	...
Kansas	(3)	(3)	(3)	(3)	(3)	(3)
Kentucky	...	...	...	1	...	1
Louisiana	...	...	...	...	...	...
Maine	9	3	6	4	2	2
Maryland	2	2	...	2	2	...
Massachusetts	(4)	(4)	(4)	(4)	(4)	(4)
Michigan	...	...	...	...	...	...
Minnesota	(4)	(4)	(4)	(4)	(4)	(4)
Mississippi	2	2	...	...	...	...
Missouri	(3)	(3)	(3)	1	1	...
Montana	1	1	...	...	...	...
Nebraska	...	...	...	...	...	...
Nevada	1	...	1	2	...	2
New Hampshire	2	1	1	2	1	1
New Jersey	...	...	...	...	...	...
New Mexico	...	...	...	2	1	1
New York	636	636	...	440	440	...
North Carolina	1	...	1	1	1	...
North Dakota	12	12	...	10	9	1
Ohio	1	1	...	2	2	...
Oklahoma	...	...	...	...	...	...
Oregon	1	1	...	...	...	...
Pennsylvania	1	...	1	1	...	1
Rhode Island	1	1	...	...	...	...
South Carolina	1	1	...	4	4	...
South Dakota	...	...	...	...	...	...
Tennessee	2	1	1	...	...	...
Texas	91	91	...	122	122	...
Utah	(4)	(4)	(4)	(4)	(4)	(4)
Vermont	1	1	...	...	...	...
Virgin Islands	...	...	...	1	1	...
Virginia	1	1	...	6	3	3
Washington	1	1	...	6	6	...
West Virginia	...	...	...	...	...	...
Wisconsin	3	3	...	4	4	...
Wyoming	(4)	(4)	(4)	(4)	(4)	(4)

[1] Includes those being licensed for the first time and those previously licensed in another state or territory of the U.S.
[2] Includes some foreign nurses required to write the SBTP examination but licensed through the endorsement procedure.
[3] Information not available.
[4] Not reported.

SOURCE: American Nurses' Association, Research and Policy Analysis Department, Statistics Unit, special tabulations from licensure table update sheets, 1980.

Table IV-E-6. Citation and Chronology of Separate Nursing Practice Acts for Practical Nurses, 1980

State or territory	Citation	Year first law enacted	Amendments to first law	Year of repeal and enactment of new law	Amendments to new law
California	Vocational Nursing Practice Act, Business and Professional Code, Division 2, Chapter 6.5-September 1951.	1951	1954, '56, '57, '59, '61, '63, '64, '65, '67, '68, '69, '70, '71, '72, '73, '74, '75, '77	...	...
Colorado	Colorado Revised Statutes, 1963, as amended. Chapter 97, Article 4.	1957	1961, '63	1967	1977
District of Columbia	Public law 86-708.	1960	1966	...	...
Georgia	Act No. 351, p. 333, Georgia Laws 1953.	1953	1974, '77	...	...
Louisiana	Louisiana Revised Statutes of 1950, Title 37, Chapter 11, Part 11.	1948	1950, '54, '68, '76, '77	...	...
Minnesota	Minnesota Statutes, Sections 148.171-148.299. (1976).	1947	1955, '61, '65, '67, '69, '71, '73, '75, '76	...	...
North Dakota	Laws of State of North Dakota Relating to Practical Nursing, N.D. Century Code, 43-21.1.	1947	1958, '63, '71, '77	...	...
Pennsylvania	Practical Nurse Law, 63 P.S. 651 et seq.	1919	1923, '27, '35, 45	1956	1961, '66, '68, '72
Texas	Article 4528c of Vernon's Texas Civil Statutes, Section 8A, as amended 1954, 1957, 1963, 1967, 1971, and 1973.	1951	1954, '57, '63, '67, '71, '73	...	...
Washington	Chapter 222, Laws of 1949.	1949	1961, '63, '67, '71	...	...
West Virginia	Chapter 30, Code of West Virginia 1931, amended 1957, Article 7A.	1957	...	1967	1973

SOURCE: American Nurses' Association, Research and Policy Analysis Department, Statistics Unit, special tabulations from licensure table update sheets, 1980.

Table IV-E-7. Nursing Practice Acts for Practical Nurses, 1979

State or territory	Year first law enacted	Separate law[1]	State or territory	Year first law enacted	Separate law[1]
Alabama	1945	No	Montana	1953	No
Alaska	1953	No	Nebraska	1955	No
Arizona	1952	No	Nevada	1949	No
Arkansas	1947	No	New Hampshire	1951	No
California	1951	Yes	New Jersey	1947	No
Colorado	1957	Yes	New Mexico	1953	No
Connecticut	1935	No	New York	1938	No
Delaware	1955	No	North Carolina	1947	No
District of Columbia	1960	Yes	North Dakota	1947	Yes
Florida	1919	No	Ohio	1956	No
Georgia	1953	Yes	Oklahoma	1953	No
Guam	1952	No	Oregon	1949	No
Hawaii	1947	No	Pennsylvania	1919	Yes
Idaho	1947	No	Rhode Island	1948	No
Illinois	1951	No	South Carolina	1947	No
Indiana	1921	No	South Dakota	1949	No
Iowa	1949	No	Tennessee	1945	No
Kansas	1949	No	Texas	1951	Yes
Kentucky	1950	No	Utah	1949	No
Louisiana	1948	Yes	Vermont	1951	No
Maine	1945	No	Virgin Islands	1945	Yes
Maryland	1922	No	Virginia	1946	No
Massachusetts	1941	No	Washington	1949	Yes
Michigan	1952	No	West Virginia	1957	Yes
Minnesota	1947	Yes	Wisconsin	1943	No
Mississippi	1954	No	Wyoming	1955	No
Missouri	1953	No			

[1] For the citation of the acts which are not separate from the registered nurse acts, refer to table in Chapter I, Section H. For the citation of the acts which are separate from the act covering registered nurses in the state, see Table IV-E-6 in this section.

SOURCE: American Nurses' Association, Research and Policy Analysis Department, Statistics Unit, special tabulations from licensure table update sheets, 1980.

Table IV-E-8. Type of Agency Administering Practical Nurse Licensure, 1980

State or territory	Administered by: State board of nursing	Administered by: Separate board	State or territory	Administered by: State board of nursing	Administered by: Separate board
Alabama	X	...	Montana	X	...
Alaska	X	...	Nebraska	X	...
Arizona	X	...	Nevada	X	...
Arkansas	X	...	New Hampshire	X	...
California	...	X	New Jersey	X	...
Colorado	...	X	New Mexico ...	X	...
Connecticut	X	...	New York	...	X
Delaware	...	X	North Carolina	X	...
District of Columbia	X	...	North Dakota ...	X	...
Florida	X	...	Ohio	X	...
Georgia	...	X	Oklahoma	X	...
Guam	X	...	Oregon	X	...
Hawaii	X	...	Pennsylvania ...	X	...
Idaho	X	...	Rhode Island ...	X	...
Illinois	X	...	South Carolina	X	...
Indiana	X	...	South Dakota ...	X	...
Iowa	X	...	Tennessee	X	...
Kansas	X	...	Texas	...	X
Kentucky	X	...	Utah	X	...
Louisiana	...	X	Vermont	X	...
Maine	X	...	Virgin Islands ...	X	...
Maryland	X	...	Virginia	X	...
Massachusetts	X	...	Washington	...	X
Michigan	X	...	West Virginia ...	...	X
Minnesota	X	...	Wisconsin	X	...
Mississippi	X	...	Wyoming	X	...
Missouri	X	...			

SOURCE: American Nurses' Association, Research and Policy Analysis Department, Statistics Unit, special tabulations from licensure table update sheets, 1980.

Table IV-E-9. Minimum Age and Citizenship Requirement of Nursing Practice Acts for Practical Nurses, 1979

State or territory	Minimum age	Citizenship	State or territory	Minimum age	Citizenship
Alabama	...	...	Montana	...	...
Alaska	18	...	Nebraska	18	...
Arizona	...	...	Nevada	18	...
Arkansas	...	...	New Hampshire	...	...
California	17	...	New Jersey	18	...
Colorado	...	Yes	New Mexico	...	...
Connecticut	...	...	New York	17	...
Delaware	...	...	North Carolina	...	...
District of Columbia	18	...	North Dakota	...	...
Florida	...	...	Ohio	18	...
Georgia	18	...	Oklahoma	...	...
Guam	...	...	Oregon	...	...
Hawaii	...	...	Pennsylvania	...	...
Idaho	...	...	Rhode Island	...	...
Illinois	18	Yes[1]	South Carolina	18	...
Indiana	...	...	South Dakota	...	Yes[2]
Iowa	...	...	Tennessee	...	...
Kansas	...	...	Texas	18	Yes[1]
Kentucky	18	...	Utah	...	...
Louisiana	...	Yes	Vermont	18	...
Maine	...	...	Virgin Islands	...	...
Maryland	...	...	Virginia	...	...
Massachusetts	...	...	Washington	18	...
Michigan	...	...	West Virginia	...	...
Minnesota	...	...	Wisconsin	18	Yes[1]
Mississippi	...	...	Wyoming	...	...
Missouri	18	...			

[1] Citizenship requirement still included in Act but not enforced based on Supreme Court ruling.
[2] Or registered "resident alien."

SOURCE: American Nurses' Association, Research and Policy Analysis Department, Statistics Unit, special tabulations from licensure table update sheets, 1980.

Table IV-E-10. Expiration Dates[1] for Renewal of License or Registration for Practical Nurses, 1980

State or territory	Expiration date	State or territory	Expiration date
Alabama	December 31[2]	Montana	December 31
Alaska	June 30[2]	Nebraska	December 31
Arizona	December 31	Nevada	February 28[2]
Arkansas	April 30[2]	New Hampshire	Birthdate[2]
California	Birthdate[2]	New Jersey	December 31[2]
Colorado	June 30[2]	New Mexico	Birthdate[2]
Connecticut	December 31	New York	August 31[2]
Delaware	December 31[2]	North Carolina	December 31[2]
District of Columbia	June 30	North Dakota	December 31
Florida	March 31	Ohio	August 31
Georgia	December 31[2]	Oklahoma	June 30
Guam	June 30	Oregon	March 31[2]
Hawaii	June 30[2]	Pennsylvania	June 30[2]
Idaho	June 30[2]	Rhode Island	March 1
Illinois	May 1[2]	South Carolina	December 31
Indiana	December 31[2]	South Dakota	Birthdate[2]
Iowa	June 30	Tennessee	December 31[2]
Kansas	Birthdate[2]	Texas	August 31
Kentucky	October 31	Utah	December 31
Louisiana	December 31	Vermont	April 30[2]
Maine	June 30	Virgin Islands	June 30
Maryland	January 31[2]	Virginia	Birthdate
Massachusetts	Birthdate[2]	Washington	Birthdate
Michigan	March 31	West Virginia	June 30
Minnesota	December 31	Wisconsin	June 30[2]
Mississippi	December 31[2]	Wyoming	June 30
Missouri	June 30		

[1] Excludes grace period.
[2] Biennial renewal.

SOURCE: American Nurses' Association, Research and Policy Analysis Department, Statistics Unit, special tabulations from licensure table update sheets, 1980.

Table IV-E-11. Selected Fees Charged for Licensure of Practical Nurses, 1980

State or territory	Examination	Endorsement	Renewal[1]	Verification of original license to other boards
Alabama	$45.00	$35.00	[2]$12.00	$ 5.00
Alaska	30.00	30.00	[2]15.00	...
Arizona	50.00	45.00	10.00	...
Arkansas	25.00	25.00	[2]10.00	15.00
California	25.00	25.00	[2]25.00	...
Colorado	30.00	30.00	[2]10.00	5.00
Connecticut	25.00	25.00	5.00	2.00
Delaware	30.00	30.00	[2]10.00	2.00
District of Columbia	(3)	(3)	(3)	(3)
Florida	40.00	20.00	6.00	6.00
Georgia	30.00	30.00	[2]10.00	5.00
Guam	40.00	40.00	8.00	10.00
Hawaii	15.00	15.00	10.00	5.00
Idaho	50.00	50.00	[2]25.00	5.00
Illinois	15.00	15.00	[2]10.00	...
Indiana	25.00	20.00	[2]10.00	...
Iowa	30.00	25.00	6.00	5.00
Kansas	25.00	25.00	[2]12.00	5.00
Kentucky	30.00	35.00	10.00	4.00
Louisiana	25.00	17.00	5.00	2.00
Maine	30.00	30.00	10.00	2.00
Maryland	20.00	20.00	[2]2.00	2.00
Massachusetts	30.00	50.00	[2]6.00	2.00
Michigan	45.00	25.00	5.00	...
Minnesota	40.00	25.00	7.00	5.00
Mississippi	35.00	35.00	[2]8.00	6.00
Missouri	20.00	20.00	5.00	...
Montana	35.00	35.00	10.00	...
Nebraska	35.00	35.00	7.00	5.00
Nevada	40.00	30.00	[2]15.00	...
New Hampshire	30.00	30.00	[2]8.00	5.00
New Jersey	25.00	15.00	[2]10.00	5.00
New Mexico	45.00	38.00	[2]15.00	5.00
New York	60.00	40.00	[2]10.00	10.00
North Carolina	27.00	30.00	[2]12.00	10.00
North Dakota	35.00	35.00	8.00	5.00
Ohio	20.00	20.00	3.00	...
Oklahoma	50.00	50.00	10.00	...
Oregon	35.00	25.00	[2]15.00	...
Pennsylvania	5.00	5.00	[2]2.00	...
Rhode Island	25.00	25.00	5.00	3.00
South Carolina	30.00	30.00	10.00	5.00
South Dakota	25.00	25.00	[2]15.00	5.00
Tennessee	30.00	30.00	[2]8.00	...
Texas	25.00	25.00	5.00	...
Utah	25.00	25.00	7.50	...
Vermont	34.00	25.00	[2]10.00	...
Virgin Islands	5.00	...	1.00	...
Virginia	35.00	30.00	5.00	5.00
Washington	25.00	25.00	8.00	2.00
West Virginia	32.00	25.00	7.50	25.00
Wisconsin	50.00	50.00	[2]25.00	10.00
Wyoming	40.00	40.00	6.00	5.00

[1]Renewal applies to annual registration unless otherwise indicated.
[2]Biennial renewal.
[3]Not reported.

SOURCE: American Nurses' Association, Research and Policy Analysis Department, Statistics Unit, special tabulations from licensure table update sheets, 1980.

Chapter IV, Section F
NATIONAL PRACTICAL NURSING ASSOCIATION

The National Federation of Licensed Practical Nurses is a federation of 39 state associations. In addition, American Samoa is a NFLPN constituent. Practical nursing students may also belong to the NFLPN; however, they are excluded from the basic membership counts. Federation membership totaled 14,412 licensed practical nurses in 1979, 100 of whom were individual members in states where there was no organized group.

Table IV-F-1. Membership in the National Federation of Licensed Practical Nurses, by State or Territory, as of December 31, 1979

State or territory	Number of members	Delegate quota	State or territory	Number of members	Delegate quota
Total	14,412	270			
Alabama	259	6	Nebraska	463	8
Alaska	12	3	Nevada	55	4
American Samoa	48	1	New Hampshire..	79	4
Colorado	128	3	New Mexico ...	88	4
Connecticut	381	7	New York	112	3
Florida	780	11	North Carolina...	890	12
Georgia	473	8	North Dakota ...	186	5
Hawaii	115	3	Ohio	98	4
Idaho	300	6	Oklahoma	633	9
Illinois	1,603	19	Oregon	496	8
Indiana	510	8	Rhode Island ...	122	4
Iowa	364	7	South Carolina...	392	7
Kansas	328	6	Tennessee	805	11
Kentucky	593	8	Texas	66	2
Louisiana	1,229	15	Virginia	529	8
Maine	131	4	West Virginia[1]....	217	1
Maryland	449	7	Wisconsin	663	10
Massachusetts[1]....	87	2	Wyoming	36	3
Minnesota	74	4			
Mississippi	276	6	Individual members[2]	100	2
Missouri	38	3	NFLPN board	[3]15	15
Montana	204	5	NFLPN past presidents ...	[3]4	4

[1]Group.
[2]Individual members in states where there is no organized constituent.
[3]Included in membership count.
SOURCE: National Federation of Licensed Practical Nurses, Inc., 1980. Unpublished data.

Chapter V, Section A
FACILITIES AND UTILIZATION

Annual statistics on hospitals are collected by the American Hospital Association. Trend data are based upon all U.S. hospitals registered with the AHA and excludes information on a small number of nonregistered hospitals. In 1978, about 215 hospitals (3 percent of the total) were not registered with the AHA; however, these hospitals accounted for a very small percentage of the utilization, financial, and personnel indicators, in most cases not exceeding 1 percent.

Recent years have witnessed declining trends in the number of the nation's hospitals. Hospitals totaled 7,015 in 1978, down 0.9 percent since 1976. Concomitantly, there were shifts in utilization trends. Admissions, the total number of times individuals are admitted to hospitals during the year, were on the rise, from 36,775,770 in 1976 to 37,243,182 in 1978. The overall gain was mainly attributable to increases in admissions to short-term facilities, with short-term psychiatric admissions up 7.8 percent and short-term general and other special hospital admissions up 1.5 percent since 1978. On the other hand, admissions to long-term hospitals in each category declined in the same period, with the largest losses observed in long-term general and other special facilities (24.4 percent), followed by long-term tuberculosis (14.5 percent) and long-term psychiatric hospitals (6.8 percent).

The average daily census, a measure of the average number of inpatients receiving care each day, showed a yearly decrease for every year since 1965, when an average of 1,403,000 inpatients were in hospitals per day. The 1978 average daily census figure was 1,041,936, reflecting a 4.4 percent decrease since 1976. The reduction in the average daily census continued to exceed the decline in the number of beds, a fact reflected by the decrease in the national bed occupancy rate. The bed occupancy rate is the rate of average daily patient census to hospital beds. Continuing a 10-year trend, the bed occupancy rate declined to 75.5 percent in 1978. It was 82.9 percent in 1968 and 76.0 percent in 1976. Nongovernment for-profit hospitals had the lowest proportion of occupied beds in 1978, over 10 percentage points below the national average. Long-term general and long-term psychiatric hospitals reported higher occupancy rates, while the tuberculosis hospitals had the lowest.

The 1978 Health Interview Survey, conducted by the National Center for Health Statistics, reports the distribution of persons with short-stay hospital episodes during the past year. Overall, 89.6 percent of the population reported not having a short-term stay in the hospital. About 12.1 percent of the women sampled and 8.5 percent of the men had one or more hospital episodes in 1978. Those in the younger age groups were less likely to have hospital stays than those in the older age group.

The American Osteopathic Hospital Association reported that in 1979 there were 198 osteopathic hospitals, a 3.9 percent decrease from the previous year. The percentage decline in the number of beds was not as great, decreasing 1.2 percent to 24,752. Among the states with the largest number of osteopathic hospitals were Michigan, Texas, and Missouri.

In 1976, there were 20,185 nursing care and related homes in the United States, as determined by the National Center for Health Statistics. This figure reflects a 7.6 percent decline since 1973, when there were 21,834 such homes. The decrease in the aggregate number of facilities was the net result of declines in the numbers of facilities with fewer than 50 beds and gains in the numbers of homes with 50 or more beds. Examination of the trends showed that from 1973 to 1976 there was actually a 6.0 percent increase in the number of beds, from 1,327,704 to 1,406,778 beds. In terms of the distribution of facilities, about 65.9 percent of the nursing care and related homes were nursing care homes and 34.1 percent were personal care and other homes.

In the National Nursing Home Survey, the National Center for Health Statistics also reported that 89.4 percent of nursing home residents in 1976 were in nursing homes with Medicare and/or Medicaid certification. In 1976 there were 1,367,400 admissions to nursing homes. The annual occupancy rate was 89.0 percent.

A health maintenance organization is a health care plan that delivers comprehensive, coordinated medical services to voluntarily enrolled members on a prepaid basis. In 1980, the Office of HMOs of the Public Health Service reported 230 HMOs were in existence, serving 8.9 million people. Membership in HMOs had increased 154 percent since 1971, when there were 39 HMOs serving 3.5 million people.

Table V-A-1. Hospitals in the United States, 1959-1978

Year	Number of hospitals
1978	7,015
1977	7,099
1976	7,082
1975	7,156
1974	7,174
1973	7,123
1972	7,061
1971	7,097
1970	7,123
1969	7,144
1968	7,137
1967	7,172
1966	7,160
1965	7,123
1964	7,127
1963	7,138
1962	7,028
1961	6,923
1960	6,876
1959	6,845

SOURCES: "Guide Issue" of *Hospitals*, Journal of the American Hospital Association, Part II, August 1, 1965, p. 448, American Hospital Association, *Hospital Statistics 1979*, p. 4.

Table V-A-2. Facilities and Utilization of Hospitals in Each State, 1978

State	Hospitals	Beds	Admissions	Average daily census	Percentage of beds occupied
Total	7,015	1,380,645	37,243,182	1,041,936	75.5
Alabama	148	25,242	752,371	19,118	75.7
Alaska	26	1,697	55,026	1,047	61.7
Arizona	78	11,339	381,835	8,287	73.1
Arkansas	96	12,650	437,193	9,016	71.3
California	613	114,836	3,329,040	79,381	69.1
Colorado	101	14,666	461,016	10,373	70.7
Connecticut	64	18,791	453,400	14,587	77.6
Delaware	15	4,099	83,440	3,434	83.8
District of Columbia	19	9,003	206,323	7,613	84.6
Florida	245	54,211	1,608,248	39,922	73.6
Georgia	189	31,146	953,571	21,926	70.4
Hawaii	27	3,813	115,985	2,924	76.7
Idaho	51	3,737	134,023	2,450	65.6
Illinois	285	75,484	2,044,793	57,951	76.8
Indiana	135	33,816	884,030	25,763	76.2
Iowa	141	21,613	576,577	15,125	70.0
Kansas	164	18,161	462,395	12,990	71.5
Kentucky	121	18,815	637,963	14,256	75.8
Louisiana	159	25,128	765,584	17,234	68.6
Maine	53	7,324	182,640	5,348	73.0
Maryland	85	25,210	562,144	20,262	80.4
Massachusetts	189	45,456	936,260	36,085	79.4
Michigan	244	50,661	1,475,922	39,457	77.9
Minnesota	188	31,051	721,385	22,274	71.7
Mississippi	114	16,234	480,422	12,112	74.6
Missouri	167	35,437	972,727	26,286	74.2
Montana	65	5,652	142,825	3,614	63.9
Nebraska	108	11,674	304,679	7,893	67.6
Nevada	25	3,234	112,072	2,095	64.8
New Hampshire	33	4,995	139,011	3,588	71.8
New Jersey	139	44,157	1,085,874	35,386	80.1
New Mexico	54	6,503	193,010	4,424	68.0
New York	368	134,425	2,739,053	114,449	85.1
North Carolina	158	33,774	922,044	25,811	76.4
North Dakota	60	5,830	147,421	4,014	68.9
Ohio	241	64,158	1,846,100	50,674	79.0
Oklahoma	141	17,482	512,410	11,946	68.3
Oregon	85	11,568	372,915	7,607	65.8
Pennsylvania	313	86,474	1,983,899	68,862	79.6
Rhode Island	21	6,700	146,925	5,524	82.4
South Carolina	88	16,919	472,960	12,895	76.2
South Dakota	70	5,676	144,660	3,750	66.1
Tennessee	160	31,008	933,101	24,104	77.7
Texas	565	79,071	2,465,947	55,837	70.6
Utah	41	5,084	204,164	3,581	70.4
Vermont	19	3,036	76,649	2,300	75.8
Virginia	135	32,138	794,746	24,369	75.8
Washington	127	16,138	584,327	11,187	69.3
West Virginia	80	14,170	395,285	10,886	76.8
Wisconsin	171	28,630	779,079	20,327	71.0
Wyoming	31	2,529	69,713	1,592	62.9

SOURCE: American Hospital Association, *Hospital Statistics 1979*, pp. 40-141.

Table V-A-3. Facilities and Utilization of Hospitals, by Type of Service and Control, 1978

Type of service and control	Hospitals	Beds	Admissions	Average daily census	Percentage of beds occupied
Total	7,015	1,380,645	37,243,182	1,041,936	75.5
Federal	370	121,859	1,997,176	95,585	78.4
State and local	2,232	462,187	7,712,300	348,046	75.3
Nongovernment nonprofit	3,532	704,202	24,545,959	538,428	76.5
Nongovernment for profit	881	92,397	2,987,747	59,877	64.8
Long-term psychiatric	375	237,234	440,931	193,812	81.7
Federal	24	23,158	72,362	19,855	85.7
State and local	250	202,640	318,144	164,161	81.0
Nongovernment nonprofit	47	6,274	20,731	5,881	93.7
Nongovernment for profit	54	5,162	29,694	3,915	75.8
Short-term psychiatric	175	20,834	211,633	15,970	76.7
Federal	...	...	...	...	...
State and local	43	12,225	88,800	9,753	79.8
Nongovernment nonprofit	47	3,504	50,293	2,842	81.1
Nongovernment for profit	85	5,105	72,540	3,375	66.1
Long-term tuberculosis	13	2,641	9,112	1,580	59.8
Federal	...	...	...	...	...
State and local	12	2,542	8,676	1,540	60.6
Nongovernment nonprofit	1	99	436	40	40.4
Nongovernment for profit	...	...	...	...	...
Short-term tuberculosis	2	142	1,895	88	62.0
Federal	...	...	...	...	...
State and local	1	63	1,109	48	76.2
Nongovernment nonprofit	1	79	786	40	50.6
Nongovernment for profit	...	...	..	...	...
Long-term general and other special	184	52,228	146,464	43,489	83.3
Federal	15	10,794	66,895	8,677	80.4
State and local	83	29,960	42,792	24,960	83.3
Nongovernment nonprofit	76	10,390	30,956	8,976	86.4
Nongovernment for profit	10	1,084	5,821	876	80.8
Short-term general and other special	6,266	1,067,566	36,433,147	786,997	73.7
Federal	331	87,907	1,857,919	67,053	76.3
State and local	1,843	214,757	7,252,779	147,584	68.7
Nongovernment nonprofit	3,360	683,856	24,442,757	520,649	76.1
Nongovernment for profit	732	81,046	2,879,692	51,711	63.8

SOURCE: American Hospital Association, *Hospital Statistics 1979*, pp. 8-11.

CHART 14.

DISTRIBUTION OF HOSPITALS, BY TYPE OF SERVICE
1978

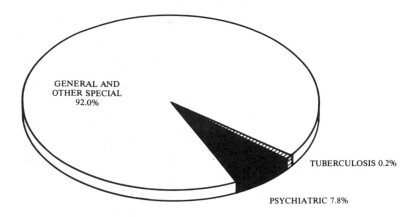

DISTRIBUTION OF HOSPITAL BEDS, BY TYPE OF SERVICE
1978

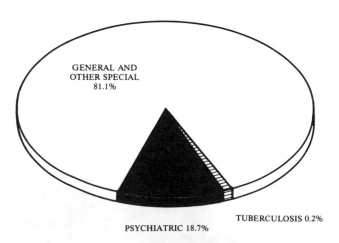

SOURCE: American Hospital Association, *Hospital Statistics 1979*.

Prepared by American Nurses' Association, Research and Policy Analysis Department, Statistics Unit, 1980.

Table V-A-4. Facilities and Utilization of Hospitals, by Type of Control and Size, 1978

Type of control and number of beds	Hospitals	Beds	Admissions	Average daily census	Percentage of beds occupied
Total	7,015	1,380,645	37,243,182	1,041,936	75.5
Under 25 beds	347	6,499	211,674	3,095	47.6
25-49	1,258	45,647	1,445,640	24,452	53.6
50-99	1,660	118,852	3,793,300	75,732	63.7
100-199	1,590	225,024	7,388,090	157,168	69.8
200-299	804	194,453	6,731,480	148,178	76.2
300-399	462	157,497	5,165,637	123,190	78.2
400-499	304	135,007	4,226,109	107,769	79.8
500 and over.....................	590	497,666	8,281,252	402,352	80.8
Federal	370	121,859	1,997,176	95,585	78.4
Under 25 beds	38	629	32,264	335	53.3
25-49	66	2,277	99,089	1,196	52.5
50-99	41	2,832	129,876	1,753	61.9
100-199	45	7,360	212,645	5,233	71.1
200-299	35	8,193	180,321	6,307	77.0
300-399	27	9,530	215,224	7,213	75.7
400-499	31	13,823	257,329	10,979	79.4
500 and over	87	77,215	870,428	62,569	81.0
State and local	2,232	462,187	7,712,300	348,046	75.3
Under 25 beds	144	2,796	81,858	1,220	43.6
25-49	555	20,159	618,299	10,151	50.4
50-99	613	43,280	1,404,047	27,043	62.5
100-199	372	52,572	1,513,422	37,140	70.6
200-299	148	35,841	1,081,220	27,017	75.4
300-399	89	30,980	676,779	24,206	78.1
400-499	67	30,093	649,113	23,328	77.5
500 and over	244	246,466	1,687,562	197,941	80.3
Nongovernment nonprofit	3,532	704,202	24,545,959	538,428	76.5
Under 25 beds	106	2,014	57,784	970	48.2
25-49	450	16,293	500,529	8,971	55.1
50-99	752	54,546	1,702,028	35,780	65.6
100-199	904	127,915	4,511,864	91,260	71.3
200-299	531	129,575	4,751,471	100,448	77.5
300-399	332	112,439	4,107,163	88,396	78.6
400-499	200	88,469	3,221,362	71,416	80.7
500 and over	257	172,951	5,693,758	141,187	81.6
Nongovernment for profit	881	92,397	2,987,747	59,877	64.8
Under 25 beds	59	1,060	39,768	570	53.8
25-49	187	6,918	227,723	4,134	59.8
50-99	254	18,194	557,349	11,156	61.3
100-199	269	37,177	1,150,159	23,535	63.3
200-299	90	20,844	718,468	14,406	69.1
300-399	14	4,548	166,471	3,375	74.2
400-499	6	2,622	98,305	2,046	78.0
500 and over	2	1,034	29,504	655	63.3

SOURCE: American Hospital Association, *Hospital Statistics 1979*, pp. 8-11.

Table V-A-5. Number of Hospital Beds, by Type of Service, 1969-1978

			Hospital beds					
Year	Total	Yearly percent change	General and other special	Yearly percent change	Psychiatric	Yearly percent change	Tuberculosis	Yearly percent change
1978	1,380,645	−1.9	1,119,794	+0.1	258,068	− 9.6	2,783	−16.0
1977	1,407,097	−1.8	1,118,441	+0.4	285,341	− 9.7	3,315	− 7.7
1976	1,433,515	−2.2	1,114,045	+1.0	315,878	−11.6	3,592	−38.6
1975	1,465,828	−3.1	1,102,622	+1.0	357,360	−13.4	5,846	−28.4
1974	1,512,684	−1.4	1,091,941	+1.9	412,581	− 8.8	8,162	−22.0
1973	1,534,726	−1.0	1,071,771	+2.3	452,494	− 7.6	10,461	−18.2
1972	1,549,665	−0.4	1,047,426	+1.6	489,453	− 3.4	12,786	−28.1
1971	1,555,560	−3.7	1,031,363	+0.4	506,424	−10.9	17,773	−10.9
1970	1,615,771	−2.0	1,027,445	+1.6	568,389	− 8.0	19,937	− 4.0
1969	1,649,663	−0.8	1,011,163	+1.7	617,721	− 4.5	20,779	− 7.4
Percent change 1969-1978	−16.3		+10.7		−58.2		−86.6	

SOURCE: "Guide Issue" of *Hospitals*, Journal of the American Hospital Association. Part II, August 1, 1970-1971: *Hospital Statistics 1979*, and previous years

Table V-A-6. Percentage of Beds Occupied, by Type of Service, 1969-1978

			Percentage of beds occupied					
Year	Total	Yearly percent change	General and other special	Yearly percent change	Psychiatric	Yearly percent change	Tuberculosis	Yearly percent change
1978	75.5	−0.3	74.2	−0.2	81.3	+0.1	59.9	−0.5
1977	75.8	−0.2	74.4	−0.6	81.2	+1.5	60.4	+2.6
1976	76.0	−0.7	75.0	−0.5	79.7	−1.2	57.8	+0.1
1975[1]	76.7	−0.5	75.5	−0.5	80.9	+0.4	57.7	−5.5
1974	77.2	−0.3	76.0	+0.1	80.5	−1.0	63.2	+1.3
1973	77.5	−0.5	75.9	(2)	81.5	−1.6	61.9	+0.7
1972	78.0	−1.5	75.9	−1.7	83.1	−0.9	61.2	+0.5
1971	79.5	−0.8	77.6	−0.6	84.0	−0.7	60.7	−1.2
1970	80.3	−1.3	78.2	−1.2	84.7	−1.0	61.9	−2.7
1969	81.6	−1.3	79.4	+0.4	85.7	+3.8	64.6	−0.5
Percent change 1969-1978	−6.1		−5.2		−4.4		−4.7	

1 Revised.
2 Less than 0.1 percent.

SOURCES: "Guide Issue" of *Hospitals*, Journal of the American Hospital Association. Part II, August 1, 1970-1971: *Hospital Statistics 1979*, and previous years.

Table V-A-7. Hospital Admissions, by Type of Service, 1969-1978

Year	Total	Yearly percent change	General and other special	Yearly percent change	Admissions Psychiatric	Yearly percent change	Tuberculosis	Yearly percent change
1978	37,243,182	+0.5	36,579,611	+0.5	652,564	− 1.3	11,007	−11.8
1977	37,059,782	+0.8	36,386,363	+0.8	660,946	− 1.3	12,473	+ 5.5
1976	36,775,770	+1.7	36,094,590	+1.8	669,357	− 1.4	11,823	−30.0
1975	36,156,516	+1.8	35,460,769	+1.9	678,849	+1.4	16,898	−20.3
1974	35,506,190	+3.4	34,815,483	+3.4	669,499	+1.3	21,208	−18.0
1973	34,352,149	+3.3	33,665,669	+3.3	660,604	+0.2	25,876	− 8.1
1972	33,264,898	+1.8	32,577,689	+2.0	659,037	−4.4	28,172	−17.3
1971	32,663,691	+2.8	31,940,507	+2.9	689,117	+3.1	34,067	− 7.5
1970	31,759,124	+3.4	31,053,879	+3.3	668,411	+5.4	36,834	+ 0.1
1969	30,728,775	+3.2	30,058,176	+3.2	633,816	+4.2	36,783	− 0.5
Percent change 1969-1978		+21.2		+21.7		+3.0		−70.1

SOURCES: "Guide Issue" of *Hospitals*, Journal of the American Hospital Association, Part II, August 1, 1970-1971; *Hospital Statistics 1979*, and previous years.

Table V-A-8. Average Daily Census, by Type of Service, 1969-1978

Year	Total	Yearly percent change	General and other special	Yearly percent change	Average daily census Psychiatric	Yearly percent change	Tuberculosis	Yearly percent change
1978	1,041,936	−2.3	830,486	−0.2	209,782	− 9.4	1,668	−16.6
1977	1,065,946	−2.2	832,333	−0.4	231,612	− 8.0	2,001	− 3.6
1976	1,089,671	−3.1	835,923	+0.4	251,673	−12.9	2,075	−38.5
1975	1,124,877	−3.6	832,399	+0.3	289,102	−13.0	3,376	−34.6
1974	1,167,353	−1.8	830,035	+2.0	332,156	− 9.9	5,162	−20.3
1973	1,189,049	−1.6	813,817	+2.4	368,759	− 9.3	6,473	−17.2
1972	1,208,863	−2.3	794,522	−0.8	406,520	− 4.4	7,821	−27.5
1971	1,236,802	−4.7	800,796	−0.4	425,213	−11.7	10,793	−12.6
1970	1,297,708	−3.6	803,994	+0.1	481,368	− 9.1	12,346	− 8.0
1969	1,346,347	−2.3	803,235	+2.3	529,684	− 8.5	13,428	− 8.1
Percent change 1969-1978		−22.6		+3.4		−60.4		−87.6

SOURCES: "Guide Issue" of *Hospitals*, Journal of the American Hospital Association, Part II, August 1, 1970-1971; *Hospital Statistics 1979*, and previous years.

Table V-A-9. Distribution of Persons with Short-stay Hospital Episodes During Past Year, by Sex and Age, 1978[1]
(Number of persons in thousands)

Sex and age	Population		Number of hospital episodes							
			None		One		Two		Three or more	
	Number	Percent	Number	Percent	Number	Percent	Number	Percent	Number	Percent
Total[2]	213,828	100.0	191,540	89.6	18,308	8.6	2,952	1.4	1,029	0.5
Under 17 years	59,012	100.0	55,871	94.7	2,746	4.7	287	0.5	107	0.2
17-24	31,731	100.0	28,360	89.4	2,937	9.3	342	1.1	93	0.3
25-34	33,012	100.0	28,908	87.6	3,605	10.9	408	1.2	92	0.3
35-44	23,883	100.0	21,571	90.3	1,931	8.1	285	1.2	96	0.4
45-64	43,403	100.0	38,148	87.9	4,050	9.3	856	2.0	349	0.8
65 and over	22,788	100.0	18,682	82.0	3,039	13.3	774	3.4	292	1.3
Male	103,174	100.0	94,389	91.5	7,188	7.0	1,139	1.1	458	0.4
Under 17 years	30,096	100.0	28,416	94.4	1,487	4.9	141	0.5	52	0.2
17-24	15,443	100.0	14,482	93.8	844	5.5	84	0.5	(3)	(3)
25-34	16,028	100.0	14,959	93.3	924	5.8	112	0.7	(3)	(3)
35-44	11,480	100.0	10,647	92.7	687	6.0	100	0.9	46	0.4
45-64	20,734	100.0	18,297	88.2	1,905	9.2	374	1.8	159	0.8
65 and over	9,393	100.0	7,589	80.8	1,341	14.3	329	3.5	134	1.4
Female	110,655	100.0	97,152	87.8	11,119	10.0	1,813	1.6	571	0.5
Under 17 years	28,916	100.0	27,456	95.0	1,259	4.4	147	0.5	55	0.2
17-24	16,288	100.0	13,878	85.2	2,093	12.8	258	1.6	59	0.4
25-34	16,985	100.0	13,949	82.1	2,681	15.8	296	1.7	58	0.3
35-44	12,404	100.0	10,925	88.1	1,244	10.0	184	1.5	50	0.4
45-64	22,668	100.0	19,851	87.6	2,145	9.5	482	2.1	191	0.8
65 and over	13,394	100.0	11,093	82.8	1,698	12.7	446	3.3	158	1.2

[1] Data are based on household interviews of the civilian, noninstitutionalized population that were conducted in 1978.
[2] Individual items may not add to totals due to rounding.
[3] Figure does not meet standards of reliability or precision.

SOURCE: U.S. Department of Health, Education, and Welfare, Public Health Service, Office of Health Research, Statistics, and Technology, National Center for Health Statistics, *Current Estimates from the Health Interview Survey: United States-1978*, DHEW Publication No. (PHS) 80-1551, p. 26.

Table V-A-10. Number of Osteopathic Hospitals by State, 1976-1979

State	1976 Hospitals	1976 Beds	1977 Hospitals	1977 Beds	1978 Hospitals	1978 Beds	1979 Hospitals	1979 Beds
Total	207	24,593	205	24,957	206	25,045	198	24,752
Arizona	5	737	5	833	5	633	5	637
California	1	46	2	96	11	1,069	10	932
Colorado	5	626	5	658	5	622	4	365
Delaware	1	100	1	100	1	97	1	97
Florida	17	2,441	16	2,421	17	2,179	17	2,439
Georgia	2	234	1	226	1	181	1	181
Illinois	3	340	3	341	3	431	3	467
Indiana	3	256	3	256	3	262	3	247
Iowa	4	349	3	434	3	413	3	413
Kansas	2	155	2	154	2	154	2	164
Maine	3	315	3	339	3	344	3	297
Massachusetts ...	1	155	1	155	1	80	1	80
Michigan	31	5,065	31	5,191	31	5,110	32	5,127
Missouri	23	2,211	24	2,137	23	2,285	22	2,287
New Jersey	7	1,172	7	1,176	7	1,160	7	1,147
New Mexico	3	45	3	159	2	137	1	112
New York	4	624	4	624	3	430	3	470
Ohio	16	2,838	16	2,928	16	2,995	15	2,905
Oklahoma	6	747	6	741	6	680	6	709
Oregon	5	214	5	214	5	214	4	164
Pennsylvania	18	2,614	17	2,576	17	2,562	17	2,595
Rhode Island	1	80	1	80	1	77	1	77
South Dakota	1	39	1	39	1	37	1	37
Tennessee	1	27	1	25	1	25	1	25
Texas	32	2,411	32	2,299	28	2,193	26	2,113
Washington	4	201	4	204	4	195	4	193
West Virginia	4	121	4	121	3	67	2	59
Wisconsin	4	430	4	430	3	413	3	413

SOURCES: American Osteopathic Hospital Association, 1978, unpublished data; *1979 Directory of the American Osteopathic Hospital Association* and *1980 Directory of the American Osteopathic Hospital Association.*

Table V-A-11. Number[1] and Percent of Nursing Care and Related Homes, by Home Size and Type of Care Provided, 1976

Home size	Total homes		Nursing care		Personal care and other homes[2]	
	Number	Percent	Number	Percent	Number	Percent
Total	20,185	100.0	13,312	100.0	6,873	100.0
Less than 25 beds	5,558	27.5	1,114	8.4	4,444	64.7
25-49	3,874	19.2	2,766	20.8	1,108	16.1
50-74	3,544	17.6	3,021	22.7	523	7.6
75-99	2,355	11.7	2,109	15.8	246	3.6
100-199	3,999	19.8	3,572	26.9	427	6.2
200-299	600	3.0	523	3.9	77	1.1
300-499	188	0.9	151	1.1	37	0.5
500 beds or more	67	0.3	56	0.4	11	0.2

[1] Preliminary data.
[2] Includes personal care homes with nursing, personal care homes without nursing, and domiciliary care homes.

SOURCE: U.S. Department of Health, Education, and Welfare, Public Health Service, Office of Health Research, Statistics, and Technology, National Center for Health Statistics, *Health Resources Statistics: Health Manpower and Health Facilities*, 1976-77 ed., DHEW Publication No. (PHS) 79-1509, p. 335.

Table V-A-12. Number[1] of Nursing Care and Related Homes and Beds, by State and Type of Care Provided, 1976

State	Total		Nursing care		Personal care and other homes[2]	
	Homes	Beds	Homes	Beds	Homes	Beds
United States	20,185	1,406,778	13,312	1,173,519	6,873	233,259
Alabama	214	19,281	192	17,460	22	1,821
Alaska	11	782	10	690	1	92
Arizona[3]	71	5,914	67	5,448	4	466
Arkansas	213	18,722	200	17,632	13	1,090
California	3,440	139,054	1,278	107,213	2,162	31,841
Colorado[3]	241	22,708	207	20,517	34	2,191
Connecticut	350	24,374	220	19,795	130	4,579
Delaware	29	2,228	22	1,898	7	330
District of Columbia	71	2,872	28	2,261	43	611
Florida.................	331	32,859	280	29,099	51	3,760
Georgia	324	29,641	313	29,179	11	462
Hawaii	140	3,172	36	2,523	104	649
Idaho[3]	67	4,823	54	3,981	13	842
Illinois	928	87,805	699	73,788	229	14,017
Indiana	490	35,935	400	31,432	90	4,503
Iowa	537	32,856	381	26,363	156	6,493
Kansas	381	22,502	320	19,770	61	2,732
Kentucky	313	20,543	177	13,710	136	6,833
Louisiana	204	19,070	193	18,156	11	914
Maine	292	8,644	129	6,463	163	2,181
Maryland	187	18,874	153	16,545	34	2,329
Massachusetts[3]	869	50,940	527	38,868	342	12,072
Michigan[3]	699	66,416	479	50,817	220	15,599
Minnesota[3]	517	43,036	398	36,441	119	6,595
Mississippi	144	8,939	128	8,483	16	456
Missouri[3]	472	33,628	366	28,366	106	5,262
Montana	105	5,299	81	4,699	24	600
Nebraska[3]	281	23,022	239	21,326	42	1,696
Nevada	35	1,574	21	1,369	14	205
New Hampshire	114	6,256	85	5,669	29	587
New Jersey	468	34,463	290	28,880	178	5,583
New Mexico	66	3,042	37	2,438	29	604
New York	996	102,591	537	76,459	459	26,132
North Carolina[3]	711	24,432	173	13,193	538	11,239
North Dakota	102	6,753	68	5,258	34	1,495
Ohio	937	64,096	813	57,732	124	6,364
Oklahoma	353	26,103	328	24,901	25	1,202
Oregon	279	15,906	189	12,829	90	3,077
Pennsylvania[3]	666	64,090	570	57,934	96	6,156
Rhode Island[3]	120	7,330	80	5,908	40	1,422
South Carolina	118	8,642	105	8,144	13	498
South Dakota	153	7,840	106	6,238	47	1,602
Tennessee[3]	289	20,074	253	18,387	36	1,687
Texas[3]	1,099	101,418	954	88,907	145	12,511
Utah	102	4,569	85	3,993	17	576
Vermont[3]	263	5,130	50	2,964	213	2,166
Virginia[3]	341	28,479	169	19,791	172	8,688
Washington	366	30,079	291	26,440	75	3,639
West Virginia	127	5,575	75	4,391	52	1,184
Wisconsin[3]	530	52,606	433	47,225	97	5,381
Wyoming	29	1,791	23	1,546	6	245

[1] Preliminary data.
[2] Includes personal care homes with nursing, personal care homes without nursing, and domiciliary care homes.
[3] States reporting 1976 data in the Cooperative Health Statistics System. Data may not always agree with individual state reports, usually because of variations in imputation procedures or in time period over which the data were collected.

SOURCE: U.S. Department of Health, Education, and Welfare, Public Health Service, Office of Health Research, Statistics, and Technology, National Center for Health Statistics, *Health Resources Statistics: Health Manpower and Health Facilities*, 1976-77 ed., DHEW Publication No. (PHS) 79-1509, pp. 330 and 332.

Table V-A-13. Distribution[1] of Nursing Homes, Beds, and Residents, by Certification Status of Nursing Home, 1976

Certification status of nursing homes	Nursing homes		Beds		Residents	
	Number	Percent	Number	Percent	Number	Percent
All types of certification	18,900	100.0	1,402,400	100.0	1,303,100	100.0
Skilled nursing facility only	3,600	19.2	294,000	21.0	269,600	20.7
Medicare and Medicaid	2,100	11.3	204,500	14.6	190,300	14.6
Medicare	700	3.7	27,000	1.9	17,800	1.4
Medicaid	800	4.2	62,600	4.5	61,500	4.7
Skilled nursing facility and intermediate care facility	4,600	24.2	549,400	39.2	527,800	40.5
Medicare SNF and Medicaid SNF and ICF ...	2,300	12.3	319,500	22.8	303,700	23.3
Medicaid SNF and ICF	2,100	10.8	218,700	15.6	213,800	16.4
Medicare SNF and Medicaid ICF	200	1.1	11,300	0.8	10,300	0.8
Intermediate care facility only	6,000	31.6	391,600	27.9	368,200	28.3
Not certified	4,700	25.0	167,400	11.9	137,500	10.6

[1] Figures may not add to totals due to rounding.

SOURCE: U.S. Department of Health, Education, and Welfare, Public Health Service, Office of Health Research, Statistics, and Technology, National Center for Health Statistics, *The National Nursing Home Survey: 1977 Summary for the United States*, Vital and Health Statistics, Series 13, No. 43, DHEW Publication No. (PHS) 79-1794, 1979, p. 8.

Table V-A-14. Selected Measures of Nursing Home Utilization, by Certification Status of Nursing Homes, 1976

Certification status of nursing homes	Measures of utilization for 1976				
	Admissions	Annual occupancy rate[1]	Discharges[3]		
			Number[2]	Percent	
				Live	Dead
All types of certification	1,367,400	89.0	1,117,500	73.9	25.9
Skilled nursing facility only	390,300	92.0	379,000	77.5	22.2
Skilled nursing facility and intermediate care facility	639,700	88.6	448,400	71.6	28.2
Intermediate care facility only	222,800	87.3	210,400	70.2	29.8
Not certified	114,600	89.1	79,600	79.3	20.6

[1] The annual occupancy rate is computed as follows: (Aggregate number of days of care provided to residents in 1976 × 100) ÷ (Estimated number of beds in 1976 × 366).
[2] Includes a small number of unknowns.
[3] Figures may not add to totals due to rounding.

SOURCE: U.S. Department of Health, Education, and Welfare, Public Health Service, Office of Health Research, Statistics, and Technology, National Center for Health Statistics, *The National Nursing Home Survey: 1977 Summary for the United States*, Vital and Health Statistics, Series 13, No. 43, DHEW Publication No. (PHS) 79-1794, 1979, p. 9.

Chapter V, Section B
OTHER HEALTH PERSONNEL

The Bureau of Health Professions, formerly the Bureau of Health Manpower estimated there were 395,200 professionally active physicians in the United States and outlying U.S. areas in 1977, representing a gain of 1.2 percent between 1976 and 1977. Of this group of physicians, 380,200 were doctors of medicine (M.D.s) and 15,000 were doctors of osteopathy (D.O.s). The 1976-1977 growth in the number of active D.O.s was larger than their counterparts in medicine, 3.4 percent versus 1.1 percent, respectively. There were 17.9 active physicians per 10,000 population in 1977. The bureau further projected that by 1990 there would be 594,000 or about 50 percent more active physicians.

The American Medical Association reported 437,486 M.D.s, active and inactive, were in the United States and U.S. outlying territories in 1978. The AMA indicated the average annual growth rate of M.D.s was 3.0 percent since 1970; the observed change between 1976 and 1978 was 6.8 percent. Over 93 percent of all M.D.s were civilian (nonfederal), the majority of whom were established in direct patient care practices. Almost three-quarters (73.3 percent) of those 325,783 M.D.s in patient care had office-based practices, while 26.7 percent were in hospital settings. Federally employed M.D.s numbered 20,242. About 83.6 percent of the M.D.s in federal services were involved in patient care. These federal M.D.s were primarily engaged in hospital-based practice. The AMA provided more detailed information on the 375,811 M.D.s who could be located for the survey and who were professionally active in the United States and its possessions. This count, then, specifically excludes those 26,831 who were inactive, 9,291 with unknown addresses, and 25,553 for whom information was not available.

While the preponderance of all active M.D.s are in specialty practices, a slightly larger proportion were in general and family practice in 1978 as contrasted to 1976, 20.4 percent versus 19.7 percent. Among the M.D.s in specialty practices, the surgical areas accounted for the largest group (39.0 percent), followed by medical specialties (36.7 percent) and psychiatry and neurology (11.2 percent).

The 1977 data from the National Center for Health Statistics showed more than three out of four D.O.s to be in office-based practices. With respect to area of practice, general practice ranked first, with 52.7 percent choosing this area.

Data from the NCHS 1976-77 Health Interview Survey indicated the average number of physician visits to be 4.9 per year. There was a direct correspondence between the average number of physician visits and age of the patient, with those in the higher age brackets recording more visits. The relationship between visits and racial/ethnic background of the patient varied among the age groups.

NCHS also provided 1978 data on physician and dental visits. In 1978 the average annual physician visits per person was 4.8. Women reported more physician visits than men, averaging 5.4 visits versus 4.0 visits.

NCHS also reported there were 115,000 active dentists in the United States in 1976, of whom 110,000 were civilians engaged in dentistry. The total number of active dentists increased 12.5 percent, and the number of civilian dentists increased by 15.0 percent since 1970. There were 51.4 active civilian dentists per 100,000 civilian population. State-by-state comparisons indicate the number of dentists per 100,000 civilian population ranged from 30 in Mississippi to 93 in the District of Columbia.

Annually, dental visits averaged 1.6 times per person nationally. A general increase in the average number of dental visits was associated with higher age groups.

Table V-B-1. Estimates and Projections of Active Physicians (M.D.s and D.O.s) in Relation to Population, United States and Outlying Areas, Selected Years, 1950-1990

Year	Number of physicians			Active physicians per 10,000 population
	Total	M.D.s	D.O.s	
Projections				
1990	594,000	564,200	29,800	24.4
1985	519,000	495,700	23,300	22.3
1980	444,000	426,300	17,700	20.0
Estimates				
1977	395,200	380,200	15,000	17.9
1976	390,600	376,100	14,500	17.9
1975	378,600	364,500	14,100	17.4
1974	362,500	348,900	13,600	16.8
1973	350,100	337,000	13,100	16.4
1972	345,000	332,400	12,600	16.3
1971	334,100	322,000	12,100	15.9
1970	323,200	311,200	12,000	15.5
1960	259,500	247,300	12,200	14.2
1950	219,900	209,000	10,900	14.2

NOTES: Population for selected years 1950-1977 includes residents in the 50 states, District of Columbia, civilians in Puerto Rico and other U.S. outlying areas; U.S. citizens in foreign countries; and the Armed Forces in the United States and abroad. For years 1980-1990, the Series II projections of the total population from the U.S. Bureau of the Census were used. Estimation and projection methods of the Bureau of Health Manpower were used. The number of M.D.s differs from the American Medical Association figures because a variant proportion of the physicians not classified by specialty is allocated into the total.

SOURCE: U.S. Department of Health, Education, and Welfare, Public Health Service, Office of Health Research, Statistics, and Technology, National Center for Health Statistics, *Health United States 1979*, pre-publication copy, DHEW Publication No. (PHS) 80-1232, 1980, p. 213.

Table V-B-2. Distribution of Active Nonfederal Physicians (M.D.s),[1] Providing Patient Care, by Type of Practice, 1978

| | | M.D.s providing patient care | | |
| | | | Hospital-based practice | |
State or territory	Total	Office-based practice	Residents[2]	Full-time physician staff
Total	325,783	238,943	57,205	29,635
United States, total	322,835	237,071	56,866	28,898
Alabama	3,833	2,981	645	207
Alaska	378	349	9	20
Arizona	3,732	2,847	629	256
Arkansas	2,165	1,749	294	122
California	41,296	32,754	5,752	2,790
Colorado	4,548	3,454	798	296
Connecticut	6,054	4,098	1,294	662
Delaware	805	601	119	85
District of Columbia	2,576	1,626	725	225
Florida	13,584	10,990	1,557	1,037
Georgia	6,090	4,691	975	424
Hawaii	1,447	1,154	198	95
Idaho	847	780	23	44
Illinois	16,602	11,856	2,760	1,986
Indiana	5,807	4,614	806	387
Iowa	3,035	2,355	548	132
Kansas	2,938	2,197	505	236
Kentucky	3,873	2,946	704	223
Louisiana	4,833	3,615	555	663
Maine	1,378	1,111	139	128
Maryland	7,808	5,207	1,731	870
Massachusetts	11,517	7,703	2,396	1,418
Michigan	11,688	8,164	2,535	989
Minnesota	6,369	4,371	1,631	367
Mississippi	2,179	1,781	254	144
Missouri	6,150	4,315	1,194	641
Montana	878	818	14	46
Nebraska	1,898	1,442	389	67
Nevada	758	701	11	46
New Hampshire	1,190	962	145	83
New Jersey	11,029	7,987	1,720	1,322
New Mexico	1,434	1,116	200	118
New York	36,307	23,282	7,788	5,237
North Carolina	6,777	5,067	1,197	513
North Dakota	707	608	59	40
Ohio	14,477	10,220	3,069	1,188
Oklahoma	3,120	2,424	465	231
Oregon	3,615	2,965	441	209
Pennsylvania	17,883	12,335	3,645	1,903
Rhode Island	1,609	1,120	271	218
South Carolina	3,159	2,342	592	225
South Dakota	611	509	69	33
Tennessee	5,614	4,073	1,156	385
Texas	16,540	12,619	2,957	964
Utah	1,829	1,388	357	84
Vermont	841	614	161	66
Virginia	6,958	5,193	1,227	538
Washington	5,553	4,476	799	278
West Virginia	2,123	1,556	322	245
Wisconsin	5,999	4,592	1,026	381
Wyoming	394	353	10	31
Outlying areas, total	2,948	1,872	339	737
Canal Zone	36	7	23	6
Pacific Islands	79	64	1	14
Puerto Rico	2,764	1,758	312	694
Virgin Islands	69	43	3	23

[1]Excludes 29,786 nonfederal M.D.s in other professional activities, 26,831 in inactive status, 8,858 with addresses temporarily unknown to AMA, and 25,553 unclassified.
[2]Effective in 1975, includes interns.
SOURCE: American Medical Association, Center for Health Services Research and Development, Department of Statistical Analysis, *Physician Distribution and Medical Licensure in the U.S., 1978*, NEA 79-468:12/79:1.5.

Table V-B-3. Physicians (M.D.s)[1] by Type of Practice, Selected Years, 1969-1978

Type of practice	1969	1972	1976	1978
Total	324,942	356,534	409,446	437,486
Nonfederal	293,397	325,789	373,111	407,953
Patient care	247,508	269,095	294,730	325,783
Office-based practice	184,355	198,974	214,710	238,943
General and family practice[2]	54,698	52,091	50,331	52,956
Other full-time primary specialty	129,657	146,883	164,379	185,987
Hospital-based practice	63,153	70,121	80,020	86,840
Training programs[3]	45,744	49,511	58,924	57,205
Full-time hospital staff	17,409	20,610	21,096	29,635
Other professional activity[4]	25,994	24,228	26,135	29,786
Inactive	19,895	20,110	22,117	26,831
Not classified[5]	...	12,356	30,129	25,553
Federal	29,464	27,580	27,578	20,242
Patient care	23,229	23,115	23,682	16,931
Office-based practice	3,811	2,328	1,823	923
General and family practice[2]	1,864	981	717	306
Other full-time primary specialty	1,947	1,347	1,106	617
Hospital-based practice	19,418	20,787	21,859	16,008
Training programs[3]	6,072	4,040	4,122	3,405
Full-time hospital staff	13,346	16,747	17,737	12,603
Other professional activity[4]	6,235	4,465	3,896	3,311
Address unknown	2,081	3,165	8,757	9,291

[1] Includes nonfederal physicians (M.D.s) in 50 states, District of Columbia, Puerto Rico, and other U.S. outlying areas (American Samoa, Canal Zone, Guam, Pacific Islands, and Virgin Islands); those whose address is temporarily unknown to AMA; and federal physicians (M.D.s) in the United States and abroad. Excludes physicians (M.D.s) with temporary foreign addresses.
[2] Includes physicians reporting "no specialty" and other specialties not listed on AMA list of specialty designations.
[3] Includes interns and residents.
[4] Includes medical teaching, administration, research, and other activities.
[5] Not classified as to their specialty.

SOURCES: U.S. Department of Health, Education, and Welfare, Public Health Service, Office of Health Research, Statistics, and Technology, National Center for Health Statistics, *Health Resources Statistics: Health Manpower and Health Facilities*, 1976-77 ed., DHEW Publication No. (PHS) 79-1509, 1979, p. 144, and American Medical Association, Center for Health Services Research and Development, Department of Statistical Analysis, *Physician Distribution and Medical Licensure in the U.S., 1978*, NEA 79-468:12/79:1.5.

Table V-B-4. Type of Practice and Primary Specialty of Active Physicians (M.D.s), 1978

Primary specialty	Total active[1]	Type of practice			
		Office-based practice	Hospital-based practice		Other professional activity[2]
			Training programs	Full-time physician staff	
Total	375,811	239,866	60,610	42,238	33,097
General and family practice[3]	76,771	53,262	10,921	7,645	4,943
Specialty practice	299,040	186,604	49,689	34,593	28,154
Medical specialties	109,743	64,860	20,719	11,361	12,803
Allergy	1,537	1,383	...	46	108
Cardiovascular diseases	8,506	6,188	...	914	1,404
Dermatology	5,105	3,902	612	323	268
Gastroenterology	3,314	2,379	...	282	653
Internal medicine	62,641	33,772	15,244	6,524	7,101
Pediatrics[4]	25,570	15,521	4,863	2,690	2,496
Pulmonary diseases	3,070	1,715	...	582	773
Surgical specialties	116,660	83,414	19,030	9,485	4,731
Anesthesiology	14,246	9,774	1,645	1,943	884
Colon and rectal surgery	679	616	24	22	17
General surgery	32,059	20,422	7,319	3,057	1,261
Neurological surgery	3,098	2,229	479	256	134
Obstetrics and gynecology	23,963	17,517	3,888	1,557	1,001
Ophthalmology	11,933	9,603	1,387	494	449
Orthopedic surgery	12,657	9,355	2,042	880	380
Otolaryngology	6,117	4,721	785	413	198
Plastic surgery	2,624	2,088	335	126	75
Thoracic surgery	2,042	1,480	206	222	134
Urology	7,242	5,609	920	515	198
Psychiatry and neurology	33,445	18,464	4,751	6,115	4,115
Child psychiatry	2,926	1,736	227	440	523
Neurology	4,923	2,553	991	613	766
Psychiatry	25,596	14,175	3,533	5,062	2,826
Other specialties	39,192	19,866	5,189	7,632	6,505
Aerospace medicine	584	195	47	126	216
General preventive medicine ...	756	236	64	67	389
Occupational medicine	2,351	1,588	16	91	656
Pathology[5]	12,854	5,137	2,272	3,209	2,236
Physical medicine and rehabilitation	1,900	796	275	645	184
Public health	2,340	490	34	157	1,659
Radiology[6]	18,407	11,424	2,481	3,337	1,165

[1]Excludes 9,291 M.D.s with addresses unknown and 25,553 unclassified M.D.s.
[2]Includes medical teaching, administration, research, and other activities.
[3]Includes no specialty reported and other specialties not listed.
[4]Includes pediatric allergy and pediatric cardiology.
[5]Includes forensic pathology.
[6]Includes diagnostic radiology and therapeutic radiology.

SOURCE: American Medical Association, Center for Health Services Research and Development, Department of Statistical Analysis, *Physician Distribution and Medical Licensure in the U.S.*, 1978, NEA 79-468:12/79:1.5, p. 46.

Table V-B-5. Distribution of Nonfederal Physicians (M.D.s) by Major Professional Activity, 1978

State or territory	Total nonfederal physicians	Total providing patient care	Major professional activity							
			Patient care					Other professional activity	Inactive	Not classified
			Office-based practice				Hospital-based practice			
			General practice	Medical specialties	Surgical specialties	Other specialties				
Total	407,953	325,783	45,148	64,624	73,540	55,631	86,840	29,786	26,831	25,553
United States, total	404,190	322,835	44,649	64,125	73,045	55,252	85,764	29,555	26,698	25,102
Alabama	4,554	3,833	623	702	1,051	605	852	306	191	224
Alaska	460	378	99	69	114	67	29	21	15	46
Arizona	4,918	3,732	551	752	900	644	885	272	689	225
Arkansas	2,610	2,165	586	322	507	334	416	132	187	126
California	52,194	41,296	5,715	8,877	9,490	8,672	8,542	3,756	4,303	2,839
Colorado	5,600	4,548	632	949	1,016	857	1,094	411	352	289
Connecticut	7,705	6,054	477	1,398	1,254	969	1,956	722	483	446
Delaware	972	805	104	158	194	145	204	52	61	54
District of Columbia	3,491	2,576	126	538	469	493	950	469	169	277
Florida	18,353	13,584	1,924	2,956	3,600	2,510	2,594	931	2,897	941
Georgia	7,259	6,090	814	1,163	1,691	1,023	1,399	424	334	411
Hawaii	1,808	1,447	182	336	367	269	293	124	138	99
Idaho	1,010	847	252	146	257	125	67	37	82	44
Illinois	20,628	16,602	2,398	3,230	3,452	2,776	4,746	1,496	924	1,606
Indiana	6,993	5,807	1,388	891	1,290	1,045	1,193	399	444	343
Iowa	3,635	3,035	744	442	694	475	680	232	211	157
Kansas	3,618	2,938	569	489	620	519	741	226	233	221
Kentucky	4,699	3,873	780	658	904	604	927	274	244	308
Louisiana	5,955	4,833	709	823	1,324	759	1,218	377	280	465
Maine	1,752	1,378	234	285	344	248	267	83	190	101
Maryland	10,390	7,808	671	1,604	1,611	1,321	2,601	1,141	539	902
Massachusetts	14,985	11,517	893	2,516	2,340	1,954	3,814	1,614	836	1,018
Michigan	14,290	11,688	1,306	2,271	2,625	1,962	3,524	949	777	876
Minnesota	7,676	6,369	1,162	1,168	1,113	928	1,998	514	464	329
Mississippi	2,571	2,179	534	333	579	335	398	101	135	156

Missouri	7,839	6,150	670	1,250	1,450	945	1,835	663	391	635
Montana	1,024	878	215	173	263	167	60	30	59	57
Nebraska	2,338	1,898	473	292	401	276	456	167	140	133
Nevada	925	758	145	152	232	172	57	46	65	56
New Hampshire	1,542	1,190	197	251	298	216	228	103	166	83
New Jersey	13,820	11,029	1,120	2,510	2,586	1,771	3,042	902	950	939
New Mexico	1,869	1,434	197	311	352	256	318	136	173	126
New York	47,021	36,307	2,998	7,734	6,922	5,628	13,025	4,239	2,563	3,912
North Carolina	8,428	6,777	1,013	1,391	1,705	958	1,710	721	494	436
North Dakota	825	707	162	131	175	140	99	35	45	38
Ohio	17,325	14,477	1,992	2,715	3,081	2,432	4,257	1,013	959	876
Oklahoma	3,650	3,120	534	581	760	549	696	193	197	140
Oregon	4,546	3,615	633	720	980	632	650	286	354	291
Pennsylvania	22,149	17,883	2,511	3,371	3,748	2,705	5,548	1,702	1,318	1,246
Rhode Island	1,967	1,609	130	390	372	228	489	133	117	108
South Carolina	3,873	3,159	642	465	777	458	817	237	233	244
South Dakota	723	611	174	94	149	92	102	29	46	37
Tennessee	6,808	5,614	764	1,016	1,424	869	1,541	456	310	428
Texas	20,143	16,540	2,771	2,976	3,984	2,888	3,921	1,406	1,042	1,155
Utah	2,225	1,829	252	346	444	346	441	166	118	112
Vermont	1,075	841	109	185	189	131	227	92	105	37
Virginia	8,653	6,958	987	1,376	1,625	1,205	1,765	594	539	562
Washington	6,981	5,553	1,014	1,018	1,323	1,121	1,077	511	521	396
West Virginia	2,565	2,123	349	364	558	285	567	145	146	151
Wisconsin	7,271	5,999	1,017	1,171	1,334	1,070	1,407	465	430	377
Wyoming	479	394	107	66	107	73	41	22	39	24
Outlying areas	*3,763*	*2,948*	*499*	*499*	*495*	*379*	*1,076*	*231*	*133*	*451*
Canal Zone	42	36	2	2	2	1	29	2	...	4
Pacific Islands	87	79	17	16	24	7	15	5	1	2
Puerto Rico	3,543	2,764	473	472	453	360	1,006	219	119	441
Virgin Islands	91	69	7	9	16	11	26	5	13	4

¹Excludes 8,858 nonfederal physicians with addresses temporarily unknown to AMA.

SOURCE: American Medical Association, Center for Health Services Research and Development, Department of Statistical Analysis, *Physician Distribution and Medical Licensure in the U.S., 1978*, NEA 79-468:12/79:1.5.

Table V-B-6. Type of Practice and Major Professional Activity of Physicians (D.O.s) Providing Patient Care, 1977

Activity	Total	Office-based practice	Hospital-based practice	Other professional activity
Total D.O.s providing patient care [1]	15,088	11,482	515	260
General practice	7,948	7,889	7	52
Specialties	953	888	12	53
Internal medicine	522	494	5	23
Pediatrics	195	171	3	21
Obstetrics and gynecology	236	223	4	9
Surgical specialties	806	784	5	17
General surgery	540	525	5	10
Obstetrical and gynecological surgery	114	110	...	4
Orthopedic surgery	152	149	...	3
Other specialties	1,500	1,353	89	58
Anesthesiology	378	359	4	15
Ophthalmology and otorhinolaryngology	253	248	...	5
Pathology	123	88	27	8
Proctology	184	181	...	3
Psychiatry	159	145	4	10
Radiology and roentgenology	403	332	54	17
All other specialties	1,050	568	402	80

[1] Includes 2,831 D.O.s not indicating type of specialty.

SOURCE: U.S. Department of Health, Education, and Welfare, Public Health Service, Office of Health Research, Statistics, and Technology, National Center for Health Statistics, *Health Resources Statistics: Health Manpower and Health Facilities*, 1976-77 ed., DHEW Publication No. (PHS) 79-1509, 1979, p. 155.

Table V-B-7. Active Dentists in Relation to Population, Selected Years 1950-1976[1]

Selected years	Total population[2] (in thousands)	Active dentists	Active dentists per 100,000 population
1976	215,869	115,000	53.2
1970	206,070	102,220	49.6
1960	182,290	90,040	49.4
1950	153,620	76,940	50.1

Selected years	Resident civilian population (in thousands)	Active civilian dentists	Active civilian dentists per 100,000 civilians
1976	213,860	110,000	51.4
1970	203,110	95,680	47.1
1960	179,740	84,500	47.0
1950	151,240	75,310	49.8

[1] All data as of December 31.
[2] Includes all persons in the United States and in the armed forces overseas.

SOURCE: U.S. Department of Health, Education, and Welfare, Public Health Service, Office of Health Research, Statistics, and Technology, National Center for Health Statistics, *Health Resources Statistics: Health Manpower and Health Facilities*, 1976-77 ed., DHEW Publication No. (PHS) 79-1509, 1979, p. 69.

Table V-B-10. Number of Active Civilian Dentists and Ratio per 100,000 Civilians, December 31, 1976

Location	Civilian population in thousands[1]	Active civilian dentists	Active civilian dentists per 100,000 civilians
United States	212,976	110,000	52
Alabama	3,640	1,168	32
Alaska	357	184	52
Arizona	2,243	1,085	48
Arkansas	2,099	668	32
California	21,234	13,743	65
Colorado	2,535	1,488	59
Connecticut	3,106	1,978	64
Delaware	576	256	44
District of Columbia	693	644	93
Florida	8,326	3,806	46
Georgia	4,912	1,894	39
Hawaii	831	530	64
Idaho	824	418	51
Illinois	11,191	5,716	51
Indiana	5,295	2,073	39
Iowa	2,869	1,293	45
Kansas	2,283	1,010	44
Kentucky	3,390	1,276	38
Louisiana	3,815	1,449	38
Maine	1,059	455	43
Maryland	4,099	2,277	56
Massachusetts	5,797	3,868	67
Michigan	9,090	4,578	50
Minnesota	3,962	2,334	59
Mississippi	2,331	694	30
Missouri	4,750	2,160	45
Montana	747	414	55
Nebraska	1,541	853	55
Nevada	600	307	51
New Hampshire	818	428	52
New Jersey	7,306	4,465	61
New Mexico	1,152	481	42
New York	18,057	12,642	70
North Carolina	5,370	1,867	35
North Dakota	631	279	44
Ohio	10,675	4,826	45
Oklahoma	2,734	1,044	38
Oregon	2,326	1,547	67
Pennsylvania	11,852	6,093	51
Rhode Island	922	462	50
South Carolina	2,778	948	34
South Dakota	680	298	44
Tennessee	4,193	1,901	45
Texas	12,331	5,043	41
Utah	1,223	771	63
Vermont	476	260	55
Virginia	4,887	2,238	46
Washington	3,556	2,461	69
West Virginia	1,820	623	34
Wisconsin	4,607	2,526	55
Wyoming	386	178	46

[1] State figures do not add to totals due to rounding. Civilian population as of July 1, 1976.

SOURCE: U.S. Department of Health, Education, and Welfare, Public Health Service, Office of Health Research, Statistics, and Technology, National Center for Health Statistics, *Health Resources Statistics: Health Manpower and Health Facilities*, 1976-77 ed., DHEW Publications No. (PHS) 79-1509, 1979, p. 70.

Table V-B-9. Total Number of Physician Visits and Average Number per Person per Year, by Age and Sex, 1978[1] (number of visits in thousands)

Age	Total		Male		Female	
	Number of visits	Average visits per person	Number of visits	Average visits per person	Number of visits	Average visits per person
Total	1,016,647	4.8	417,278	4.0	599,370	5.4
Under 17 years	242,441	4.1	125,626	4.2	116,816	4.0
17-24	134,897	4.3	45,866	3.0	89,030	5.5
25-44	266,438	4.7	94,604	3.4	171,834	5.8
45-64	229,439	5.3	96,538	4.7	132,901	5.9
65-74	91,203	6.2	35,057	5.5	56,145	6.8
75 and over	52,230	6.4	19,587	6.4	32,643	6.4

[1]Data are based on household interviews of the civilian, noninstitutionalized population conducted in 1978.
SOURCE: U.S. Department of Health, Education, and Welfare, Public Health Service, Office of Health Research, Statistics, and Technology, National Center for Health Statistics, *Current Estimates from the Health Interview Survey: United States, 1978*, DHEW Publication No. (PHS) 80-1551, p. 30.

Table V-B-10. Total Number of Dental Visits and Average Number per Person per Year, by Age and Sex, 1978[1] (Number of visits in thousands)

Age	Total		Male		Female	
	Number of visits	Average visits per person	Number of visits	Average visits per person	Number of visits	Average visits per person
Total	342,472	1.6	149,348	1.4	193,124	1.7
Under 17 years	95,022	1.6	44,079	1.5	50,943	1.8
17-24	48,386	1.5	21,053	1.4	27,333	1.7
25-44	95,490	1.7	41,393	1.5	54,096	1.8
45-64	75,834	1.7	33,335	1.6	42,499	1.9
65 and over	27,740	1.2	9,487	1.0	18,253	1.4

[1]Data are based on household interviews of the civilian, noninstitutionalized population conducted in 1978.
SOURCE: U.S. Department of Health, Education, and Welfare, Public Health Service, Office of Health Research, Statistics, and Technology, National Center for Health Statistics, *Current Estimates from the Health Interview Survey: United States, 1978*, DHEW Publication No. (PHS) 80-1551, p. 28.

Table V-B-11. Average Annual Number of Physician and Dental Visits
by Age and Racial/Ethnic Background, in the United States, 1976-77

Age and racial/ethnic background	Population in thousands	Physician visits		Dental visits	
		Number per person per year	One or more visits Percent	Number per person per year	One or more visits Percent
Total[1]	211,400	4.9	75.3	1.6	49.2
White	160,129	5.0	76.1	1.8	53.2
Black	23,066	4.6	74.3	0.9	34.1
Hispanic	11,913	4.2	69.4	1.2	34.1
Under 17 years	60,399	4.1	74.5	1.5	50.6
White	42,740	4.3	76.5	1.7	55.9
Black	7,992	2.9	69.1	0.7	35.6
Hispanic	4,854	3.7	67.9	1.1	33.1
17-44	85,662	4.6	75.0	1.7	53.9
White	64,281	4.6	75.6	1.8	58.3
Black	9,373	5.2	76.6	1.1	38.4
Hispanic	4,957	4.1	68.9	1.3	36.5
45-64	43,306	5.6	74.8	1.8	47.6
White	34,999	5.5	74.7	1.9	51.2
Black	3,893	5.8	77.4	1.0	28.8
Hispanic	1,597	5.7	71.8	1.4	33.3
65 and over	22,033	6.7	79.8	1.3	30.6
White	18,109	6.8	79.9	1.4	32.9
Black	1,807	6.9	79.0	0.6	17.1
Hispanic	505	5.5	79.8	0.7	21.0

[1] Includes other races not shown separately. The categories white, black, and Hispanic are mutually exclusive.

SOURCE: U.S. Department of Health, Education, and Welfare, Public Health Service, Office of Health Research, Statistics, and Technology, National Center for Health Statistics, *Health United States 1979*, prepublication copy, DHEW Publication No. (PHS) 80-1232, 1980, p. 40.

Chapter V, Section C
EXPENDITURES FOR HEALTH CARE

According to the Bureau of Labor Statistics, the annual average Consumer Price Index increased 6.5 percent between 1976 and 1977. Medical care costs exceeded gains in all other items in the CPI, rising 9.6 percent from 1976 to 1977. Transportation costs increased 7.1 percent; housing, 7.0 percent; personal care, 6.5 percent; and food, 6.3 percent.

Within the medical care component of the CPI, hospital service charges, and particularly operating room charges, rose sharply between 1976 and 1977. The increase in hospital services was recorded at 10.4 percent and operating room charges at 13.3 percent. The next largest gain was an increase of 9.3 percent in physicians' fees, followed by an 8.5 percent increase in X-ray, diagnostic series, and upper gastrointestinal series.

National expenditures for health in 1977 totaled $16.3 billion, amounting to 8.8 percent of the nation's gross national product. The proportion of the GNP spent on health has been rising over the decade. Hospital care costs were the largest categorical components of the total health expenditures, followed by physician service charges, 40.4 percent and 19.8 percent, respectively.

Americans were spending more on health care in 1977 than they were the previous year, even when the per capita expenditures were adjusted for general price changes. In 1977 the per capita health expenditure was $736.92. Adjusted for aggregate changes in prices for the economy as a whole, this figure represented a 1.4 percent gain over the previous fiscal year. Information supplied by the Social Security Administration on the amounts spent on health care by the sources of funds indicated that in 1977 59.9 percent of the $142.6 billion personal health care expenditures was paid from private sources. Approximately 27.9 percent was provided by federal sources, and 12.1 percent was from state and local governments.

The percentages of consumer expenditures for health care met by private insurance companies were increasing over the decade. In 1976 46.3 percent of the expenditures were provided by private insurance. Private insurance policies paid 85.8 percent of hospital care costs, 45.9 percent of physician services, and 18.4 percent of out-of-hospital dental costs. Private insurance for dental services appeared to be growing substantially in recent years. The number of persons holding various types of insurance protection has generally increased from 1976 to 1977; however, decreases were noted in the number of persons having surgical and physician expense coverage.

Table V-C-1. Consumer Price Index for All Items and Major Components, 1973 to 1977 (1967=100)

Item	Annual averages				
	1973	1974	1975	1976	1977
All items	133.1	147.7	161.2	170.5	181.5
Food	141.4	161.7	175.4	180.8	192.2
Housing	135.0	150.6	166.8	177.2	189.6
Apparel and upkeep	126.8	136.2	142.3	147.6	154.2
Transportation	123.8	137.7	150.6	165.5	177.2
Medical care	137.7	150.5	168.6	184.7	202.4
Personal care	125.2	137.3	150.7	160.5	170.9
Reading and recreation	125.9	133.8	144.4	151.2	157.9
Other goods and services[1] ...	129.0	137.2	147.4	153.3	159.2

[1]Includes tobacco, alcoholic beverages, legal services, banking fees, burial services, etc.

SOURCE: U.S. Department of Labor, Bureau of Labor Statistics, *Handbook of Labor Statistics, 1978,* Bulletin 2000, p. 398.

Table V-C-2. Consumer Price Index for Medical Care Items, 1973 to 1977 (1967=100)

Medical care items	Annual averages				
	1973	1974	1975	1976	1977
Total medical care	137.7	150.5	168.6	184.7	202.4
Drugs and prescriptions	105.9	109.6	118.8	126.0	134.1
Physicians' fees	138.2	150.9	169.4	188.5	206.0
Optometric examination and dispensing of eyeglasses ...	129.5	138.6	149.6	158.9	168.2
Routine laboratory tests	122.8	135.4	151.4	160.5	169.4
Hospital service charges[1]	105.6	115.1	132.3	148.7	164.1
Operating room charges	179.1	201.3	239.4	274.8	311.3
X-ray, diagnostic series, upper G.I.	131.8	140.6	156.2	174.6	189.4

[1]January 1972=100.

SOURCE: U.S. Department of Labor, Bureau of Labor Statistics, *Handbook of Labor Statistics, 1978,* Bulletin 2000, pp. 422-424.

Table V-C-3. Total Health Expenditures, by Object of Expenditure, Fiscal Years 1972-73 to 1976-77
(in millions)

Object of expenditure	Fiscal year ending in June				Fiscal year ending in September[1]		
	1972-73[2]	1973-74[2]	1974-75[2]	1975-76[3]	1974-75	1975-76	1976-77
Total health expenditures ...	$95,384	$106,321	$123,716	[3]$139,312	$127,719	$145,102	$162,627
Health services and supplies ...	88,941	99,330	116,111	131,022	119,771	136,368	153,887
Hospital care	36,155	41,020	48,376	55,400	49,973	57,497	65,627
Physicians' services	17,995	19,742	23,839	26,350	24,553	28,504	32,184
Dentists' services	6,101	6,870	7,870	8,600	8,034	8,987	10,020
Other professional services	1,781	1,929	2,378	2,400	2,463	2,849	3,212
Drug and drug sundries	[4]8,987	[4]9,416	[4]10,357	[4]11,168	10,582	11,472	12,516
Eyeglasses and appliances	1,986	1,674	1,751	1,980	1,822	1,986	2,086
Nursing home care	6,650	7,450	9,342	10,600	9,620	10,834	12,618
Expenses for prepayment and administration ...	4,299	5,483	5,768	7,336	6,016	6,628	7,572
Government public health activities	2,152	2,531	2,960	3,255	3,091	3,522	3,729
Other health activities ...	2,835	3,214	3,469	3,933	3,616	4,088	4,322
Research and medical facilities construction ...	6,443	6,991	7,605	8,290	7,947	8,734	8,739
Research	[4]2,298	[4]2,527	[4]2,972	[4]3,327	[5]3,132	[5]3,623	[5]3,684
Construction	4,145	4,464	4,633	4,963	4,815	5,111	5,055

[1] The federal fiscal year was changed in 1977 to end on September 30; estimates for fiscal years 1975 and 1976 are adjusted to conform to the same fiscal year (ending in September) and presented along with preliminary estimates for fiscal year 1977 to allow annual comparisons to be made.

[2] Revised estimates.

[3] Revised estimate for "total health expenditures" is $141,013. Revised estimates for breakdown not available.

[4] Research expenditures of drug companies are included in "drug and drug sundries" and excluded from "research expenditures."

[5] Research and development expenditures of drug companies and other manufacturers and providers of medical equipment and supplies excluded from "research expenditures" but included in the expenditure class in which the product falls.

SOURCE: U.S. Department of Health, Education, and Welfare, Social Security Administration, Office of Research and Statistics, Social Security Bulletin, February 1976, Vol. 39, No. 2, p. 12; Social Security Bulletin, July 1978. Vol. 41. No. 7. pp. 3. 6 and 15: and individual releases.

Table V-C-4. Total National Health Expenditures and Percent of
Gross National Product, Fiscal Years 1968-69 to 1976-77

Fiscal year	Gross national product (in billions)	National health expenditures (in millions)	Expenditure as a percent of gross national product
Ending September[1]			
1976-77	$1,838.0	$162,627	8.8
1975-76	1,667.4	145,102	8.7
1974-75	1,487.1	127,719	8.6
Ending June			
1975-76[2]	1,625.4	141,013	8.7
1974-75[2]	1,454.5	123,716	8.5
1973-74	1,361.2	106,321	7.8
1972-73	1,238.6	95,383	7.7
1971-72	1,111.8	86,687	7.8
1970-71	1,019.8	77,162	7.6
1969-70	960.2	69,201	7.2
1968-69	904.2	60,617	6.7

[1] The federal fiscal year was changed in 1977 to end on September 30; estimates for fiscal years 1975 and 1976 are adjusted to conform to the same fiscal year (ending in September) and presented along with preliminary estimates for fiscal year 1977 to allow annual comparisons to be made.
[2] Revised estimate.
SOURCE: U.S. Department of Health, Education, and Welfare, Social Security Administration, Office of Research and Statistics, *Social Security Bulletin*, July 1978, Vol. 41, No. 7, p. 5.

Table V-C-5. Per Capital National Health Expenditures, Fiscal Years 1972-73 to 1976-77

Source of funds and object of expenditure	Fiscal year ending in June				Fiscal year ending in September[3]		
	1972-73[2]	1973-74[2]	1974-75[2]	1975-76[2]	1974-75	1975-76	1976-77
Total health expenditures ...	$447.31	$495.01	$571.21	$645.76	$588.48	$663.06	$736.92
Total health expenditures based on 1977 prices[4]	657.48	665.71	685.72	707.64	706.46	726.60	736.92
Source of funds							
Public...............	171.96	193.27	241.79	275.60	251.03	281.22	310.13
Private	275.35	301.74	329.42	370.16	337.45	381.84	426.78
Selected objects of expenditure							
Hospital care	169.55	186.06	215.12	(5)	230.25	262.74	297.38
Physicians' services	84.39	91.12	102.02	(5)	113.13	130.25	145.84
Nursing home care	31.19	34.69	41.55	(5)	44.33	49.51	57.18

[1] Based on January 1 data from the Bureau of the Census for total U.S. population (including armed forces and federal civilian employees overseas and the civilian population of outlying areas).

[2] Revised estimates.

[3] The federal fiscal year was changed in 1977 to end on September 30; estimates for fiscal years 1975 and 1976 are adjusted to conform to the same fiscal year (ending in September) and presented along with preliminary estimates for fiscal year 1977 to allow annual comparisons to be made.

[4] Based on medical care components of the BLS Consumer Price Index.

[5] Information not available.

SOURCE: U.S. Department of Health, Education, and Welfare, Social Security Administration, Office of Research and Statistics, *Social Security Bulletin*, July 1978, Vol. 41, No. 7, pp. 5, 7-9; and individual releases.

Table V-C-6. Estimated Personal Health Care Expenditures, by Type of Expenditure, Age Group, and Source of Funds, Fiscal Year 1977[1] (in millions)

Type of expenditure and age group	Total expenditures[2]	Source of funds		
		Federal	State and local	Private
Total, all ages	$142,586	$39,823	$17,299	$85,465
Hospital care	65,637	25,715	10,484	29,427
Physicians' services	32,184	5,808	2,016	24,360
Dentists' services	10,020	310	190	9,520
Other professional services	3,212	683	241	2,288
Drug and drug sundries ...	12,516	614	529	11,373
Eyeglasses and appliances	2,086	66	64	1,956
Nursing home care	12,618	4,204	2,980	5,434
Other health services	4,322	2,424	793	1,105
Total, under 19 years ...	17,909	3,186	2,331	12,392
Hospital care	6,333	1,777	1,108	3,448
Physicians' services ...	4,924	440	304	4,180
Dentists' services	2,144	124	96	1,925
Other professional services	305	84	52	169
Drug and drug sundries	2,319	91	67	2,161
Eyeglasses and appliances	270	15	7	248
Nursing home care	341	98	81	162
Other health services ...	1,272	558	616	98
Total, 19-64 years	83,422	13,244	10,729	59,449
Hospital care	41,109	9,172	8,096	23,840
Physicians' services ...	20,115	1,249	1,575	17,291
Dentists' services	6,854	154	80	6,620
Other professional services	2,091	139	158	1,794
Drug and drug sundries	7,338	283	266	6,790
Eyeglasses and appliances	1,505	44	56	1,405
Nursing home care	1,741	592	412	737
Other health services ...	2,669	1,610	85	973
Total, 65 and over	41,256	23,393	4,239	13,624
Hospital care	18,185	14,766	1,280	2,140
Physicians' services ...	7,145	4,119	137	2,889
Dentists' services	1,022	32	15	976
Other professional services	816	460	31	325
Drug and drug sundries	2,859	240	197	2,423
Eyeglasses and appliances	312	7	2	303
Nursing home care	10,536	3,514	2,487	4,535
Other health services ...	381	256	91	33

[1]The federal fiscal year was changed in 1977 to end on September 30. Preliminary estimates.
[2]Individual items may not add to totals due to rounding.
SOURCE: U.S. Department of Health, Education, and Welfare, Social Security Administration, Office of

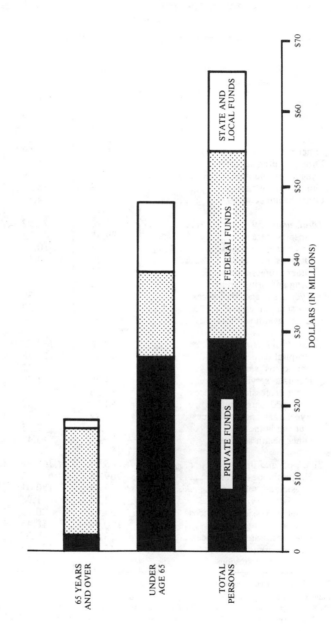

CHART 15. ESTIMATED HEALTH EXPENDITURES FOR HOSPITAL CARE BY AGE GROUP, AND SOURCE OF FUNDS, FISCAL YEAR 1977

SOURCE: U.S. Department of Health, Education and Welfare, Social Security Administration, *Social Security Bulletin*, January 1979, Vol. 42, No. 1.

Prepared by American Nurses' Association, Research and Policy Analysis Department, Statistics Unit, 1980.

Table V-C-7. Estimated Per Capita Personal Health Care Expenditures, by Type of Expenditure, Age Group, and Source of Funds, Fiscal Year 1977[1] (in millions)

Type of expenditure and age group	Total expenditures[2]	Source of funds	
		Public	Private
Total, all ages	*$646.11*	*$258.84*	*$387.27*
Hospital care	297.38	164.03	133.35
Physicians' services	145.84	35.45	110.39
Dentists' services	45.41	2.27	43.14
Other professional services	14.56	4.19	10.37
Drug and drug sundries	56.72	5.18	51.54
Eyeglasses and appliances	9.45	.59	8.86
Nursing home care	57.18	32.55	24.62
Other health services	19.59	14.58	5.01
Total, under 19 years	*252.96*	*77.92*	*175.03*
Hospital care	89.45	40.76	48.70
Physicians' services	69.55	10.51	59.05
Dentists' services	30.29	3.10	27.19
Other professional services	4.31	1.92	2.39
Drug and drug sundries	32.76	2.23	30.52
Eyeglasses and appliances	3.81	.30	3.51
Nursing home care	4.81	2.52	2.29
Other health services	17.97	16.58	1.39
Total, 19-64 years	*660.78*	*189.89*	*470.89*
Hospital care	325.62	136.78	188.83
Physicians' services	159.33	22.37	136.96
Dentists' services	54.29	1.86	52.43
Other professional services	16.56	2.36	14.21
Drug and drug sundries	58.13	4.35	53.78
Eyeglasses and appliances	11.92	.79	11.13
Nursing home care	13.79	7.95	5.84
Other health services	21.14	13.43	7.71
Total, 65 and over	*1,745.17*	*1,168.84*	*576.33*
Hospital care	769.25	678.73	90.52
Physicians' services	302.23	180.01	122.23
Dentists' services	43.24	1.96	41.28
Other professional services	34.51	20.75	13.77
Drug and drug sundries	120.94	18.46	102.48
Eyeglasses and appliances	13.20	.37	12.83
Nursing home care	445.68	253.86	191.82
Other health services	16.12	14.71	1.41

[1] The federal fiscal year was changed in 1977 to end on September 30. Preliminary estimates.

[2] Individual items may not add to totals due to rounding.

SOURCE: U.S. Department of Health, Education, and Welfare, Social Security Administration, Office of Research and Statistics, *Social Security Bulletin*, January 1979, Vol. 42, No. 1, p. 5.

Table V-C-8. Percentage of Consumer Expenditures for Health Care Met by Private Insurance Benefits, 1966-1976

Year	Total	Hospital care	Physicians' services	Prescribed drugs (out-of-hospital)	Dental care (out-of-hospital)	Other[1]
1976	46.3	85.9	45.9	8.1	18.4	9.6
1975	45.0	86.8	46.8	6.9	13.9	8.3
1974[1]	42.9	77.8	50.7	6.2	11.5	9.8
1973[1]	39.9	75.9	46.1	6.0	8.6	6.8
1972[1]	39.9	77.6	45.7	5.4	7.3	6.0
1971	39.8	82.5	43.9	5.5	6.3	4.6
1970	38.5	77.9	43.8	4.5	5.3	5.2
1969	36.6	74.3	41.1	(2)	(2)	16.0
1968	36.3	76.9	40.7	(2)	(2)	13.9
1967	33.5	73.3	35.9	(2)	(2)	13.8
1966	32.3	69.0	33.9	(2)	(2)	9.8

[1] Revised percentages.
[2] Information not available.

SOURCE: U.S. Department of Health, Education, and Welfare, Social Security Administration, Office of Research and Statistics, *Social Security Bulletin*, September 1978, Vol. 41, No. 9, p. 14.

Table V-C-9. Number of Persons with Health Insurance Protection, by Type of Coverage,[1] 1968-1977 (in thousands)

Year	Type of coverage[2]				Disability income		Dental expense[4]
	Hospital expense	Surgical expense	Physicians' expense	Major medical expense[3]	Short-term	Long-term	
1977	178,968	167,220	160,429	139,362	64,627	19,364	53,510
Under 65	165,051	156,050	149,997	(5)	(5)	19,364	(5)
65 and over	13,917	11,170	10,432	(5)	(5)	....	(5)
1976	176,581	167,432	163,094	134,992	62,250	17,779	46,936
Under 65	164,027	156,852	152,867	(5)	(5)	17,779	(5)
65 and over	12,554	10,580	10,227	(5)	(5)	....	(5)
1975	177,980	168,895	161,854	134,092	62,971	18,396	34,729
Under 65	165,357	158,518	152,157	(5)	(5)	18,396	(5)
65 and over	12,623	10,377	9,697	(5)	(5)	....	(5)
1974	173,140	166,434	158,170	131,438	65,282	17,799	32,810
Under 65	161,604	156,846	149,291	(5)	65,282	17,799	(5)
65 and over	11,536	9,588	8,879	(5)	....	....	(5)
1973	168,455	162,644	151,680	124,627	64,168	17,011	21,927
1972	164,098	154,687	140,873	113,837	61,548	14,538	18,678
1971	161,849	153,093	139,399	108,813	59,280	12,284	16,276
1970	158,847	151,440	138,658	103,544	58,089	10,966	12,908
1969	155,025	147,774	131,792	95,528	57,770	9,282	8,858
1968	151,947	143,625	126,233	87,641	55,636	7,836	5,867

[1] For 1975 and later, data include the number of persons covered in Puerto Rico and other U.S. territories and possessions. The data refer to the net total of people protected, i.e. duplication among persons protected by more than one kind of insuring organization or more than one insurance company policy providing the same type of coverage has been eliminated.

[2] The "disability income" category represents coverage by insurance companies, formal paid sick leave plans, and coverage through employee organizations. All other categories represent coverage by insurance companies, Blue Cross, Blue Shield, medical society-approved plans, and other plans.

[3] Data are revised from previous editions to include data for all private health insurers; previously, only coverage by insurance companies were reported.

[4] Revised data for 1968 through 1975.

[5] Information not available.

SOURCE: Health Insurance Institute. *Source Book of Health Insurance Data 1976-77*, p. 22; and *Source Book of Health Insurance Data 1978-79*, p. 9.

Chapter V, Section D
VITAL STATISTICS

An estimated 220,099,000 persons resided in the United States in 1979, an estimated increase of 8.3 percent, or 16,797,000 persons, since the 1970 census. Including the armed forces overseas, the 1979 U.S. population totaled 220,584,000 persons. The yearly percentage increases have not exceeded 1 percent since 1971.

The 1979 data revealed a slight but unabating trend for a larger portion of the population to be in the 65 years of age and older group. In 1979, 11.2 percent of the total U.S. population was over 64 years of age, while only 4 years earlier, in 1975, 10.5 percent of the population was in that age bracket. The U.S. birth rate has been climbing in recent years. In 1979, the birth rate was 15.8 births per 1,000 population, up one percentage point from 1975.

The past decade has shown a downward trend in the death rate. In 1979 there were 8.7 deaths per 1,000 population. Similar data for 1970 showed the death rate to be 9.5 deaths per 1,000 population. Diseases of the heart were the leading causes of death, with 37.8 percent of all deaths in 1978 attributed to heart disease. There has been little variation in this over the past 5 years. The proportion of persons dying from malignant neoplasms has not been so stagnant over the interval from 1974 to 1978. In 1974 18.6 percent of deaths were related to malignant neoplasms; by 1978, 20.6 percent of deaths were associated with this disease. The next leading cause of death was cerebro-vascular disease, followed by deaths from accidents.

Table V-D-1. Estimated Resident Population[1] by State, for Selected Years as of July 1 (in thousands)

State	Resident population						
	1970[2]	1977	Percent change 1970-77	1978	Percent change 1970-78	1979[3]	Percent change 1970-79[4]
United States, total[5] ...	203,302	216,383	+ 6.4	218,228	+ 7.3	220,099	+ 8.3
Alabama	3,444	3,691	+ 7.2	3,728	+ 8.2	3,769	+ 9.4
Alaska	303	413	+36.3	411	+35.6	406	+34.3
Arizona	1,775	2,305	+29.9	2,373	+33.7	2,450	+38.0
Arkansas	1,923	2,152	+11.9	2,167	+12.7	2,180	+13.4
California	19,971	21,887	+ 9.6	22,314	+11.7	22,696	+13.6
Colorado	2,210	2,625	+18.8	2,706	+22.4	2,772	+25.5
Connecticut	3,032	3,107	+ 2.5	3,116	+ 2.8	3,115	+ 2.7
Delaware	548	582	+ 6.2	584	+ 6.6	582	+ 6.2
District of Columbia	757	685	− 9.5	671	−11.4	656	−13.4
Florida	6,791	8,466	+24.7	8,661	+27.5	· 8,860	+30.5
Georgia	4,588	5,041	+ 9.9	5,075	+10.6	5,118	+11.5
Hawaii	770	891	+15.7	902	+17.1	915	+18.8
Idaho	713	856	+20.1	882	+23.7	905	+26.9
Illinois	11,110	11,228	+ 1.1	11,238	+ 1.2	11,230	+ 1.1
Indiana	5,195	5,350	+ 3.0	5,386	+ 3.7	5,400	+ 3.9
Iowa	2,825	2,888	+ 2.2	2,906	+ 2.9	2,903	+ 2.7
Kansas	2,249	2,320	+ 3.2	2,347	+ 4.4	2,369	+ 5.3
Kentucky	3,221	3,468	+ 7.7	3,490	+ 8.4	3,527	+ 9.5
Louisiana[6]	3,645	3,930	+ 7.8	3,986	+ 9.4	4,026	+10.5
Maine	994	1,084	+ 9.1	1,092	+ 9.9	1,097	+10.4
Maryland	3,924	4,137	+ 5.4	4,148	+ 5.7	4,149	+ 5.7
Massachusetts	5,689	5,777	+ 1.5	5,771	+ 1.4	5,769	+ 1.4
Michigan	8,882	9,148	+ 3.0	9,181	+ 3.4	9,208	+ 3.7
Minnesota	3,806	3,980	+ 4.6	4,024	+ 5.7	4,060	+ 6.7
Mississippi[6]	2,217	2,386	+ 7.6	2,400	+ 8.3	2,406	+ 8.5
Missouri	4,678	4,822	+ 3.1	4,847	+ 3.6	4,868	+ 4.1
Montana	694	766	+10.4	780	+12.4	786	+13.2
Nebraska	1,485	1,555	+ 4.7	1,569	+ 5.7	1,574	+ 6.0
Nevada	489	637	+30.3	666	+36.2	702	+43.6
New Hampshire	738	850	+15.2	869	+17.8	887	+20.2
New Jersey	7,171	7,338	+ 2.3	7,315	+ 2.0	7,332	+ 2.2
New Mexico	1,017	1,196	+17.6	1,215	+19.5	1,241	+22.1
New York	18,241	17,932	− 1.7	17,746	− 2.7	17,649	− 3.2
North Carolina	5,084	5,515	+ 8.5	5,571	+ 9.6	5,606	+10.3
North Dakota	618	650	+ 5.2	653	+ 5.7	657	+ 6.3
Ohio	10,657	10,696	+ 0.4	10,732	+ 0.7	10,731	+ 0.7
Oklahoma	2,559	2,817	+10.1	2,842	+11.1	2,892	+13.0
Oregon	2,092	2,385	+14.0	2,452	+17.2	2,527	+20.8
Pennsylvania	11,801	11,796	−(7)	11,763	− 0.3	11,731	− 0.6
Rhode Island	950	937	− 1.4	932	− 1.9	929	− 2.1
South Carolina	2,591	2,878	+11.1	2,902	+12.0	2,932	+13.2
South Dakota	666	688	+ 3.3	690	+ 3.6	689	+ 3.4
Tennessee	3,926	4,292	+ 9.3	4,333	+10.4	4,380	+11.6
Texas	11,199	12,806	+14.3	13,050	+16.5	13,385	+19.5
Utah	1,059	1,270	+19.9	1,316	+24.3	1,367	+29.0
Vermont	445	482	+ 8.3	487	+ 9.4	493	+10.9
Virginia[6]	4,651	5,095	+ 9.5	5,177	+11.3	5,197	+11.7
Washington	3,413	3,681	+ 7.9	3,793	+11.1	3,926	+15.0
West Virginia	1,744	1,853	+ 6.3	1,861	+ 6.7	1,878	+ 7.7
Wisconsin	4,418	4,644	+ 5.1	4,683	+ 6.0	4,720	+ 6.8
Wyoming	332	406	+22.3	425	+28.0	450	+35.3

[1] Includes estimated armed force personnel residing in each state.
[2] April 1, 1980 census data, which includes recognized changes through September 1979.
[3] Provisional.
[4] Percentages based on unrounded numbers.
[5] Items may not add to totals due to rounding.
[6] Because of a late data change for Mississippi, estimate shown may be revised upward about 10,000 for 1978 and 20,000 for 1979. Data revisions for Louisiana and Virginia may result in declines in 1978 and 1979.
[7] Less than 0.1 percent.
SOURCE: U.S. Department of Commerce, Bureau of the Census, *Current Population Reports*, December 1978, Series P-25, No. 790, p. 2, and November 1979, Series P-25, No. 868, p. 2.

Table V-D-2. Estimates of U.S. Population, 1968-1979, as of July 1
(in thousands)

Year	Total population	Yearly percentage increase	Resident population[1]	Yearly percentage increase	Civilian resident population[2]	Yearly percentage increase
1979	220,584	0.9	220,099	0.9	218,497	0.9
1978	218,717	0.8	218,228	0.8	216,600	0.9
1977	216,880	0.8	216,400	0.8	214,746	0.8
1976[3] ...	215,152	0.7	214,680	0.8	213,011	0.8
1975[3] ...	213,559	0.8	213,051	0.8	211,373	0.8
1974[3] ...	211,901	0.7	211,389	0.7	209,683	0.8
1973[3] ...	210,410	0.7	209,859	0.8	208,102	0.8
1972[3] ...	208,846	0.9	208,234	1.0	206,461	1.1
1971[3] ...	207,053	1.1	206,219	1.2	204,258	1.3
1970[4] ...	204,878	1.1	203,810	1.2	201,722	1.3
1969	202,677	1.0	201,385	1.0	199,145	1.0
1968	200,706	1.0	199,399	1.0	197,113	0.9

[1] Excludes armed forces overseas.
[2] Excludes armed forces in U.S. and overseas.
[3] Revised estimates.
[4] Census count of resident population: April 1, 1970—203,235,298.

SOURCES: U.S. Department of Commerce, Bureau of the Census, *Current Population Reports*, May 1979, Series P-25, No. 802, p. 12 and 13; and January 1980, Series P-25, No. 874.

Table V-D-3. Estimates of the U.S. Population,[1] by Age, 1975-1979, as of July 1, (in thousands)

Age	1979 Number	1979 Percent	1978 Number	1978 Percent	1977 Number	1977 Percent	1976 Number	1976 Percent	1975 Number	1975 Percent
Total[2]	220,584	100.0	218,717	100.0	216,880	100.0	215,152	100.0	213,631	100.0
Under 5 years	15,649	7.1	15,378	7.0	15,248	7.0	15,345	7.1	15,896	7.4
5 to 9 years	16,493	7.5	16,895	7.7	17,169	7.9	17,355	8.1	17,334	8.1
10 to 14 years	18,071	8.2	18,589	8.5	19,203	8.9	19,819	9.2	20,418	9.6
15 to 19 years	20,918	9.5	21,074	9.6	21,169	9.8	21,214	9.9	21,028	9.9
20 to 24 years	20,726	9.4	20,461	9.4	20,077	9.3	19,630	9.1	19,242	9.0
25 to 29 years	18,441	8.4	18,057	8.3	17,742	8.2	17,808	8.3	16,941	7.9
30 to 34 years	16,584	7.5	15,915	7.3	15,420	7.1	14,241	6.6	13,994	6.6
35 to 39 years	13,614	6.2	13,079	6.0	12,342	5.7	11,919	5.5	11,630	5.5
40 to 44 years	11,522	5.2	11,330	5.2	11,202	5.2	11,161	5.2	11,195	5.2
45 to 49 years	11,222	5.1	11,370	5.2	11,512	5.3	11,661	5.4	11,790	5.5
50 to 54 years	11,735	5.3	11,829	5.4	11,880	5.5	11,980	5.6	11,981	5.6
55 to 59 years	11,367	5.2	11,241	5.1	11,036	5.1	10,753	5.0	10,537	4.9
60 to 64 years	9,585	4.3	9,436	4.3	9,367	4.3	9,313	4.3	9,243	4.3
65 to 69 years	8,688	3.9	8,576	3.9	8,450	3.9	8,282	3.8	8,099	3.8
70 to 74 years	6,584	3.0	6,364	2.9	6,143	2.8	5,917	2.8	5,775	2.7
75 to 79 years	4,274	1.9	4,171	1.9	4,072	1.9	4,055	1.9	4,001	1.9
80 to 84 years	2,780	1.3	2,748	1.3	2,764	1.3	2,728	1.3	2,649	1.2
85 years and over	2,332	1.1	2,206	1.0	2,085	1.0	1,972	0.9	1,877	0.9

[1]Includes armed forces overseas.
[2]Items may not add to totals, due to rounding.

SOURCES: U.S. Department of Commerce, Bureau of the Census, *Current Population Reports*, November 1975, Series P-25, No. 614, and January 1980, P-25, No. 870, pp. 7-12.

Table V-D-4. Live Birth Rates and Death Rates in the United States per 1,000 Population, 1970-1979

Year	Rate per 1,000 population	
	Birth	Death[1]
1979	[2]15.8	[2]8.7
1978	[2]15.3	[2]8.8
1977	15.4	8.8
1976	14.8	8.9
1975	14.8	[3]8.9
1974	[3]14.9	[3]9.2
1973	[3]14.9	9.4
1972	15.6	9.4
1971	17.2	9.3
1970	18.4	9.5

[1] Excludes fetal deaths.
[2] Provisional data.
[3] Revised.

SOURCE: U.S. Department of Health, Education, and Welfare, Public Health Service, Office of Health Research, Statistics, and Technology, National Center for Health Statistics, *Monthly Vital Statistics Report*, August 13, 1979, Vol. 27, No. 13, p. 1, and February 8, 1980, Vol. 28, No. 11, p. 1.

Table V-D-5. Estimated Death Rates[1] for the Ten Leading Causes of Death[2] in the United States, 1974-1978

Rank	Cause of death	Death rate				
		1978[3]	1977	1976	1975	1974
	All causes	*882.3*	*878.1*	*889.6*	*888.5*	*915.1*
1	Diseases of heart	333.9	332.3	337.2	336.2	349.2
2	Malignant neoplasms, including neoplasms of lymphatic and hemato- poietic tissues	181.6	178.7	175.8	171.7	170.5
3	Cerebrovascular diseases	79.1	84.1	87.9	91.1	98.1
4	Accidents	49.5	47.7	46.9	48.4	49.5
5	Influenza and pneumonia	26.7	23.7	28.8	26.1	25.9
6	Diabetes mellitus	15.0	15.2	16.1	16.5	17.7
7	Cirrhosis of liver	13.7	14.3	14.7	14.8	15.8
8	Arteriosclerosis	13.4	13.3	13.7	13.6	15.3
9	Suicide	12.6	13.3	12.5	12.7	12.1
10	Certain causes of mortality in early infancy	10.1	10.8	11.6	12.5	13.6
	All other causes	146.7	144.7	144.4	144.9	147.4

Rank	Cause of death	Percent[4] of total deaths				
		1978[3]	1977	1976	1975	1974
	All causes	*100.0*	*100.0*	*100.0*	*100.0*	*100.0*
1	Diseases of heart	37.8	37.8	37.9	37.8	38.2
2	Malignant neoplasms, including neoplasms of lymphatic and hemato- poietic tissues	20.6	20.4	19.8	19.3	18.6
3	Cerebrovascular diseases	9.0	9.6	9.9	10.3	10.7
4	Accidents	5.6	5.4	5.3	5.4	5.4
5	Influenza and pneumonia	3.0	2.7	3.2	2.9	2.8
6	Diabetes mellitus	1.7	1.7	1.8	1.9	1.9
7	Cirrhosis of liver	1.6	1.6	1.7	1.7	1.7
8	Arteriosclerosis	1.5	1.5	1.5	1.5	1.7
9	Suicide	1.4	1.5	1.4	1.4	1.3
10	Certain causes of mortality in early infancy	1.1	1.2	1.3	1.4	1.5
	All other causes	16.6	16.5	16.2	16.3	16.1

[1] Rates per 100,000 population.
[2] Data refers only to deaths occurring within the U.S., excluding fetal deaths.
[3] Based on a 10 percent sample of deaths.
[4] Percentages may not add to 100.0 due to rounding.

SOURCES: U.S. Department of Health, Education, and Welfare, Public Health Service, Office of Health Research, Statistics, and Technology, National Center for Health Statistics, *Monthly Vital Statistics Report*, August 13, 1979, Vol. 27, No. 13, p. 5, and U.S. Department of Commerce, Bureau of the Census, *Statistical Abstract of the United States: 1979* (100th edition) Washington D.C., 1979, p. 76.

Chapter VI

The **American Nurses' Association, Inc.,** 2420 Pershing Road, Kansas City, Missouri 64108, is the professional association for registered nurses. It was organized in 1896.

The purposes of the American Nurses' Association are to foster high standards of nursing practice, promote the professional and educational advancement of nurses, and promote the welfare of nurses so all people may have better health care. These purposes are unrestricted by considerations of nationality, race, religion, or sex. ANA represents nurses and serves as their spokesman with allied national and international organizations, governmental bodies, and the public.

The American Nurses' Association includes 53 constituent nurses' associations in the 50 states, the District of Columbia, Guam, and the Virgin Islands. These constituent associations are, in turn, composed of more than 800 district nurses' associations.

ANA's policies and programs are established by the membership through representation in a House of Delegates, which is the highest authority in the association; the Board of Directors; the commissions; the Congress for Nursing Practice; the divisions on practice; the standing committees; and special committees and task forces.

BOARD OF DIRECTORS

During the interim between the biennial conventions, the Board of Directors transacts the general business of the association. The board is also responsible for establishing the major policies governing the affairs of the association and for implementing measures for the association's growth and development.

COMMISSIONS

Five commissions are responsible for developing and implementing programs of activity designed to carry out specific functions and to obtain recognition and acceptance of the association's concern, influence, and accomplishments in their respective areas of responsibility.

The *Commission on Economic and General Welfare* is responsible for planning and implementing the economic and general welfare program of the association. The commission develops general economic standards and devises methods of implementation; formulates policy and recommends action related to federal and state economic security legislation interests; advises and assists constituent associations in the development of their programs in economic and general welfare; and develops and implements an economic education program. The commission studies and evaluates the economics of health care generally, as well as the economics of nursing.

ANA's economic and general welfare program is based on the principle that nurses have the right and responsibility to participate in the determination of their employment conditions. The collective bargaining process is viewed as an effective vehicle through which to establish conditions conducive to the delivery of quality nursing care.

The aim of the program is to have nurses speaking for nursing, to protect and advance the economic and professional status of nurses, and to involve nurses in the decisions affecting the nursing care of patients. Such assurance is an essential precondition to recruiting and retaining the number of qualified nurses necessary to meet the nation's health needs. ANA advises and assists the constituent state nurses' associations, which, in turn, act as the collective bargaining representative of nurses in their employment settings. The state associations directly represent nurses' economic professional interest in various ways, including collective bargaining with employers, public and private.

The commission has established the Council of Local Unit Members, the purposes of which are to promote effective, aggressive collective bargaining; implement ANA standards; establish a strike fund; and promote exchange of ideas.

The *Commission on Human Rights* addresses and responds to the equal opportunity and human rights concerns of nurses and health care recipients, with the major focus on ethnic people of color. Through its affirmative action programming, and in conjunction with the ANA Ombudsman, the Commission on Human Rights works to prevent abridgement of rights and to overcome all vestiges of exclusion or discrimination. The primary goal of the ANA affirmative action program is to affirmatively assist all nurses to gain full equality of opportunity in nursing to the end that all may have better nursing care.

The commission evaluates social, economic, scientific, and educational changes to determine their implication for the health and welfare of nurses and consumers from minority groups. The commission promotes the inclusion of ethnic and other minority concerns in the development and application of standards for nursing education, nursing practice, and nursing research. The commission determines priorities relevant to human rights and recommends appropriate actions to structural units and constituent associations.

The Commission on Human Rights has established a Council on Intercultural Nursing. The purposes of this council are to provide direction in the development and implementation of policies and programs that relate to human rights concerns and to improve the quality of nursing care by being responsive to the cultural and ethnic variances among consumers.

The *Commission on Nursing Education* develops standards for nursing education. The commission evaluates scientific and educational developments as well as changes in health needs and practices to determine implications for nursing education. The encouragement and stimulation of research in all areas of nursing education and the formulation of policy recommendations concerning federal and state legislation in the field of education are also responsibilities of the commission. The Council on Continuing Education, under the aegis of the commission develops standards of continuing education and works toward their implementation, formulates and recommends policies and programs to fulfill the association's responsibility in relation to continuing education, provides for accreditation of continuing education, and provides a means of communication among nurses whose primary interest and responsibility lie in continuing education in nursing.

The *Commission on Nursing Research* formulates policy concerning research in nursing and recommends action for the implementation of these policies. The commission evaluates social, scientific, and educational issues in health needs and nursing practice in relation to research. The commission recommends priorities for the profession's research concerns, encourages research in all areas of nursing, provides for the conduct of nursing research forums for the ANA membership and assists in the dissemination of findings from research. The Council of Nurse Researchers is a membership group accountable to the Commission on Nursing Research. The purposes of the council are to provide for the exchange of ideas among researchers and to recognize excellence in research. The responsibility of the council relates specifically to the needs of researchers in nursing.

The commission and council also maintain a national network of nurse researchers. This network, the Legislative Action Subcommittee, is involved in legislative activities to secure a stable funding base for nursing research, as well as other legislative activities concerning nursing research. During the 1978 ANA Convention, a joint standing committee of the Commission on Nursing Research and the Council of Nurse Researchers was recommended to coordinate and direct the work of this network. This committee, the Legislative Coordinating Committee, is composed of two representatives each for the commission and the council. The charge of the committee includes (1) better communication with the Legislative Action Subcommittee, Commission on Nursing Research, and the Council of Nurse Researchers and (2) maintenance of an active Legislative Action Subcommittee.

The *Commission on Nursing Services* establishes the scope of the association's responsibility for organized nursing services. In addition to the development of standards and guidelines for organized nursing services in health agencies, the commission is responsible for evaluation of scientific and educational developments and changes in health needs and health practice for their implications for nursing manpower needs and resources. The commission works to bring about improvement in the organization and management of nursing service in all settings. The commission formulates policy and recommends action concerning federal and state legislation related to health manpower and nursing services.

Under the aegis of the Commission on Nursing Services is the Council on Nursing Administration composed of ANA members who have primary interest in and/or responsibility for enabling and advancing nursing practice within organized nursing services. The purposes of the council are to advance sound administrative practice, implement the standards for nursing sevices, promote the exchange of ideas, and recognize excellence in nursing service administration.

CONGRESS FOR NURSING PRACTICE

The Congress for Nursing Practice is responsible for advancing the practice of nursing through activities that deal with the nature and scope of nursing practice. The Congress for Nursing Practice studies ethical and legal aspects of nursing practice, provides for the public recognition of the significance of nursing practice to health care, evaluates and describes the changing scope of nursing practice; monitors scientific and educational development and trends in health care; formulates policy and recommends action concerning federal and state legislation related to nursing practice, encourages research in the practice of nursing, and ensures coordination of activities among the divisions on practice.

DIVISIONS ON PRACTICE

There are five divisions on nursing practice: Community Health Nursing Practice, Gerontological Nursing Practice, Maternal and Child Health Nursing Practice, Medical-Surgical Nursing Practice, and Psychiatric and Mental Health Nursing Practice. It is through these divisions that ANA responds to nurses' interests and concerns with their practice; to their needs for identification with clinical areas of nursing practice; to the need for standards of nursing practice; to the need to accord recognition for achievement in the performance of nursing practice; to the need for keeping abreast of new knowledge and its applications to practice through special publications, clinical institutes, and conferences, and to the need for identifying ANA's concern and involvement in major health problems. Nurses may belong to the one or two divisions that are of the greatest interest and assistance to them. Under the sponsorship of divisions on practice the following councils have been established to serve the interest of specific groups: the Council of Primary Health Care Nurse Practitioners; the Council of High-Risk Perinatal Nursing; the Council of Specialists in Psychiatric and Mental Health Nursing; and the Council of Nursing Home Nurses.

Through the Congress for Nursing Practice, the five divisions on practice and the councils on practice, as well as through other association programs, ANA works continually to improve the quality of nursing care available to the public. The profession assumes responsibility for the competence of its members, defining and interpreting the ethical principles and standards of nursing practice to which the profession is committed, and advising upon general professional and legal aspects of practice. By setting and enforcing standards that are higher than minimum legal standards, the association strives to improve the practice of its members and ensure a high quality of nursing service to the public. ANA sponsors clinical conferences to assist individual nurses to continue their professional development and improve patient care.

AMERICAN ACADEMY OF NURSING

The American Academy of Nursing was initiated in 1973 with the designation of 36 Charter Fellows by the ANA Board of Directors. Fellows are elected by the academy annually. The academy identifies and explores issues in health care, in the health professions, and in society as they affect and are affected by nurses and nursing; examines the dynamics within nursing, the interrelationships among the segments within nursing, and the interaction among nurses as all these affect the development of the nursing profession; and identifies and proposes resolutions to issues and problems confronting nursing and health.

PROGRAMS AND SERVICES

The association's administrative structure is designed to support the work of the organizational units in implementing the policies and programs established by the membership.

Accreditation—ANA has a mechanism for the accreditation of continuing education in nursing. Through designated approving bodies, the association grants public recognition to continuing education activities provided by various organizations that meet established educational standards as determined through initial and periodic evaluations.

Certification—Through its programs of certification the association recognizes the achievement of individual nurses engaged in the clinical practice of nursing or in nursing administration.

Fiscal Services—The Division of Administration is charged with three basic functions within the organizational structure of the American Nurses' Association. These functions are: (1) to protect the assets of the association, (2) to administer the financial affairs of the association, and (3) to supervise the service units, such as the telephone system, archives, the word processing unit and the processing of the mail and related services that help the association to perform its daily activities.

A major responsibility of the division is the supervision of the central billing department. The central billing department is responsible for the collection and distribution of the tri-level dues for those state nurses' associations that are a part of the central billing process.

Government Relations—Through its government relations activities ANA evaluates and promotes legislation to advance the goals of the association; monitors federal and state legislation; and studies trends in government for their implications for nursing practice, service, education, economics, and the goals of ANA. ANA maintains an office at 1030 15th Street, N.W., Washington, D.C. 20005.

Marketing/Membership Services—This department provides a marketing service for ANA and all programs and services. Through membership services, ANA programs have been devised for giving membership benefits such as insurance and travel plans and other tangible benefits.

Meetings—A biennial convention is held in the even-numbered years. The association conducts regional programs in clinical, research, and other professional areas of interest.

Public Relations—Through its public relations services, ANA programs, activities, and goals are interpreted to nurses, allied professional health groups, the government and its special agencies, and the public.

Publications—ANA publishes clinical papers; proceedings from conferences, institutes, and conventions; and other publications pertinent to nurses, the profession, and the public.

Statistics—ANA collects, analyzes, and disseminates information on nurses and nursing. Activities include the development of current and comprehensive manpower data in nursing, the compilation and maintenance of information about ANA and its membership, the provision of statistical support to ANA departments and programs, and the dissemination of information to nurses and the public through *Facts About Nursing* and other reports.

The American Nurse—The official newspaper of ANA is published 10 times a year and mailed to each ANA member. It reports a broad range of professional, economic, political, ethical and legal issues, and events that affect nursing. It provides continuing coverage of ANA affairs and highlights the accomplishments of nurses.

The **American Nurses' Foundation, Inc.**, 2420 Pershing Road, Kansas City, Missouri 64108, was established in 1955 by the American Nurses' Association. ANF is a not-for-profit organization that receives tax deductible funds to conduct projects compatible with the aims and purposes of the American Nurses' Association. ANF provides research funds for nursing research and analyzes health policy as it impacts the nursing profession.

The **National League for Nursing**, 10 Columbus Circle, New York, New York 10019, is dedicated to improving the quality of nursing education, nursing service and health care delivery in the United States. The league accomplishes its mission by identifying the nursing and health care needs of the nation and fostering programs and services to meet those needs.

NLN is a nonprofit organization comprised of a unique coalition of nurses, other health care professionals, and health care consumers. Its individual members include the deans, directors, and faculty members of educational programs in nursing; nursing service administrators, directors, supervisors, managers, and other key staff in facilities that provide nursing services; and leaders in other health professions and the community who are concerned with solving health care problems. The league's agency members are nursing educational institutions and providers of nursing and other health care services—home, community, and public health agencies.

NLN channels the expertise and concerns of its members into a broad variety of health planning and implementation activities through four components representing nursing education—associate degree programs, baccalaureate and higher degree programs, diploma programs, and practical nursing programs— and two components representing nursing service—home health agencies and community health services, and hospital and long-term care nursing services. The league provides a range of continuing education and consultation programs. Most individual NLN members also belong to one of 45 state or regional constituent leagues, which sponsor multifaceted health care service programs designed to meet community needs.

NLN is recognized by the U.S. Department of Education and by the Council on Postsecondary Accreditation as the national accrediting agency for master's, baccalaureate, associate degree, diploma, and practical nursing programs. Through a joint program with the American Public Health Association, NLN accredits home health agencies and community nursing services.

The NLN Division of Measurement provides preadmission and achievement tests to state-approved schools of nursing. It also acts as the test service for the State Board Test Pool Examinations for registered and practical nurse licensure, which are sponsored by the National Council of State Boards of Nursing.

The league is a prime source of statistical data on nursing manpower and trends. Ongoing projects of NLN's Research Division include the *Annual Survey of State-Approved Schools of Nursing*, the *Annual Survey of Employment Experiences of Newly Licensed Nurses*, the biennial *Nurse-Faculty Census*, and the longitudinal *Nurse Career-Pattern Study.*

The NLN Public Affairs Office works to ensure nursing input into health policy formulation affecting the delivery of health services to all citizens. Materials produced by the active NLN publishing program include guides to management and administration, evaluation tools for both institutions and individuals, and books and pamphlets with general and specific information about nursing education and service. *Nursing and Health Care*, a monthly referred journal, is the official organ of the National League for Nursing.

The **American Journal of Nursing Company**, 555 West 57th Street, New York, New York 10019, a publishing company incorporated under the laws of New York State, publishes five magazines and a nursing index and operates an Educational Services Division. The American Nurses' Association is the company's sole owner.

The *American Journal of Nursing*, first published in 1900, is the professional journal of the American Nurses' Association. The editorial content of this monthly journal consists largely of clinical material that enables nurses to keep up-to-date in general nursing practice or to obtain the more detailed information required for specialized practice. It emphasizes content that can be applied in all areas of nursing and presents developments within the profession and the health field at large. It is the major resource on national and international affairs that directly or indirectly affect the profession and the employment of nurses. It provides discussions of controversial issues and promotes programs of the American Nurses' Association.

Nursing Outlook was initiated in 1953. Its content emphasizes current concepts, trends, and issues in the nursing profession, especially in relation to nursing education and practice, nursing service administration, community health, and health care delivery. Issued monthly, it is directed toward nurses who are concerned with those topics and toward other health professionals and lay persons with a broad interest in nursing and health care matters.

Nursing Research was first published in 1952, when the Association of Collegiate Schools of Nursing requested the American Journal of Nursing Company to publish it as the official magazine of the ACSN. *Nursing*

Research is not the official organ of any organization at the present time. The publication is a referred journal issued bimonthly. It carries reports, articles, abstracts, and other materials to inform members of nursing and other professions of the results of scientific studies in nursing and to stimulate research in nursing.

MCN, The American Journal of Maternal Child Nursing, a bimonthly journal for nurses in the maternal child health field, was introduced in January 1976. Major classifications of editorial content are (1) new material related to clinical practice, (2) articles designed to resensitize nurses in their maternal child nursing practice, and (3) issues that professionals should understand to competently function in the field. *MCN* offers original articles by authorities on their specialties within maternal child nursing.

Geriatric Nursing: American Journal of Care for the Aging is a new journal; its first issue appeared in May 1980. It is published bimonthly and is for all health professionals providing care to the aged. Editorial content focuses on promoting the well being of the elderly as well as current and advanced concepts and practice in the clinical care of the elderly client.

International Nursing Index, prepared in cooperation with the National Library of Medicine, is a quarterly cumulation that began in 1966. The purpose of this publication is to meet the ever-increasing need of the profession for bibliographic control of its literature. The index contains references from over 200 nursing periodicals and other serials, including those of state nurses' associations, state leagues for nursing, references from periodicals of other countries, and references from non-nursing journals regularly indexed in *Index Medicus*. It also lists new nursing books published throughout the world by commercial publishers as well as those published by nursing organizations.

The *Educational Services Division* of the American Journal of Nursing Company provides publications and audiovisual materials for use in schools of nursing, continuing education programs, and individual study. Publications include original programmed instruction series and series reprinted from the *American Journal of Nursing*. The Contemporary Nursing Series is compiled from articles appearing in all four AJN Company periodicals. Audiovisual materials available include films, videotapes, filmstrips, audiotapes, and audiotape programmed instruction units. The division also conducts NBR, a nursing review course for those about to take the state board licensure examination.

The **National Student Nurses' Association, Inc.**, 10 Columbus Circle, New York, New York 10019, is the national organization for undergraduate nursing students in the United States and the largest independent student pre-professional association in this country. NSNA carried a membership of 36,000 as of October 31, 1979. NSNA consists of members in constituent associations in 50 states, the District of Columbia, Puerto Rico, Guam, and the Virgin Islands.

The purpose of the association is to assume responsibility for contributing to nursing education in order to provide for the highest quality health care; to provide programs representative of fundamental and current professional interests and concerns; and to aid in the development of the whole person, his/her professional role, and his/her responsibility for the health care of people in all walks of life. The association promotes and encourages student participation in interdisciplinary activities and activities toward improved health care and the resolution of related social issues. It speaks for nursing students to the public, institutions, organizations, governmental bodies, and legislation. Members work to influence development of relevant approaches to nursing education; they participate in nursing recruitment, especially among minority groups; and they work closely with the American Nurses' Association, the National League for Nursing, and the International Council of Nurses, as well as other nursing and health related organizations.

The Board of Directors is responsible for transacting the business of the association between meetings of the House of Delegates at the annual convention. Nine members and two consultants comprise the board, appointed by the boards of the ANA and NLN.

The NSNA magazine, *Imprint*, is published five times a year and is sent to all members. The focus of the magazine is to serve as a forum on issues facing nursing and society. One issue is the annual Career Planning Guide. In conjunction with various sponsors, NSNA awards eight scholarships annually to its members. PRN Scholarships are open to all members; Breakthrough to Nursing Scholarships for Ethnic People of Color are open to members who are ethnic students of color; and Career Mobility Scholarships are open to members who are RNs enrolled in a baccalaureate program or LPNs enrolled in programs leading to licensure as a registered nurse. In 1980, NSNA gave over $30,000 in scholarships.

In addition, a scholarship of $600 is awarded annually to a registered nurse who has formerly been a member of NSNA. This scholarship is administered by Nurses' Educational Funds, Inc. A number of state student associations have also established scholarships.

NSNA remains deeply committed to participation in legislative activities at the local, state, and national levels, and during the last few years has worked to support legislation involving nursing, nursing education, and health. Members are kept informed of such legislation by the NSNA through legislative alerts and through a regular column in *Imprint*.

NSNA Project Tomorrow workshops are continuing this year. The workshops, held in a few sites across the country, are designed to give career planning guidance to NSNA members and to give NSNA members the opportunity to speak to hospital recruiters and learn about options open to them.

The 1975 House of Delegates adopted the Student Bill of Rights and Grievance Procedures to guarantee students' rights and assist in the establishment of grievance procedures in every school of nursing. Each NSNA constituent association was urged to "make an immediate and concentrated effort to implement the Guidelines in schools in their areas."

NSNA is involved in community health projects, educational issues, and recruitment into nursing through the Breakthrough to Nursing Project.

The headquarters office of NSNA is a clearinghouse of information about student organization interests; it publishes and distributes materials to aid officers and members of the constituent associations in carrying out NSNA purposes and programs. The NSNA is financially self-supporting, with income derived from dues.

The **National Council of State Boards of Nursing, Inc.**, 303 East Ohio Street, Suite 2010, Chicago, Illinois 60611, is composed of state boards of nursing. State boards of nursing are charged with the responsibility for administering the licensure laws for nursing in each state. The National Council of State Boards of Nursing provides the means through which boards of nursing act on matters of common interest and concern affecting the public health, safety, and welfare.

Through the national council, member boards of nursing develop and regulate the use of the licensing examinations in nursing, identify and promote reasonable uniformity in standards in nursing education and nursing practice, and identify and assist in efforts to promote continued competence of practitioners in nursing.

The **American Association of Colleges of Nursing**, 11 Dupont Circle, Suite 430, Washington, D.C. 20036, is composed of 250 institutions of baccalaureate and graduate programs in nursing. The purpose of the association is to improve necessary care and its delivery in the public interest through advancing the quality of academic nursing education and strategic leadership in nursing.

The objectives of the association are to advance the quality of baccalaureate and graduate nursing programs through scholarship, research, and practice, and to advance the quality of influential leadership in academic nursing education in a variety of contexts.

Activities of the AACN include workshops, seminars, and conferences on issues of concern to members; surveys and other information from its data bank; and publications on relevant issues. A recently funded HEW project, "Continuing Education for Nurse Academic Administrators," has evolved an executive development series to train those interested in careers in academic administration in nursing. Other plans include a bibliographic service for constituents and a data bank on deans.

The **Commission on Graduates of Foreign Nursing Schools**, 3624 Market Street, Philadelphia, Pennsylvania 19104, is an independent, nonprofit, national organization incorporated in March 1977. It is jointly sponsored by the American Nurses' Association and the National League for Nursing.

The purposes of the commission are to benefit the public by (1) developing and administering a testing and evaluation program for graduates of foreign nursing schools who desire registered nurse licensure in the various states of the United States; (2) serving as a clearinghouse for authoritative information on programs in nursing education and licensure (or similar recognition) of nursing personnel in foreign countries; (3) providing a system for the evaluation of credentials of graduates of foreign nursing schools; (4) conducting and publishing studies relevant to graduates of foreign nursing schools.

The CGFNS program prevents the exploitation of graduates of foreign nursing schools who come to the United States to practice professional nursing, but are prevented from doing so when they fail to pass state licensing examinations.

The program also helps to assure the American public of safe patient care. CGFNS supports the U.N. Declaration of Human Rights, which affirms the freedom of the individual to migrate; however, CGFNS neither encourages nor discourages immigration.

The CGFNS Qualifying Examination covers proficiency in the same five areas of nursing (medical, surgical, obstetric, pediatric, and psychiatric) that nurses are taught in the United States and are covered by state licensing examinations. The CGFNS all-day examination, given in English, also includes a separate one-hour English proficiency examination. Obtaining a CGFNS Certificate means a foreign nurse graduate has obtained a passing grade in the five major nursing areas and in English comprehension, English sentence structure, and English vocabulary.

The CGFNS Certificate is required by the U.S. Immigration and Naturalization Service before it will issue a non-immigrant occupational preference visa (H-1) to foreign nurse graduates seeking to enter the United States for temporary employment. The CGFNS Certificate is required by the U.S. Department of Labor before it will issue a labor certificate to foreign nurse immigrants seeking to enter the United States permanently on an occupational preference basis (third and sixth preference). The CGFNS Certificate is already required in many states as a criterion for taking the State Board Test Pool Examination, and other state boards of nursing are moving in that direction.

The first CGFNS examination was administered in October 1978. It is given twice a year (in April and October) on the same day in over 30 countries throughout the world and in 5 centers in the United States.

The commission is governed by an 11 member Board of Trustees, which appoints various committees and which establishes policy.

The commission publishes a "Guidebook for Applicants" and issues periodic news releases, statistics, and fact sheets.

The **National Federation of Licensed Practical Nurses, Inc.**, 888 Seventh Avenue, New York, New York 10106, comprises 39 constituent state associations. It is composed of 700 local divisions and individual memberships in 11 other states. Member enrollment in 1979 was 15,000 with 3,277 student affiliates.

All state members participate in formulating the policies and programs of the NFLPN through their representatives in the national House of Delegates. These delegates are elected every year at each state's annual convention. Individual members in turn elect their own delegates during a special meeting held just prior to the opening of the national annual convention.

The primary functions of the NFLPN are to speak, act, and establish policy for it members on the local, state, and national level, in all areas where their welfare may be affected; to establish educational programs for its members through the NFLPN Education Committee in cooperation with an educational consultant; to seek betterment of all licensed practical nurses as an integral part of the health care team; and to assure the public that optimum standards of personal nursing care are observed. The NFLPN's purposes are unrestricted in terms of race, nationality, life style, or creed.

Interorganization committees help maintain practical nursing as an integral part of nursing. Liaison committees exist both with the American Nurses' Association and with the National League for Nursing. These committees are composed of board members from each organization, and serve as a means of direct communication on issues of mutual concern. The committees meet at least once annually.

Within the structure of the NFLPN there is also an Interorganization Council, composed of official representatives both of the major medical and nursing organizations and of government agencies, appointed by the federation. Other health representatives may also be appointed by the NFLPN board. The purpose of the council is to provide a national forum for the exchange of information and for discussion of mutual concerns of those issues in practical nursing service and education that are relevant to the total complex.

The Economic and General Welfare Committee is responsible for establishing guidelines and providing resource materials to those of its constituent state associations involved in collective bargaining. The federation itself, as a national organization, does no collective bargaining. Its Economic and General Welfare Committee functions in a purely advisory capacity. The NFLPN also maintains a consultant on labor relations to advise and assist in the work of the committee. These actions are based on the principle that licensed practical nurses have an earned right to participate in the development of all policies governing the conditions of their employment.

The Education Committee works cooperatively with the National Licensed Practical Nurses Educational Foundation, the research arm of the NFLPN, in developing guidelines for continuing education, and serves as an information resource to NFLPN constituents.

The NFLPN works cooperatively with the NLN and supports its efforts in the development of practical nursing education programs, accreditation, improvement of curriculum, and research in practical nursing.

The NFLPN encourages health agencies to provide continuing inservice education for licensed practical nurses on their staffs, as part of a coordinated effort for improvement of patient care.

The *Journal of Nursing Care* is the official monthly publication of the National Federation of Licensed Practical Nurses. Its circulation of more than 60,000 includes licensed practical nurses and other paramedical personnel involved in patient care; students of nursing; educators in nursing and allied health care fields; and others concerned with health care. Each month the magazine contains articles on new clinical techniques, current developments in all areas of health care, news of legislation and economic security issues, and the activities of the NFLPN.

The NFLPN is also a sponsor of the National Task Force's CEU program, and currently evaluates learning events submitted for approval by instructors. It grants CEU credits, where earned, to both members and nonmembers of the federation, and maintains complete ongoing records at its headquarters office.

This step is the latest development in the continuing education program initiated by the federation in 1968, with the founding of its Achievement Point

Program. At that time, the Licensed Practical Nurses Educational Foundation became the first in the U.S. nursing field to establish a standard for awarding recognition of continuing education.

The **National Licensed Practical Nurses Educational Foundation, Inc.**, 888 Seventh Avenue, New York, New York 10106, a tax-exempt corporation, was founded in 1962 by the National Federation of Licensed Practical Nurses, Inc., for the purposes of research, the awarding of scholarships to students enrolled in practical nursing, and the development of continuing education programs for licensed practical nurses. The foundation is supported by the members of the NFLPN and through additional contributions from members, individuals, constituents of NFLPN, and other agencies.

The **International Council of Nurses**, 37 Rue de Vermont, 1202 Geneva, Switzerland (mailing address: P.O. Box 42, CH-1211, Geneva 20 Switzerland), founded in 1899, is a federation of national nurses' associations. It provides a medium through which member associations can share their common interest in developing the contribution of nursing toward the promotion of health and the care of the sick. ICN's functions are to assist national nurses' associations to improve the standards of nursing and the competence of nurses; to promote the development of strong national nurses' associations; to serve as the authoritative voice for nurses internationally; and to assist the national nurses' associations to improve the status of nurses.

ICN is a self-governing organization. It is nonpolitical and embraces all religious faiths. Its membership is composed of registered nurses from each of 89 countries. The American Nurses' Association is an active charter member.

The highest governing body of the ICN is the Council of National Representatives, which consists of one representative from each of the 89 member associations. It meets at least once every 2 years. A Board of Directors, composed of a president, three vice-presidents, and 11 members, meets at least once annually to conduct ongoing ICN affairs. There is one standing committee, Professional Services, dealing with nursing education, nursing service, and social and economic welfare; the committee is advisory in function. Members of the Board of Directors are elected by the Council of National Representatives; members of the Professional Services Committee are elected by the board.

The ICN, on behalf of its members, has developed and maintained relationships with other international organizations in the fields of health and social welfare. The ICN is on the Consultative Register to the United Nations Economic and Social Council, which gives all members of the ICN a direct contact with the work of the United Nations and its specialized agencies. The ICN is in official relationship with the World Health Organization and has consultative status with the Council of Europe. It is included on a special list of nongovernmental organizations maintained by the International Labor Organization for consultative purposes, and is in membership with the International Hospital Federation. The ICN is in relationship with International Committee of the Red Cross; League of Red Cross Societies; World Medical Association; International Confederation of Midwives; United Nations Educational, Scientific and Cultural Organization; United Nations Internal Children's Emergency Fund; and Union of International Associations.

The **Florence Nightingale International Foundation**, 37 Rue de Vermont, 1202 Geneva, Switzerland, founded in 1934 as an independent educational trust, has been associated with the International Council of Nurses since 1949. The income from the invested trust fund of the foundation is used for special projects and other educational activities. The FNIF is administered by the Board of Directors of the ICN.

INDEX